ENDOCRINOLOGY

Internal Medicine Today: A Comprehensive Postgraduate Library

Sherman Mellinkoff, M.D.*, and *David H. Solomon, M.D.
Series Editors-in-Chief

Titles in the Series:

Rheumatology

Hematology

Oncology

Pulmonary Disease

Cardiology

Gastroenterology

Infectious Diseases

Endocrinology

Clinical Allergy and Immunology

ENDOCRINOLOGY

Edited by **Harold E. Carlson, M.D.**
Associate Professor of Medicine
University of Missouri School of Medicine
Chief, Endocrinology Section
Harry Truman Veterans Administration Hospital
Columbia, Missouri

A WILEY MEDICAL PUBLICATION
JOHN WILEY & SONS
New York • Chichester • Brisbane • Toronto • Singapore

Library of Congress Cataloging in Publication Data:

Main entry under title:

Endocrinology.

(Internal medicine today)
"A Wiley medical publication."
Includes index.
1. Clinical endocrinology. I. Carlson, Harold E.
(Harold Ernest) II. Series. [DNLM: 1. Endocrine
diseases. WK 100 E534]
RC649.E53 1983 616.4 82-17648
ISBN 0-471-09553-2

(Series statement)
Notes
L.C. subject heading Joint author entry
Title and series added entries

L.C. call no. Dewey classification no. L.C. card no.
ISBN 0-471-00000-0
ISBN 0-471-00000-0 (pbk)

Printed in the United States of America

10 9 8 7 6 5 4 3 2 1

Contributors

Gildon N. Beall, M.D., Professor of Medicine, UCLA School of Medicine, Los Angeles, California; Chief, Division of Allergy and Clinical Immunology, Harbor–UCLA Medical Center, Torrance, California

Glenn D. Braunstein, M.D., Professor of Medicine, UCLA School of Medicine; Director, Division of Endocrinology, Cedars–Sinai Medical Center, Los Angeles, California

Arnold S. Brickman, M.D., Associate Professor of Medicine, UCLA School of Medicine, Los Angeles, California; Chief, Mineral Metabolism Section, UCLA–San Fernando Valley Program, Sepulveda Veterans Administration Medical Center, Sepulveda, California

Harold E. Carlson, M.D., Associate Professor of Medicine, University of Missouri School of Medicine; Chief, Endocrinology Section, Harry Truman Veterans Administration Hospital, Columbia, Missouri

David Heber, M.D., Ph.D., Associate Professor of Medicine, UCLA School of Medicine, Los Angeles, California; Associate Director, Clinical Research Center, Endocrinology Division, Harbor–UCLA Medical Center, Torrance, California

Jerome M. Hershman, M.D., Professor of Medicine, UCLA School of Medicine; Chief, Endocrinology Section, Wadsworth Veterans Administration Medical Center, Los Angeles, California

Stanley G. Korenman, M.D., Professor of Medicine, UCLA School of Medicine, Los Angeles, California; Chief, Department of Medicine, UCLA–San Fernando Valley Program, Sepulveda Veterans Administration Medical Center, Sepulveda, California

J. Frederick Krall, Ph.D., Assistant Research Professor, UCLA School of Medicine, Los Angeles, California; Endocrinology Section, UCLA–San Fernando Valley Program, Sepulveda Veterans Administration Medical Center, Sepulveda, California

Seymour R. Levin, M.D., Professor of Medicine, UCLA School of Medicine; Chief, Special Diagnostic and Treatment Unit, Director, Diabetes Clinic, Wadsworth Veterans Administration Medical Center, Los Angeles, California

David R. Meldrum, M.D., Associate Professor of Obstetrics and Gynecology; Division of Reproductive Endocrinology, UCLA School of Medicine, Los Angeles, California

Stewart A. Middler, M.D., Ph.D., Assistant Clinical Professor of Medicine, UCLA School of Medicine, Los Angeles, California

James R. Sowers, M.D., Associate Professor of Medicine, UCLA School of Medicine, Los Angeles, California; Assistant Chief, Endocrinology Section, UCLA–San Fernando Valley Program, Sepulveda Veterans Administration Medical Center, Sepulveda, California

Ronald S. Swerdloff, M.D., Professor of Medicine, UCLA School of Medicine, Los Angeles, California; Chief, Division of Endocrinology, Harbor–UCLA Medical Center, Torrance, California

Michael L. Tuck, M.D., Associate Professor of Medicine, UCLA School of Medicine, Los Angeles, California; Chief, Endocrinology Section, UCLA–San Fernando Valley Program, Sepulveda Veterans Administration Medical Center, Sepulveda, California

Andre J. Van Herle, M.D., Professor of Medicine, Division of Endocrinology, UCLA School of Medicine, Los Angeles, California

UCLA Department of Medicine Committee on Continuing Education

Sanford Bloom, M.D., Adjunct Associate Professor of Medicine, Division of Family Practice

Glenn Braunstein, M.D., Associate Professor of Medicine, Division of Endocrinology

Robert Brook, M.D., Associate Professor of Medicine and Public Health, Division of General Internal Medicine and Health Services Research

William Cabeen, M.D., Assistant Clinical Professor of Medicine, Division of Cardiology

Harold Carlson, M.D., Associate Professor of Medicine, Division of Endocrinology

Sheryl Crowley, Program Representative, Division of Medicine, UCLA Extension

Arlene Fink, Ph.D., Associate Social Sciences Researcher, Department of Medicine

Stanley S. Franklin, M.D., Clinical Professor of Medicine, Division of Nephrology

Robert Gale, M.D., Associate Professor of Medicine and Microbiology and Immunology, Division of Hematology/Oncology

Jeffrey Galpin, M.D., Assistant Professor of Medicine, Division of Infectious Disease

Gary L. Gitnick, M.D., Professor of Medicine, Division of Gastroenterology

Ralph Gold, M.D., Clinical Instructor of Medicine, Division of Family Practice

Harvey C. Gonick, M.D., Adjunct Professor of Medicine, Division of Nephrology

Arnold Gurevitch, M.D., Adjunct Associate Professor of Medicine, Division of Dermatology

Jackie Kosecoff, Ph.D., Associate Social Sciences Researcher, Department of Medicine

Richard Meyer, M.D., Associate Professor of Medicine, Division of Infectious Disease

Linda Olt, M.A., Editor, Department of Medicine

Harold Paulus, M.D., Professor of Medicine, Division of Rheumatology

Michael Reza, M.D., Assistant Clinical Professor of Medicine, Division of Rheumatology

William Rodney, M.D., Assistant Professor of Medicine, Division of Family Practice

Gregory Sarna, M.D., Assistant Professor of Medicine, Division of Hematology/Oncology

Andrew Saxon, M.D., Associate Professor of Medicine; Chief, Division of Clinical Immunology and Allergy

Martin Shickman, M.D., Clinical Professor of Medicine; Director, Department of Continuing Education in Health Sciences, UCLA Extension; Assistant Dean for Postgraduate Medical Education, UCLA School of Medicine

Vasant Udhoji, M.D., Adjunct Professor of Medicine, Division of Cardiology

Stuart Vener, M.D., Assistant Clinical Professor of Medicine, Division of Endocrinology

Irwin Weinstein, M.D., Clinical Professor of Medicine, Division of Hematology

Thomas Yoshikawa, M.D., Associate Professor of Medicine, Division of Infectious Disease

Roy Young, M.D., Associate Professor of Medicine; Director, General Internal Medicine Residency Training Program; Division of General Internal Medicine and Health Services Research

This publication was developed in association with a course sponsored by UCLA Extension, Health Sciences Division.

Preface

This book has been designed to provide internists and other practitioners with a review and update of modern clinical endocrinology. It is not all-inclusive but focuses on the disorders most commonly seen in medical practice.

The first chapter provides an overview of recent major advances in the understanding of how hormones act and relates these observations to human endocrine dysfunction. Clinical chapters follow and are concerned with pituitary, thyroid, gonadal, and adrenal disease, as well as with disorders of glucose and calcium metabolism. The final chapter discusses autoimmune disease as it affects the endocrine system.

Each of the clinical chapters discusses the pathophysiology, practical diagnosis, and treatment of the various disorders. At the end of each chapter except the first, case examples are presented with questions and answers about diagnosis and therapy. These cases allow the reader to assess his or her comprehension of the material. This volume will also serve as a useful office reference for the practicing clinician.

H.E.C.

Contents

1

STANLEY G. KORENMAN
J. FREDERICK KRALL

Mechanisms of Hormone Action

Hormones function to convey information about the internal and external environment to tissues and to individual cells. Similarities among the mechanisms employed by a wide variety of regulatory substances, including many that act without circulating and many that are not the secretion products of traditional endocrine glands, have expanded the concept of endocrine regulation of cell function. Regulation by circulating compounds may be termed *endocrine,* by local chemical effectors *paracrine*, and by the products of the cell itself *autocrine*.

As we have seen our society turn from producing goods to producing and processing information, so we have come to the recognition that organisms expend a great deal of effort similarly engaged, employing information-bearing molecules. The cell must both recognize these compounds and transduce their signals into a response. Specific proteins called *receptors* perform these functions. They are distinguished by their linkage to the cellular response from other binding proteins such as those in the plasma and from binding to enzymes that participate in hormone metabolism. A *target cell* is defined as one containing a concentration of receptor sufficient to show a response within the physiologic range of hormone concentration.

In this review we will not discuss physiologic control by hormones of the overall function of tissues or organisms or how hormones interact to control growth or energy utilization. Rather, we will focus on the initial interactions of hormones with cells, that is, on the molecular mechanisms of hormone action, for which a theoretical framework applicable to a broad range of hormonal stimuli is being assembled.

When one considers the vast array of regulatory substances, it is reassuring that we can now characterize them in three major groups with respect to mechanism of action, which, although susceptible to further division, allow certain generalizations about hormone action. These groups are:

1. Steroid and steroid-like
2. Cell surface-active, adenylate cyclase-stimulating
3. Cell surface-active, non-adenlyate cyclase-stimulating.

Table 1 lists the principal hormones of each type. Prostaglandins are identified with both types of cell surface-active hormones because they represent a single group whose mechanism of action is diverse.

Table 1 **Hormones and Other Cell Regulators and Their Mechanisms of Action**

Steroid and Steroid-like	*Cell Surface—Adenylate Cyclase*	*Cell Surface—Other*
Estrogens	TSH	Insulin
Androgens	ACTH	Growth hormone
Progesterone	FSH	Somatomedin
Glucocorticoids	LH	Prolactin
Mineralocorticoids	PTH	α-Adrenergic catecholamine
Vitamin D	Calcitonin	Somatostatin
Thryoid	β-Adrenergic catechol-amine	Dopamine
	Vasopressin, kidney	Prostaglandins
	TRH	Acetylcholine
	GnRH	Gastrin
	Glucagon	Bombesin
	Prostaglandins	Substance P
	Secretin	Growth factors—epidermal, nerve, fibroblast, platelet-derived
	Vasoactive intestinal polypeptide	
	Histamine	

STEROID HORMONE ACTION

Hormonal steroids, sterols, and thyronines act to regulate cell function at the level of transcription, that is, by regulating the amount of specific RNA produced in the nucleus. It is important to emphasize that the most plentiful circulating hormone is not necessarily the active agent. While testosterone, 25-hydroxycholecalciferol, and thyroxine are present in the highest

Table 2 **Molecular Mechanisms of Steroid Hormone Action**

Uptake of hormone into cells
Transformation of hormone to active form
Binding to intracellular receptor
Transformation of the hormone–receptor complex
Translocation to nucleus
Binding to nuclear acceptor sites
Transcription of highly selective mRNA molecules
Processing of initial transcriptates
Translation of proteins coded by the message
Enzymatic, structural, and secretory alterations of the cell

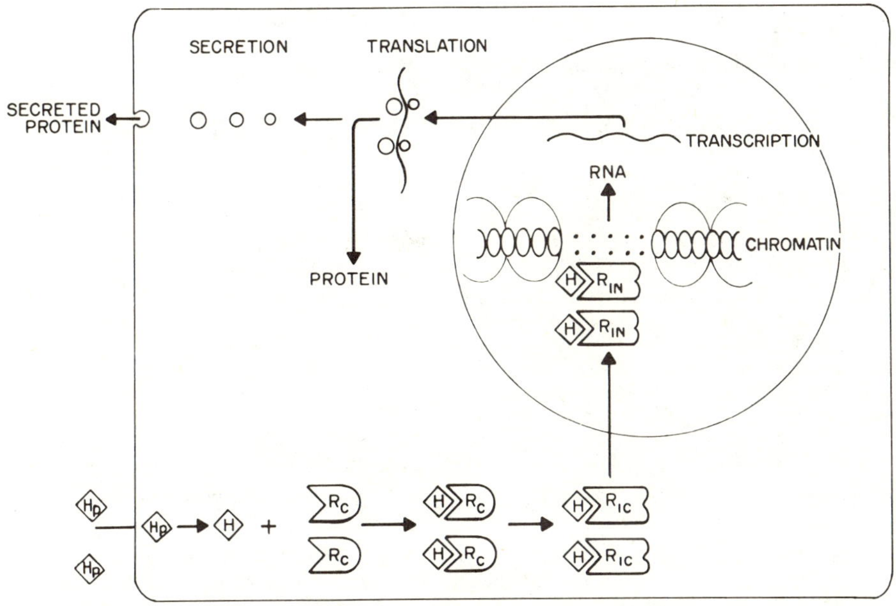

Figure 1. Hormone free in the plasma (H_p) diffuses into the target cell to form a complex with the receptor in its cytoplasmic form (R_C). After hormone binding, the receptor is transformed to an activated state ($H\,R_{IC}$). Then the hormone receptor complex is translocated to the nucleus where it associates with specific chromatin sites, initiating the transcription of target genes into RNA. mRNA is translated in the cytoplasm into proteins with either intracellular enzymatic or structural functions, or exported as a hormone-specific secretory product.

concentration in plasma, the most active hormones are 5α-dihydrotestosterone, 1,25-dihydroxycholecalciferol, and L-triiodothyronine. While 25-hydroxycholecalciferol is converted in the kidney and transported to intestinal and perhaps bone receptor sites, both testosterone and thyroxine are converted in the target tissue itself to the more active hormones.

The principal steps involved in steroid hormone action are summarized in Table 2 and illustrated in Fig. 1. Steroids appear to pass through the cell membrane without impediment, as demonstrated by the time course of radioactive hormone uptake. This is not surprising, since steroids, sterols, and thyronines are amphiphilic; that is, they have polar, water-loving regions and nonpolar, lipid-like regions.

Receptors

The current theory of steroid hormone action was generated by the discovery in 1957 that radioactive estradiol of high specific activity was concentrated and retained in the uterus and vagina, its principal target tissues, long after it was cleared from the blood. This led inexorably

Table 3 **Features of Steroid Hormone Receptors**

Near-absolute specificity for hormone, other agonists or competitive antagonists
Localization at high concentration in target tissues only
High affinity of interaction between hormone and receptor
Ability of hormone–receptor complex to be transformed to a nuclear form
Binding of hormone–receptor complex to acceptor sites on nuclear chromatin

to the conclusion that there must be receptor molecules for the steroid to account for its retention. Target tissues were found to contain nonnuclear soluble proteins that bound hormone in vivo and in vitro with great affinity and with even more remarkable specificity.

Glucocorticoids, mineralocorticoids, estrogens, androgens, progesterone, and dihydroxycholecalciferol each bind to a distinct hormone-specific soluble protein in target cell cytoplasm. The relative affinities of specific receptors for hormone analogs correlate well with their physiologic function and relative potency as a hormone or antagonist, an important criterion in verifying the role of receptors in the control of endocrine responses. So far as is known, receptors for the same hormone are indistinguishable in different target organs, and the affinity and specificity with which receptors bind are largely preserved among species.

Steroid receptors share important functional similarities (Table 3). When isotopic steroids are administered in situ, these receptor proteins with their radioactive tags translocate from the cytoplasm to the site of their long-term retention, the nucleus. Within the target cell nucleus, the receptor–hormone complex becomes associated with *chromatin* (the native state of DNA in the mammalian nucleus), presumably its subcellular site of action. Receptors for estradiol and for progesterone have been purified to near or total homogeneity. It was found that the estrogen receptor is activated or transformed to a nuclear form, which has both a greater affinity for hormone and a greater ability to bind to chromatin. It is the latter property that has profound consequences in terms of the nuclear role of the hormone–receptor complex.

The progesterone receptor has two subunits, designated A and B, which have essentially identical affinities for progesterone but differ slightly in molecular weight. Component A binds to purified DNA, whereas B binds to proteins associated with chromatin, suggesting that each plays a somewhat different role in binding the hormone–receptor complex to the proper location in the genome for selective activation of transcription. Increased synthesis of mRNA for the specific products of hormonal stimulation (transcription) has actually been demonstrated in several cases. While the progesterone receptor, unlike the estrogen receptor, apparently does not undergo transformation as a prerequisite for translocation and nuclear binding, a more subtle activation step apparently takes place involving receptor phosphorylation. Transformation does follow the interaction of dihydrotestosterone, glucocorticoids, aldosterone, and dihydroxycholecalciferol with their specific receptors before nuclear translocation. The specificity with which transformation occurs is perhaps best demonstrated by the glucocorticoid receptor which also binds progesterone with high affinity. Progesterone binding does not induce transformation, and consequently no translocation occurs, accounting for its antiglucocorticoid action.

Nuclear Actions

Chromatin Binding

One of the most intriguing problems in molecular biology is how the hormone–receptor complex recognizes specific target genes, considering the enormous size of the mammalian genome. The human diploid nucleus contains $5\frac{1}{2}$ billion nucleotides per strand of duplex molecule. If an average gene is 2,000 nucleotides in length, even if the hormone were to activate as many as 1,000 genes, this would require the complex to find and recognize as specific 0.04% of the DNA nucleotide sequences. The localization of such a few specific target genes is believed to be facilitated by the structure of DNA in the mammalian cell nucleus, by its associated basic proteins (histones), and by a heterogeneous mixture of nonhistone or acidic proteins. This complex is called chromatin when isolated and purified for subsequent characterization and is believed to be a reasonable approximation of gene structure in intact cells. The binding of a radioactive progesterone–receptor complex to chromatin from chicken oviduct disappeared as different classes of proteins were selectively removed from the chromatin. The *acceptor sites* for the progesterone–receptor complex were specifically associated with a class of nonhistone chromatin proteins. Nonhistone proteins also appear to comprise the high-affinity acceptor site for the glucocorticoid–receptor complex. Recently, the acceptor sites associated with the nonhistone proteins in chick oviduct have been found to be present in chromatin from nontarget tissues, but they appear to be unavailable. Chromatin acceptor sites for the progesterone–receptor complex are increased in immature chick oviduct by treatment with diethylstilbestrol, suggesting that acceptor site availability may be another modifier of hormone action.

Elucidation of the events following translocation of the steroid–receptor complex was facilitated by the development of a method for quantifying nuclear receptors. Following estradiol administration, there is a large influx of hormone–receptor complex into uterine nuclei. The influx is transient and decreases after 6 hours to about three times the unstimulated level. Thereafter, nuclear estradiol–receptor levels remain elevated for more than 18 hours. It is this long-term retention that is important for the estrogen-induced uterotrophic (growth) response. The long-term nuclear hormone–receptor complexes are probably more tightly bound to what appears to be 1,000 to 1,300 chromatin acceptor sites per cell. This represents retention of only 5–20% of the available cytoplasmic receptors. Thus it is envisioned that selective binding of as few as 1,000 hormone–receptor complexes to chromatin will produce by a cascading sequence of events, all the changes characterizing the cellular response to the hormone.

Initiation of Transcription

Sex steroid treatment is accompanied by an increase in *template activity*, the capacity of chromatin to form a complex among DNA, RNA polymerase, and nucleotide triphosphates, the step preliminary to synthesis of new RNA molecules. Stimulation of RNA synthesis or chromatin template activity by the direct addition of hormone–receptor complex in various states of purity has been demonstrated for uterine estradiol–receptor, prostatic dihydrotestosterone–receptor, and chick oviduct progesterone–receptor. Such experiments have been criticized because of the inadvertent addition of contaminants in receptor preparations, which stimulate RNA polymerase activity, so a causal relationship between acceptor site occupancy and transcription has not been definitely demonstrated. However, a close correlation between increased occupancy of nuclear acceptor sites after estradiol administration and an increase in chromatin initiation sites have been reported. In addition, synthesis of two species of estrogen-dependent mRNA has been correlated with receptor binding in the nucleus of the chick oviduct, strongly supporting the thesis that steroid hormones regulate transcription via binding of transformed hormone–receptor complex to acceptor sites on chromatin, followed by an increase in DNA-dependent RNA polymerase activity.

Steroid Hormone Regulation of mRNA Synthesis in Situ

Identification of sex steroid-specific proteins provided tentative evidence of the existence of hormone-specific mRNAs. The diversity of RNA species in mammalian cells proved to be an obstacle to the isolation of mRNA, which constitutes less than 1% of the total, until the discovery that most mRNAs contain a tail of 200 or more nearly homogeneous adenylic acid residues sequences, which makes possible their purification.

Table 4 is a list of target tissues in which responses mediated by hormone-specific mRNA have been demonstrated. These examples represent the best evidence of the genetic specificity with which steroids act. Ingenious purification techniques led to isolation of the mRNA for ovalbumin, growth hormone, and other proteins, leading to quantification of the rate at which these genes are transcribed following hormone treatment. It was shown that there is a lag of several hours between nuclear binding of the estrogen receptor and the accumulation of specific ovalbumin mRNA, suggesting intermediate steps subsequent to nuclear binding and preceding transcription. There is no significant lag between accumulation of mature ovalbumin mRNA and ovalbumin synthesis, indicating that ovalbumin production is regulated by mRNA synthesis. Similarly, thyroid hormone and glucocorticoids control growth hormone production in rat pituitary tumor cells by regulating growth hormone mRNA synthesis. However, induction of mRNA may not be the only mechanism through which hormones regulate protein synthesis. Casein mRNA is found in unstimulated mammary gland, and casein synthesis is initiated by treatment with prolactin using the preformed mRNA. There are many other examples of messages whose translation is dependent on another control mechanism, not necessarily hormonal.

Table 4 **Hormone-Specific mRNA**

Organ	*Protein Synthetic Response*	*Hormone(s)*
Rat liver	α_2-u-globulin	Androgen, glucocorticoids, thyroid
Rat liver	Tryptophan oxygenase	Glucocorticoids
Rat pituitary tumor	Growth hormone	Glucocorticoids, thyroid
Rat prostate	Aldolase	Androgen
Rat mammary gland	Casein	Estrogen prolactin
Rabbit uterus	Blastokinin	Progesterone
Avian liver	Egg yolk protein	Estrogen
Avian retina	Glutamine synthetase	Glucocorticoids
Avian oviduct	Ovalbumin	Estrogen
Avian oviduct	Avidin	Progesterone
Avian oviduct	Ovomucoid and lysozyme	Estrogen
Avian oviduct	Conalbumin	Estrogen

Direct comparisons of the rate of accumulation of conalbumin mRNA and ovalbumin mRNA in chicken oviduct after estrogen administration have shown that steroid target genes may have different responses to hormones. Conalbumin mRNA begins to accumulate within 30 minutes following estrogen administration, whereas ovalbumin mRNA production lags by about 3 hours. Moreover, the rate of conalbumin mRNA production was found to be directly proportional to the concentration of nuclear steroid receptors, while ovalbumin mRNA production was about 30% less sensitive. These disparities may mean that eukaryotic genes, including steroid target genes, are regulated in more than one way.

It is not surprising that steroids have multiple target genes in the same tissues (see Table 4), but there are also several cases in which it has been shown that more than one hormone interacts in the regulation of a single gene. Androgen regulation of α_2-u-globulin synthesis in rat liver is through control of the level of the mRNA for this protein. Maximal induction of α_2-u-globulin synthesis, however, requires simultaneous treatment with androgen, glucocorticoid, thyroxine, and growth hormone. In another example, the induction of casein mRNA requires both estrogen and prolactin. Synthesis of growth hormone mRNA in rat pituitary tumor cell cultures was increased 17-fold by triiodothyronine, 3-fold by dexamethasone, and 45-fold by both. The mechanism through which hormones interact to regulate mRNA synthesis in these examples is not understood, but there is evidence that some of the gene products regulated are receptors. In various target organs, estrogen or prolactin induces estrogen and progesterone receptors, testosterone induces lutenizing hormone (LH) receptors, and estrogen induces α-adrenergic catecholamine receptors after ovariectomy. Although steroidal control of receptor concentrations has not been shown definitively to be through the control of gene expression as detailed above, the implication is clear that, among the most important gene products regulated by steroids may be the specific receptors through which target cells perceive the normal milieu.

CELL SURFACE-ACTIVE HORMONES: THE HORMONE-SENSITIVE ADENYLATE CYCLASE SYSTEM

For most hormones, action begins at the cell surface (Table 1). This requires the presence of recognition sites and a mechanism for transducing the information that the hormone is present to the cellular response mechanism (Fig. 2). The response mechanism for many hormones in this class is receptor-mediated activation of adenylate cyclase, the membrane enzyme that catalyzes the formation of cyclic AMP (cAMP) from ATP. Cyclic AMP in turn binds to and activates a special class of protein-phosphorylating enzymes. It is the enzymatic phosphorylation of proteins by these enzymes that is the final mediator of the action of the hormone.

Receptors

Identification of recognition sites for cell surface hormones was difficult because their low concentrations required binding molecules of very high specific radioactivity and stabilization of the hormone–receptor complexes to achieve measurable specific binding and because of the presence of nonspecific binding sites on the cell surface. It was crucial to develop criteria for the identification of hormone uptake as binding to receptor.

The most important criterion for the identification of specific cell surface receptors is that they recognize physiologic effectors as a function of potency. Receptors were characterized for

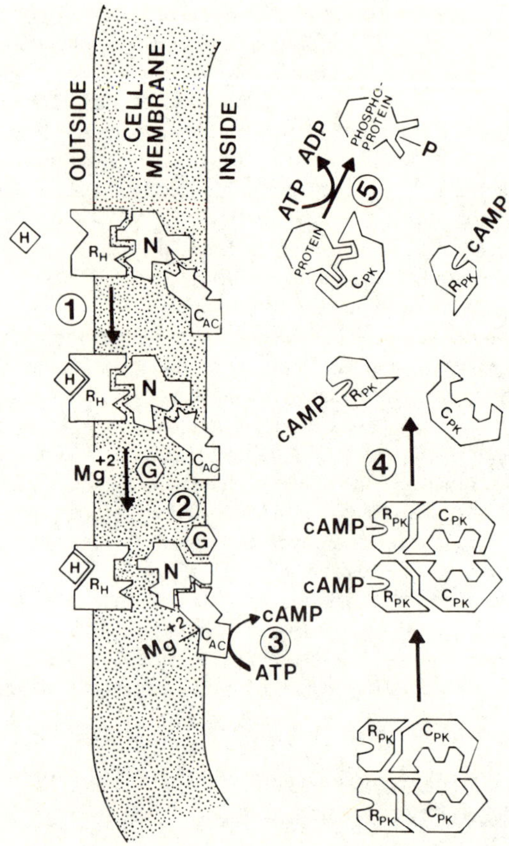

Figure 2. Mechanism of cAMP-medicated receptor function. The hormone (⟨H⟩) or agonist forms a complex with the membrane-associated target cell receptor (R_H), step ①. Formation of the hormone–receptor complex leads to step ②, GTP binding (⟨G⟩) by the coupling factor (N), and resultant activation of the MG^{2+}-sensitive catalytic subunit (C_{AC}) with an increase in the rate of cAMP production (step ③). cAMP activates the protein kinase catalytic subunit (C_{PK}) by binding to its regulatory subunit (R_{PK}) and dissociation of the tetrameric enzyme, step ④. The active catalytic subunit then transfers a phosphate from ATP to the dephosphorylated form of a specific soluble or membrane-associated protein, altering its function in a hormone-specific manner (step ⑤), thus initiating the hormone-mediated process.

a variety of cell surface-active hormones and have been shown to have certain typical characteristics (Table 5).

Extensive studies on rat testicular Leydig cells of the mechanism of LH action in cAMP-mediated steroidogenesis showed a large discrepancy among receptor occupancy, cAMP production, and steroidogenesis. This disparity gave rise to the "spare receptor hypothesis," since the physiologic response, steroidogenesis, was regulated over a hormone concentration range that permitted occupancy of only a small fraction of the total number of LH receptors. Target

Table 5 **Properties of Cell Surface Receptors**

Protein in structure
Bind agonists and antagonists as a function of their physiologic potency
Intimately associated with, yet markedly mobile in the lipid bilayer of the cell membrane
Disappear from the cell surface on protracted exposure to agonists but not antagonists

cells for many cell surface-active hormones have a similarly large reserve capacity to synthesize cAMP (and activate protein kinase), indicating a highly efficient amplification mechanism that translates the occupancy of a few receptors into a large physiologic response. The significance of this relative abundance of receptors is not established, but a high concentration of receptors relative to those required to achieve the physiologic response would be expected to increase target cell sensitivity to hormones. Consequently, small changes in receptor number could have large physiologic consequences.

Changes in receptor number and concomitant changes in target tissue sensitivity to hormonal stimulation have been demonstrated in the case of insulin-resistant diabetes, human chorionic gonadotropin (hCG) regulation of luteal cell steroidogenesis, and the regulation of smooth and cardiac muscle contractility by catecholamines.

Regulation of Cell Surface Receptor Number and Function

Ovarian follicular maturation represents an interesting example of hormonal interaction in the regulation of cell surface receptors. Granulosa cell LH receptors increase during maturation, and this increase has been shown to be follicle-stimulating hormone (FSH)-dependent. However, hypophysectomized rats receiving FSH do not show the increase unless they also receive estrogen. Estrogen administered alone actually decreases the number of granulosa cell LH receptors, so the sex steroid and FSH function synergistically, although the mechanism through which these quite different hormones interact is uncertain.

Receptors mediate changes in cellular response termed desensitization and down-regulation. *Desensitization* is defined as agonist-induced refractoriness of biologic response. *Down-regulation* is a form of desensitization due to agonist-induced reduction in the number of available hormone receptors. It has now been directly demonstrated that β-adrenergic catecholamines, insulin, and gonadotropins promote time-dependent changes in the properties of their respective receptors. In the case of the β-adrenergic catecholamine receptor, this leads first to a functional uncoupling of the receptor from adenylate cyclase, then to a reduction in the affinity for hormone, and eventually to a reduction in the cell surface concentration of receptor. Initial uncoupling may also occur with other receptors but has not been documented, while agonist-induced down-regulation is common to a variety of hormones. Some hormones shown to induce desensitization are given in Table 6.

Desensitization has two components which may or may not be present in all target tissues: a specific component by which the agonist induces refractoriness only to itself (homologous desensitization), and another nonspecific or heterologous component. Through the latter, an agonist induces refractoriness not only to itself but also to the action of different agonists whose actions are mediated by different receptors. The heterologous component is of potential clinical

Table 6 **Desensitization Demonstrated**

Hormone	*Tissue*
Insulin	Human monocyte
Calcitonin	Embryonic bone
β-Adrenergic catecholamines	Frog erythrocyte, rat uterus
Luteinizing hormone	Leydig cell and ovary
Glucagon	Fat cell
Opiates	Guinea pig smooth muscle
Parathyroid hormone	Embryonic bone
Prostaglandins E_2 and $F_{2\alpha}$	Rat uterus, embryonic bone

relevance, since it has been shown to occur in humans in vivo. Lymphocytes isolated from human subjects under infusion with the β-adrenergic agonist isoproterenol showed not only a loss of isoproterenol-dependent cAMP production but also a loss of prostaglandin-dependent cAMP synthesis. It can readily be appreciated that receptors for different cell surface-active hormones may desensitize heterologously in combinations that vary in different target tissues. Thus the physiologic response to two or more hormones or agonists could be tissue-specific and quantitatively or qualitatively different from the effects of each alone.

Adenylate Cyclase and cAMP

Binding of hormone to these classes of cell surface receptors results in the formation of an active complex that stimulates conversion of ATP to cAMP by adenylate cyclase. Mere binding to the receptor, however, does not result in an active complex, since hormone antagonists such as propranolol bind with high affinity. The precise mechanism of stimulation is just becoming understood. The β-adrenergic catecholamine receptor appears to be a highly mobile membrane protein capable of migrating substantial distances over the cell surface to activate the catalytic subunit of adenylate cyclase exposed to the inner cell surface. A mechanism exists that couples the receptor to adenylate cyclase.

GTP-Mediated Coupling

A complex GTP-requiring mechanism couples cell surface receptors with the adenylate cyclase catalytic subunit on the inside of the plasma membrane. Of pivotal importance in the functioning of the mechanism is a discrete class of GTP-binding "coupling" proteins termed variously N, G, or G/F proteins. The binding of hormone to receptor promotes formation of a GTP–coupling protein complex which activates the catalytic subunit of adenylate cyclase, leading to increased cAMP production. Hydrolysis of bound GTP to GDP and its subsequent dissociation from the coupling protein leads to inactivation of the catalytic subunit. GTP binding to the coupling protein alters the receptor, lowering its affinity for agonist binding but not antagonist binding. It is possible, but so far uncertain, that the GTP and coupling protein concentrations are the loci at which hormone responsiveness is regulated.

cAMP-Dependent Protein Kinase

It is currently believed that all physiologic actions of cAMP are mediated through the activation of protein kinases. Correlations between cAMP-dependent protein kinase activity and physiologic responses to cAMP support this hypothesis. Protein kinases are enzymes that transfer the terminal phosphate of ATP to serine or threonine residues of specific proteins, and while a variety of these enzymes are probably present in most tissues, only a few are cAMP-responsive. These have a common structure and are made up of two cAMP-binding regulatory subunits and two inactive catalytic subunits. cAMP binding by the regulatory subunits dissociates the complex, activating the catalytic subunits. Two principal species of cAMP-dependent protein kinase are present, and the relative content of these forms appears to be tissue-specific.

The action of protein kinases in the phosphorylation of specific substrates has been well documented in a few examples of physiologic regulation.

Induction of Lipolysis by Lipolytic Hormones in Fat Cells

Lipolytic hormones such as ACTH, glucagon, and epinephrine all raise cytoplasmic cAMP levels with the subsequent activation of protein kinase. Activated protein kinase phosphorylates hormone-sensitive triglyceride lipase, converting it from its inactive to its active form, thereby stimulating the release of free fatty acids. Lipolysis is further augmented by the cAMP-dependent protein kinase-mediated activation of glycogen phosphorylase and deactivation of glycogen synthetase.

Glycogen Metabolism in Liver

The rate-limiting steps in glycogen synthesis and breakdown are catalyzed by glycogen synthetase and glycogen phosphorylase. The active and inactive forms by both these enzymes are interconvertible through phosphorylation by protein kinase. Hormone-mediated elevations of cAMP in liver lead to protein kinase activation followed by (1) deactivation of glycogen synthetase, and (2) activation of phosphorylase kinase which then activates phosphorylase by phosphorylation. Phosphorylase mediates glycogenolysis. Alternate mechanisms of phosphorylase kinase activation exist, providing non-cAMP-mediated mechanisms for regulation of hepatic glycogen metabolism. In fact, the mechanism of epinephrine's effects on liver glycogenolysis, elucidation of which led to the discovery of cAMP as the mediator of β-adrenergic receptor function, is now recognized as an α-adrenergic receptor-mediated effect of this mixed agonist in vivo. In this instance, phosphorylase kinase is activated not by cAMP-dependent phosphorylation but by α-adrenergic receptor-mediated mobilization of Ca^{2+} from intracellular sources.

Other Responses

Besides these specific examples, however, protein kinase-dependent phosphorylation of other regulatory proteins has been shown to alter their properties. Phosphoprotein substrates for protein kinase that regulate basic target cell functions known to be altered by hormone treatment include the following.

RNA Synthesis. The cell nucleus contains a number of protein kinases, both cAMP-dependent and -independent, some of which are associated with the chromatin regions most active in RNA synthesis. These enzymes may regulate the rate of RNA synthesis, as both RNA polymerase activity and chromatin template activity are increased by phosphorylation. In some target tissues, hormones that elevate cAMP directly induce translocation of protein kinase from the cytoplasm to the nucleus.

Membrane Properties. Protein kinases associated with membranes have been described in a variety of tissues. Phosphorylation of specific membrane proteins by these enzymes has been correlated with changes in membrane transport rates or permeability in fat cells, erythrocytes, toad bladder, and heart muscle and with changes in electrical excitability in neuronal tissue. Phosphorylation of red blood cell membrane proteins has recently been implicated in ATP-dependent changes in erythrocyte shape, suggesting that some cellular properties as basic as form may be regulated by protein kinase activity. Hormone treatment has been shown to cause redistribution of soluble cytoplasmic protein kinase to a membrane fraction of uterine smooth muscle. Thus, induced translocation to specific subcellular compartments may be a ubiquitous mechanism by which hormones increase protein kinase activity in the vicinity of their specific substrates.

cGMP Protein Kinase

There are numerous reports that target cell cGMP levels, like cAMP levels, fluctuate with hormone treatment. Unlike adenylate cyclase, direct hormone effects on guanylate cyclase activity have been difficult to demonstrate, and the hypothesis to date is that cGMP levels are indirectly modulated by hormones and other physiologically active agents. It has been shown that guanylate cyclase is directly stimulated by oxides and peroxides, so it is possible that cGMP levels are most responsive to changes in cell metabolism.

cGMP, like cAMP, is believed to exert its effects through activation of a specific protein kinase. cGMP-sensitive protein kinase is distinct from the cAMP-activated enzyme, chiefly in that the cyclic nucleotide-binding part of the molecule is not dissociable from the catalytic part, but the two forms of cyclic nucleotide-sensitive protein kinase may have evolved from a common progenitor. Specific substrates for cGMP-dependent protein kinase have been described, but the only proteins of defined function whose activity is altered by phosphorylation by purified cGMP-dependent protein kinase are cAMP-dependent protein kinase substrates. In light of the proposed common origin of cyclic nucleotide-dependent protein kinases, it is not surprising that both the cAMP- and cGMP-dependent enzymes have similar substrate specificities.

Other Protein Kinases

An interesting new class of protein kinases that phosphorylate tyrosine rather than serine or threonine amino acid residues have recently been discovered, and the activity of some of them is actually inhibited by cAMP. Each of these protein kinases is a substrate for phosphorylation by one or more of the others, and the phosphorylated form of one of them may regulate Na^+, K^+-ATPase (the cellular Na^+-K^+ pump enzyme) activity. At least one peptide hormone (epidermal growth factor, EGF) activates one of the tyrosine protein kinases in a non-cAMP-mediated fashion. Because of the central role of ion transport in cell excitability, this new class of protein-phosphorylating enzymes may be of immense importance in the mechanism of action of some hormones.

Phosphodiesterase

Intracellular cAMP levels are regulated not only by adenylate cyclase-catalyzed synthesis of the cyclic nucleotide but also by its rate of breakdown to the inactive 5′-AMP. This is the specific function of phosphodiesterase. The importance of cAMP hydrolysis is emphasized by the observation that many responses to cAMP are mimicked when tissues are treated with phosphodiesterase inhibitors.

Norepinephrine, insulin, growth hormone, and glucocorticoids have been implicated in the regulation of phosphodiesterase activity in some target organs. With the exception of cortisol, which has a direct inhibitory effect on phosphodiesterase, the mechanisms are uncertain. The enzyme is modulated by changes in intracellular concentrations of Ca^{2+} which, when bound to the protein calmodulin, activates phosphodiesterase. cAMP may regulate its own intracellular levels to some extent through a feedback mechanism involving activation of phosphodiesterase by the calmodulin–Ca^{2+} complex.

Receptor Interaction

The adenylate cyclase-activating function of cell surface receptors for many hormones is antagonized by the inhibitory action of receptors for completely different agonists. For example, adenylate cyclase stimulation by series-E prostaglandins in the brain is antagonized by the opiate receptor, and glucagon-dependent adenylate cyclase in the liver is inhibited by the receptor for adenosine. The mechanisms by which these interactions occur are not well understood, but the antagonistic functions require GTP binding. Heterologous desensitization, discussed above, may be a special case of these inhibitory interactions, or the mechanism by which they occur.

In view of the extreme specificity of many of these interacting agonists for their respective receptors, it is unlikely that competition for the same binding sites is the basis of inhibition. Direct interaction between different kinds of receptors cannot, however, be excluded. For instance, in the brain the receptor for γ-aminobutyric acid (GABA) decreases the rate of dissociation of benzodiazepine drugs from their receptor. While many examples of inhibitory interactions are known, there are few documented examples of facilitation.

OTHER CELL SURFACE-ACTIVE HORMONES

A number of cell surface-active hormones that do not themselves activate adenylate cyclase, such as acetylcholine, opiates, α-adrenergic catecholamines, somatostatin, and some prostaglandins, may react directly to inhibit this system through interactions at the cell surface. On the other hand, the principal anabolic hormones, growth hormone, somatomedin, insulin, prolactin, and the growth factors act in a different and yet unknown manner to stimulate protein synthesis, cell growth, and cell division in their respective targets.

Insight into the possible mechanisms of action of this diverse class of hormones is perhaps to be gained, however, by improved understanding of how the epidermal growth factor (EGF)–receptor complex stimulates mitosis in many kinds of cells. Exposure of target cells for many hours is required for EGF to induce cell division. Initially, however, there is a disappearance of the EGF–receptor complex from the cell surface as it is transported intracellularly (internalized) within small plasma membrane vesicles (endocytosis). Each vesicle contains clusters of complexes, since EGF binding promotes aggregation of these mobile receptors. Even though this internalization process ends well short of the time required for EGF exposure to have its growth effects, it may be an important step in its action, since the intact hormone in its intracellular form ultimately becomes associated with numerous subcellular compartments including lysosomes, the Golgi apparatus, endoplasmic reticulum, and the nucleus. Consequently interaction at the cell surface between hormone and receptor could be the initial step in translocating the complex to an intracellular site of action.

In contrast, the metabolic effects of insulin have been related specifically to binding of the cell surface and have been shown not to be related to internalization. It is not known whether the growth effects of insulin are initiated simply by binding to a receptor.

RELATION OF HORMONE ACTION TO CLINICAL MEDICINE

Steroid Hormones

Understanding of the mechanism of action of steroid and steroid-like hormones has led to a much clearer picture of the pathogenesis of a number of relatively uncommon diseases.

Androgen Resistance

The syndromes of androgen resistance are characterized by partial or complete inability to respond to a normal or increased secretion of testosterone. Since these are genetic diseases, they are expressed during fetal development.

5α-Reductase Deficiency

The enzyme responsible for converting testosterone to dihydrotestosterone is absent or nonfunctional. This is an autosomal recessive disorder expressed only in males. Structures derived from the Wolffian duct, which are testosterone-dependent (epididymis, vas deferens, and seminal vesicle), develop normally, while the prostate and external genitalia, which depend on dihydrotestosterone, fail to differentiate. These individuals thus have female external genitalia and normal Wolffian structures ending in a vagina. They have labial, scrotal, or abdominal testes. At the time of puberty the external genitalia mature variably, sexual hair develops, testosterone secretion rises, and male sexual orientation ensues. Gonadotropin levels are only slightly elevated, and gynecomastia is never seen. Facial and body hair are not quite normal in amount, acne is not seen, and the prostate is not palpable. Deficient or abnormal 5α-reductase activity can be demonstrated in fibroblasts from affected individuals.

Androgen Receptor Defects

Complete testicular feminization, type I (TFM-I) describes a group of X-linked disorders characterized by an absence of or a severe defect of androgen receptors. The individuals differentiate as females. Müllerian tissues regress so there is no uterus, and after an apparent normal puberty patients have primary amenorrhea. The testes, located intraabdominally or in the inguinal canal, secrete ample testosterone, and estrogen levels are in the female range. There is a near absence of sexual hair.

Incomplete testicular feminization refers to a heterogeneous group of syndromes—see Table 7 for clinical manifestations—with a diminished receptor concentration, an abnormal (heat-

Table 7 **Partial TFM-I Syndromes**

Stage	*Eponym*	*Characteristics*
I	Complete	Complete failure of male sexual differentiation. Female phenotype, near absence of sexual hair, blind-ending vagina
II	Lubs	Partial Wolffian development, partial labioscrotal fusion, pubic and axillary hair, masculine skeleton
III	Gilbert-Dreyfus	Small phallus, hypospadias, incomplete Wolffian structures, gynecomastia
IV	Reifenstein	Hypospadias, bifid scrotum, gynecomastia
V	Rosenwater	Sterility, gynecomastia

sensitive) receptor, or a normal apparent receptor concentration but a defective androgenic function in which the expression of normal or elevated androgen concentrations is defective.

No receptor defect demonstrating resistance to other steroid hormones has been characterized.

Vitamin D Resistance

A defect of the intestinal vitamin D receptor might be expected to cause some cases of familial vitamin D-resistant rickets, but no such cases have been described. The principal syndrome is apparently due to defective conversion of 25-hydroxycholecalciferol to 1,25-dihydroxycholecalciferol.

CELL SURFACE-ACTIVE-HORMONES

Receptor Diseases

With the development of information about protein receptors on the cell surface, there came a simultaneous realization that receptor diseases may exist. Three disorders, Graves' disease, myasthenia gravis, and several forms of insulin-resistant diabetes mellitus have been characterized as receptor diseases. Some features of these disorders are summarized in Table 8.

Table 8 **Receptor Diseases**

	Graves'	*Insulin-Resistant Diabetes*	*Myasthenia Gravis*
Receptor involved	TSH	Insulin	Acetylcholine of neuromuscular junction
Antibody involved	Yes	Sometimes	Yes
Antibody effect	Stimulation	Blocking	Destructive
Competes with agonist	Yes	Yes	?

Graves' Disease

Graves' disease is a multisystem illness with three principal manifestations—hyperthyroidism, infiltrative ophthalmopathy, and infiltrative dermopathy—known to be associated with other autoimmune diseases. The discovery of long-acting thyroid stimulator (LATS) in a substantial percentage of patients with Graves' disease turned attention from thyroid-stimulating hormone (TSH) in its pathogenesis. LATS was shown to be an IgG that stimulated thyroid adenylate cyclase similarly to TSH. LATS and other thyroid-stimulating immunoglobulins have been shown to compete with TSH for thyroid membrane receptor sites and to activate the thyroid gland.

Insulin Receptor and Diabetes Mellitus

Abnormalities of the insulin receptor have been found in obesity, in lipoatrophic diabetes, and in the syndromes of insulin resistance and acanthosis nigricans (Table 9).

The insulin receptor has a unique feature in that receptor affinity as well as number is sensitive to exposure to insulin. In obesity and in adult-type diabetes with obesity (type II diabetes), there is substantial insulin resistance and reduced binding to receptor, resulting in hyperglycemia and hyperinsulinism. Acute and chronic severe food intake restriction returns the receptor concentration to normal in association with the decline in insulin concentration. In theory then, whether an obese subject develops clinical diabetes depends on his or her insulin secretory reserve in the face of reduced cell surface receptor affinity and concentration. Certain thin, type II diabetics have similar features. However, in studies relating insulin receptors and insulin concentration to its action in large and small fat cells, it has been shown that the lesion is not primarily an insulin-binding defect but that defective action of the enzymes is involved in glucose metabolism beyond uptake and phosphorylation.

Recently the syndromes of severe insulin resistance and of acanthosis nigricans were described, in which acanthosis nigricans is accompanied by severe endogenous hyperinsulinemia and extreme resistance to exogenous insulin. Other causes of insulin resistance such as antiinsulin antibodies, severe obesity, lipoatrophy, Cushing's syndrome, and acromegaly are absent. Type

Table 9 **Insulin Receptor Disorders**[a]

	Resistance and Obesity	*Resistance and Lipoatrophy*	*Resistance and Acanthosis Nigricans*	
			Type A	*Type B*
Endogenous insulin	↑	↑↑	↑↑	↑↑
Sensitivity to exogenous insulin	↓	↓	↓	↓
Receptor number	↓	↓	↓ or N	↓ N or ↑
Mean receptor affinity	↓	↓	N	↓
Antireceptor antibody	No	No	No	Yes
Recovery of receptor with starvation	Yes	?	No	No

[a]Normal; ↑, increased; ↓, decreased; ↑ ↑, increased greatly.

A is found in women with polycystic ovarian disease, and these patients have an unexplained basis for their insulin resistance. Type-B patients have a high incidence of other autoimmune diseases and are found to have circulating antibodies to insulin receptor. This results in a marked reduction in mean insulin receptor affinity in whatever cells are studied. The defect was produced by treating normal cells with the antibody. The antisera inhibited insulin-stimulated glucose oxidation. The antibody had a small degree of agonist activity when tested alone, reminescent of the situation in Graves' disease.

In lipoatrophic diabetes, the well-known syndrome of glucose intolerance, absence of subcutaneous fat, and extreme insulin resistance has been reported to be associated with extreme endogenous hyperinsulinemia and severe receptor deficiency, particularly of the highest-affinity binding sites. The role of the receptor defect in the pathogenesis of this syndrome is unknown.

Acetylcholine Receptor and Myasthenia Gravis

When a pure acetylcholine receptor isolated from the electric organ of certain eels was employed to generate antisera, a disorder similar to myasthenia gravis was produced in the immunized rabbits. Immunization with antibody to eel acetylcholine receptor will make an animal weak for as long as 90 days. The disorder starts with acute intensive myasthenic symptoms with low antibody titers and proceeds to a situation with high antibody titers and destruction of 80–90% of the postsynaptic neuromuscular junctions. The loss of receptors appears to be the main reason for the muscle weakness.

In human myasthenia gravis there is a profound deficiency of acetylcholine receptors at neuromuscular junctions. Serum from human myasthenics causes a similar syndrome in mice by passive immunization. The active factor is an IgG enhanced by the C_3 component of complement, indicating that autoimmunity to the acetylcholine receptor of the neuromuscular junction is pathogenic in myasthenia and that the antibody to receptor destroys the receptor. Removal of antibody by plasmapheresis has resulted in marked improvement in a group of patients with progressive myasthenia gravis.

Disorders of Coupling

One variety of pseudohypoparathyroidism has been demonstrated to be associated with a substantial decrease in cellular capacity for coupling receptor occupancy to cAMP generation. It is characterized by hypocalcemia and tetany, a diminished responsiveness to elevated parathyroid hormone levels, and a variety of skeletal abnormalities of variable penetrance. Patients with the disease also have a less then normal complement of membrane coupling proteins. Recent studies have tended to demonstrate a reduced physiologic response to a variety of hormonal stimuli normally expressed via cAMP generation.

SUGGESTED READING

Baxter JD, Funder JW: Hormone receptors. *N Eng J Med* 301:1149–1161, 1979.

Catt KJ, Harwood JP, Aguilero G, Dufau ML: Hormonal regulation of peptide receptors and target cell responses. *Nature* 280:109–115, 1979.

Clark JH, Peck EJ: *Female Sex Steroids Receptors and Function.* Berlin, Springer-Verlag, 1979.

Levitzki A: Negative cooperativity at the insulin receptor. *Nature* 289:442–443, 1981.

Oppenheimer JH: Thyroid hormone action at the cellular level. *Science* 203:971–979, 1979.

Rodbell M: The role of hormone receptors and GTP-regulatory proteins in membrane transduction. *Nature* 284:17–21, 1980.

Ross EM, Gillman AG: Biochemical properties of hormone-sensitive adenylate cyclase. *Ann Rev Biochem* 49:533–564, 1980.

2 HAROLD E. CARLSON

Pituitary Diseases

The pituitary, by virtue of its trophic effect on the thyroid, adrenals, and gonads, is frequently involved in endocrine disorders, either primarily or secondarily. Because pituitary hormones are now readily measurable by radioimmunoassay methods and their control reasonably well understood, the investigation and treatment of patients with pituitary disorders is particularly logical and satisfying. This chapter will deal with hypofunction and hyperfunction of the anterior pituitary gland (the adenohypophysis), reviewing the pathophysiology of the various disorders and suggesting an economical approach to diagnosis and therapy.

NORMAL PITUITARY PHYSIOLOGY

The normal adenohypophysis secretes six well-characterized hormones; a seventh hormone, β-lipotropin, is secreted by corticotropic cells and synthesized along with adrenocorticotropin (ACTH) as part of a large precursor molecule known as pro-opiomelanocortin. The physiologic control and action of β-lipotropin are still poorly understood; under some circumstances, it may serve as a precursor of endogenous opiate peptides (endorphins) or may stimulate adrenal function. The existence of a distinct melanocyte-stimulating hormone (MSH) in humans is unclear; ACTH has moderate MSH activity and may account for most of the skin darkening seen in Addison's disease or Nelson's syndrome (see Chapter 8).

Thyroid-stimulating hormone (TSH, thyrotropin), adrenocorticotropin (ACTH), and the two gonadotropins, luteinizing hormone (LH) and follicle-stimulating hormone (FSH), act on end-organ target glands to stimulate the secretion of hormones that exert a restraining negative feedback effect on their respective pituitary trophic cells. Thus TSH secretion is largely controlled by the inhibitory feedback effects of circulating thyroxine (T_4) and triiodothyronine (T_3) on the pituitary; similar relationships hold for ACTH and cortisol, and for LH-FSH and gonadal steroids. In contrast, prolactin (PRL) and growth hormone (GH) have no well-defined peripheral product that exerts a feedback effect (although there is some evidence that somatomedins, a group of GH-dependent growth-promoting peptides, can inhibit GH secretion). In addition to feedback effects of end-organ products, the hypothalamus exerts a measure of control over pituitary secretion by means of releasing and inhibiting factors secreted into the hypothalamopituitary portal circulation and carried to the adenohypophysis where they influence hormone release. Several factors have been identified to date: Thyrotropin-releasing hormone (TRH, protirelin) releases TSH and PRL from the pituitary; gonadotropin-releasing hormone (GnRH) releases both LH and FSH; somatostatin inhibits GH (and, to some extent, TSH) secretion; dopamine, a potent inhibitor of PRL release, is probably the main factor physiologically regulating this hormone. It has been assumed that end-organ hormones may exert their feedback effects on the hypothalamus as well as directly on the pituitary, but this is still unproven.

HYPOPITUITARISM

As the reader may gather from the above discussion, hypofunction of the pituitary may arise as a consequence of disease either of the pituitary itself or of the hypothalamus (Table 1). In most cases, the end result is the same: decreased secretion of pituitary hormones with consequent effects on the function of the remainder of the organism. Thus TSH deficiency produces hypothyroidism without goiter; ACTH deficiency leads to hypoadrenalism and poor tanning of the skin; LH and FSH deficiency produces hypogonadism; PRL deficiency results in failure of postpartum lactation; and GH deficiency produces short stature, fine facial wrinkles, and occasionally fasting hypoglycemia in children.

In the cases of TSH, ACTH, LH, and FSH, the diagnosis of secondary (i.e., pituitary-hypothalamic) end-organ hypofunction can be easily established by demonstrating low serum levels of the appropriate pituitary hormone concurrent with low levels of the target organ hormone. Thus a low serum TSH level in the presence of clinical hypothyroidism with a low serum free T_4 index suggests a diagnosis of secondary rather than primary hypothyroidism. To separate hypothalamic from pituitary causes of hypofunction, as well as to diagnose GH or PRL deficiency, specific pituitary stimulation tests are needed. In some cases, however, it is of no practical importance to distinguish hormonally pituitary and hypothalamic disorders, since the endocrine therapy is not altered by this information.

Pituitary Function Testing

Serum GH levels are normally low or undetectable throughout most of the day in adults, rising during exercise, sleep, and stress or postprandially. More reliable stimulation tests such as insulin-induced hypoglycemia (0.05–0.15 units/kg body weight i.v.), arginine infusion (30 g over 30 minutes), or L-dopa ingestion (250–500 mg orally, with or without concurrent propranolol administration) are usually employed clinically (Fig. 1); all three of these agents act by increasing the secretion of GH-releasing factor from the hypothalamus. A serum GH value of at least 7 ng/ml at any time during the test constitutes a normal response. Obese or hypothyroid patients often have blunted responses to all GH-provocative agents. The GH responses of normal men and prepubertal children may be enhanced by 3 days of estrogen pretreatment (e.g., diethylstilbestrol, 2.5 mg orally twice daily). Since 5–10% or normal subjects fail to respond appropriately to any single testing agent, hyporesponsiveness to at least two different stimuli should be documented before GH deficiency is diagnosed.

In normal subjects, PRL secretion is usually low through much of the day, rising during sleep and stress and, perhaps, postprandially. Clinically useful provocative tests of PRL release include intravenous thyrotropin-releasing hormone (TRH) (100–500 μg i.v. bolus) which directly stimulates the lactotroph, and dopamine antagonists (i.m. or oral phenothiazine [e.g.,

Table 1 **Causes of Hypopituitarism**

Infarction
Postpartum necrosis (Sheehan's syndrome)
Vascular disease (in diabetes mellitus)
Head trauma
Neoplasms involving pituitary
Pituitary adenoma
Craniopharyngioma
Metastatic or primary carcinoma (rare)
Granulomas
Sarcoidosis
Histiocytosis X
Infections
Tuberculosis
Fungi
Pyogenic
Syphilis
Aneurysm of internal carotid artery
Hemochromatosis
Idiopathic or genetic
Deficient production of pituitary hormone
Synthesis of abnormal hormone
Primary hypothalamic disorders
Tumors (e.g., craniopharyngioma, glioma)
Granulomas (histiocytosis X, sarcoidosis)
Midline CNS structural anomalies of hypothalamus
Head trauma
Genetic or idiopathic releasing factor deficiency
Iatrogenic
Radiation
Stalk section
Hypophysectomy

perphenazine 8 mg p.o.], or oral or i.v. metoclopramide, 5–10 mg) which block endogenous PRL-inhibiting factor. A minimal normal PRL response in any of these tests consists of a doubling of baseline values with a peak of at least 12 ng/ml. PRL responses to all tests are enhanced by estrogen administration and are therefore generally larger in women. Patients with hypopituitarism will have low baseline serum PRL levels which fail to rise appropriately after administration of TRH or other stimuli. In contrast, patients with pure hypothalamic disease will have basal hyperprolactinemia, since the intact lactotrophs will have been freed from the tonic inhibitory effect of hypothalamic dopamine; PRL responses to TRH may be either blunted or normal in such patients.

Patients with pituitary or hypothalamic disease may have hypothyroidism as one component of their pituitary dysfunction. With pure pituitary disease (e.g., posthypophysectomy), serum

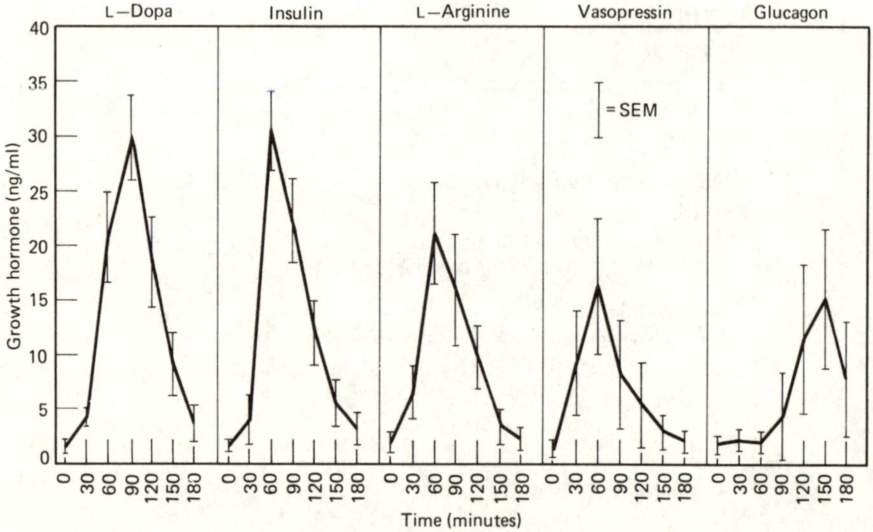

Figure 1. GH reserve is usually evaluated with oral L-dopa, insulin-induced hypoglycemia, or arginine infusion. Responses to vasopressin or glucagon are less reliable and, therefore, are not often employed. Mean ± SEM responses in 20 normal subjects are shown. Reprinted by permission of Eddy RL, Human growth hormone release, *Am J Med* 56:179–185, 1974. Copyright Technical Publishing Company.

TSH levels are low and fail to rise after intravenous administration of TRH, which directly stimulates thyrotrophs. Patients with pure hypothalamic disease may have low, normal, or even slightly elevated serum TSH levels in the presence of hypothyroidism, with a normal-sized but delayed TSH increment following TRH administration (see Chap. 4, Fig. 1), presumably reflecting TRH deficiency. Observation of the apparent paradoxical occurrence of hypothyroidism despite normal or elevated TSH levels by radioimmunoassay has been explained by the recent finding that serum TSH bioactivity is low in such patients; it has, therefore, been proposed that endogenous TRH is needed to confer full bioactivity on the TSH molecule.

Similar testing procedures may be applied to gonadotropin secretion as well. Synthetic GnRH, a direct stimulator of gonadotrophs, may be injected (100-μg i.v. bolus), and LH and FSH responses assessed. Patients with complete pituitary destruction show low baseline LH and FSH levels with no rise after GnRH injection. As expected, subjects with hypothalamic disease *do* respond to GnRH, although "priming" doses of GnRH may need to be given for several days to demonstrate the response fully (Fig. 2). Unfortunately GnRH is not commercially available in the United States at present. The gonadotropin reserve may also be assessed by testing with oral clomiphene, an estrogen antagonist. In normal men and women, clomiphene provokes a rise in both LH and FSH by blocking the inhibitory feedback effects of gonadal steroids on the hypothalamus. Although useful as a research tool, clomiphene testing has only occasional practical application.

The assessment of ACTH secretion has traditionally been indirect, because of the difficulty and expense of plasma ACTH measurements. Recent advances in ACTH radioimmunoassay techniques, however, have made the clinical use of plasma ACTH determinations much more

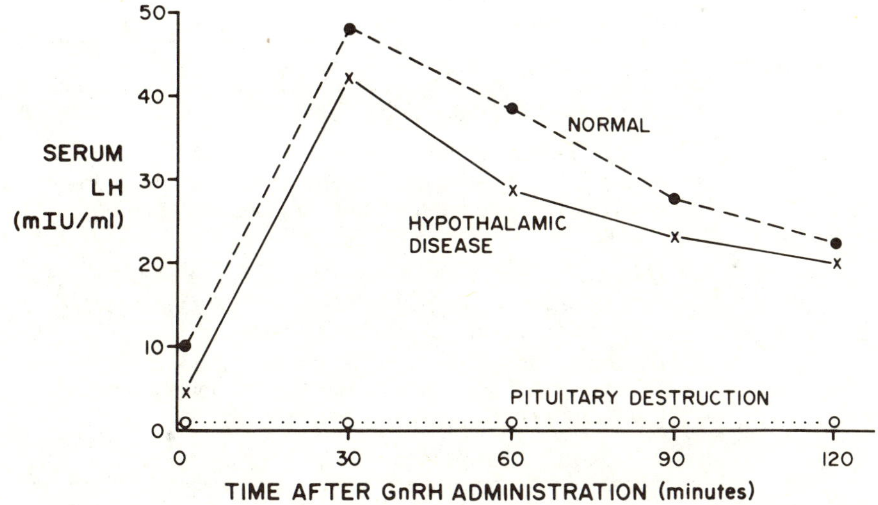

Figure 2. Serum LH responses to intravenous GnRH in patients with pituitary destruction (dotted line), patients with hypothalamic disease (solid line), and normals (dashed line). After "priming" with GnRH for 7–14 days, patients with pure hypothalamic disease respond normally to GnRH, while patients without functioning pituitary tissue continue to show no response.

widely available. Indirect assessments have utilized measurements of plasma cortisol levels, which parallel plasma ACTH levels under most circumstances, or levels of urinary free cortisol or corticosteroid metabolites (e.g., 17-hydroxycorticosteroids). In patients with obvious adrenal insufficiency, one may reliably distinguish between primary and secondary (pituitary-hypothalamic) adrenal failure by measuring plasma ACTH in the morning (6–9 AM), when levels are normally highest. In the presence of low serum cortisol concentrations, plasma ACTH levels are elevated in patients with primary adrenal failure, while low or low-normal levels are seen in patients with secondary adrenal insufficiency. Provocative testing with insulin-induced hypoglycemia or metyrapone may be used to document lesser defects in the ACTH reserve. Chapter 8 gives further details on these procedures. Pituitary β-lipotropin secretion is not usually evaluated clinically, although the regulation of this hormone is currently a subject of intense investigation.

The clinical use of detailed pituitary function testing may be summarized as follows:

1. To assist in the diagnosis of otherwise obscure pituitary or hypothalamic disease.
2. To determine the need for GH replacement therapy in children with short stature.
3. In the future, possibly to assess the feasibility of treating hypogonadism due to hypothalamic disease with GnRH.

Note that, with the exception of GH treatment for short stature and gonadotropins for infertility, the need for hormone replacement therapy is solely determined by clinical status and measurement of end-organ products (T_4, cortisol, and testosterone) rather than pituitary hormones.

Table 2 **Treatment of Hypopituitarism**

Deficient Hormone	*Therapy*
TSH	L-Thyroxine, 0.1–0.3 mg/day orally
ACTH	Oral glucocorticoid; for example, prednisone, 5 mg in the morning, 2.5 mg at noon, *or* hydrocortisone, 20 mg in the morning, 10 mg at noon. Mineralocorticoid is not usually needed.
LH or FSH	Men: Testosterone enanthate or cypionate, 200–300 mg i.m. every 2–3 weeks, *or* fluoxymesterone, 2–10 mg/day orally, *or* methyltestosterone, 10–40 mg/day orally Women: Cyclic estrogen and progesterone. For restoration of fertility in either sex, HMG and HCG are given by injection, usually for periods of several months
GH	1–3 units i.m., three times weekly

Treatment of Hypopituitarism

In most cases, the hormonal deficiencies of hypopituitarism are treated rather simply by supplying the needed end-organ hormones. Table 2 summarizes this therapy. PRL replacement therapy is rarely needed and is unavailable in any case. Replacement pituitary hormones are given in only two circumstances. First, GH is given to GH-deficient children with short stature and unfused epiphyses; human GH for treatment is available both from the National Pituitary Agency and also commercially. Second, exogenous gonadotropins may be given to stimulate gonadal function in hypopituitary patients desiring fertility; for this purpose, human chorionic gonadotropin (hCG) is used as a readily available substitute for LH, while human menopausal gonadotropin (hMG) is used to provide FSH activity. Chapters 12 and 13 give further details of this expensive therapy, which is generally undertaken only by specialists. Patients with hypopituitarism should carry or wear identification showing their hormonal status. Both patients and their families should be able to administer supplemental glucocorticoid in case of severe illness or injury.

Patients with hypopituitarism may have an intracranial mass lesion as the cause of their hormone deficiency. These tumors also require management, as outlined below.

PITUITARY TUMORS

General Considerations

Pituitary tumors, nearly always benign, account for about 10% of all intracranial neoplasms. Recent evidence based on serum radioimmunoassays, tissue electron microscopy, and immunohistochemistry has shown that nonfunctioning tumors are the single most common neoplasm, followed by PRL-secreting tumors and GH-secreting lesions (Table 3). The appearance of a pituitary tumor on hematoxylin and eosin staining bears little relationship to its functional status; "chromophobe" tumors commonly secrete PRL, GH, or other hormones, and this outmoded term should be discarded in favor of a more useful classification by hormone secretion.

Table 3 **Frequency of Pituitary Tumors**

Type of Tumor	*Relative Incidence* (%)
Nonfunctioning	35
PRL-secreting	30
GH-secreting	20
Mixed GH- and PRL-secreting	7
ACTH- or lipotropin-secreting	7
LH-, FSH-, or TSH-secreting	1

Reprinted by permission of Carlson HE, Functioning pituitary tumors, in Hershman JM (ed), *Practical Endocrinology,* New York, John Wiley and Sons, New York, 1981, p 53. Copyright John Wiley and Sons.

Both secreting and nonsecreting tumors may produce a variety of signs and symptoms because of their space-occupying characteristics and their locations. These features, such as headaches, visual impairment (classically, bitemporal hemianopsia due to compression of the optic chiasm), extraocular palsy, hydrocephalus, seizures, and cerebrospinal fluid (CSF) rhinorrhea are all more common with macroadenomas (larger than 1 cm in diameter), and tumors with extrasellar extension than with intrasellar microadenomas (less than 1 cm in diameter). Additionally, hypopituitarism and diabetes insipidus are more commonly associated with large, destructive tumors.

Radiologic procedures have a major role in the diagnosis and treatment of pituitary lesions. Plain or coned-down views of the sella may show generalized expansion or destruction of the sella when a large tumor is present. Focal depression of the sellar floor may be seen as a "double floor" on a lateral view of the skull, often with bony thinning or erosion. Hypocycloidal polytomography of the sella provides the ability to delineate more clearly these focal abnormalities produced by small intrasellar tumors; several recent reports, however, suggest that normal variants of sellar anatomy may resemble these tumor-induced changes, greatly complicating the interpretation of sellar tomograms. Computed tomography (CT) has recently led to startling improvements in the resolution of intrasellar pathology; new fourth-generation (and beyond) high-resolution machines, which permit scanning or reconstruction of images in coronal as well as axial section, have led to the routine detection of pituitary microadenomas (Fig. 3), enabled neurosurgeons to evaluate suprasellar extension of tumor, and greatly simplified the diagnosis of an "empty" sella (see page 34). To a large extent, invasive procedures such as pneumoencephalography and carotid angiography are now unnecessary in the evaluation of pituitary disease; sellar tomography may also be unnecessary if high-resolution CT scans are available.

Spontaneous hemorrhage into a pituitary tumor occurs in perhaps 5% of patients; clinically recognizable instances (pituitary apoplexy) are characterized by headache, decreased vision, extraocular palsies, and other neurologic findings. Emergency evacuation of the hematoma may be needed in severe cases, along with fluids and glucocorticoid supplements.

Management of Pituitary Tumors

In occasional elderly or terminally ill patients with pituitary tumors, no treatment other than observation and end-organ hormone replacement is indicated. Most patients, however,

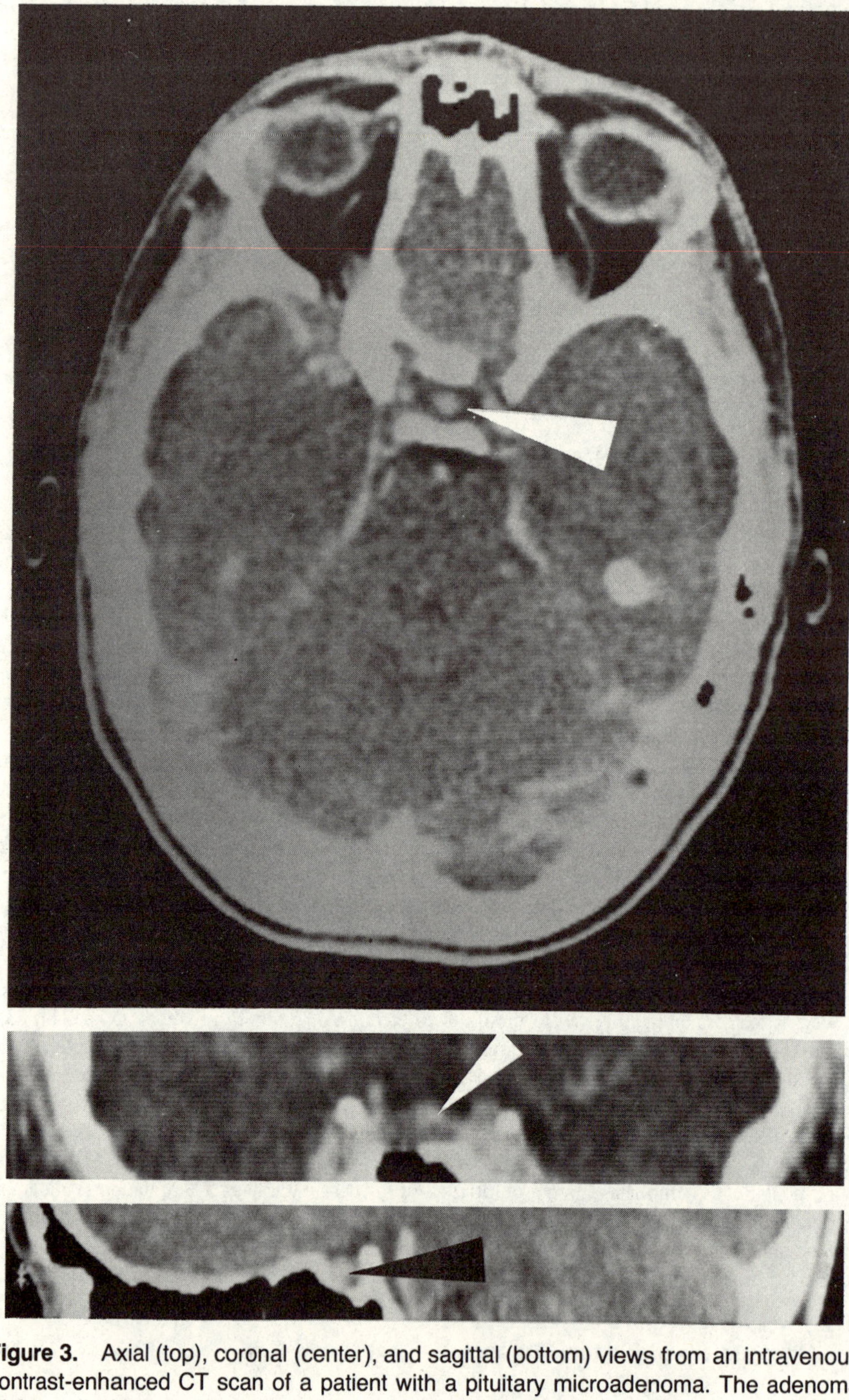

Figure 3. Axial (top), coronal (center), and sagittal (bottom) views from an intravenous contrast-enhanced CT scan of a patient with a pituitary microadenoma. The adenoma "lights up" with contrast agent on all three views (arrowheads). Scans courtesy of Huntington Memorial Hospital, Pasadena, California.

require some additional therapy to diminish hormone hypersecretion, if present, and to correct or prevent the mass effects of the intracranial neoplasm. Pituitary tumor ablation with either surgery or radiation is available for these purposes. Table 4 lists the relative merits and deficiencies of the two methods. In general, surgery is preferred when serious anatomic complications exist (e.g., visual field defects) or when immediate correction of hormone hypersecretion is

Table 4 **Choice of Surgery vs. Radiation Therapy for Pituitary Tumors**

Radiation therapy
- Appropriate for
  - Small or medium-sized tumors with minimal or modest suprasellar extension
  - Patients in whom surgery is contraindicated or refused
  - Postoperative adjunctive therapy in patients with invasive or incompletely removed tumors
- Contraindicated as sole therapy in
  - Patients with large suprasellar extensions
  - Patients with major visual field defects
  - Acromegalics with serum growth hormone levels >50 ng/ml prior to treatment
  - PRL patients who wish to restore fertility

Surgery, transfrontal approach
- Appropriate for
  - Large suprasellar extensions, especially if dumbbell-shaped with a constriction at the diaphragma sellae, or with lateral suprasellar extension
  - Patients in whom the transsphenoidal approach to the sella is relatively contraindicated (patients with chronic sinusitis or an incompletely pneumatized sphenoid sinus

Surgery, transsphenoidal approach
- Appropriate for
  - Microadenomas (less than 1 cm in diameter)
  - Tumors associated with cerebrospinal fluid rhinorrhea or extension into the sphenoid sinus
  - Tumors associated with pituitary apoplexy
  - Macroadenomas (>1 cm diameter) with minimal or modest suprasellar extension
- Contraindicated in
  - Tumors with large dumbbell-shaped or lateral suprasellar extensions
  - Patients with chronic sinusitis or incompletely pneumatized sphenoid sinus (relative, not absolute contraindications)

Reprinted by permission of Carlson HE, Pituitary diseases, in Hershman JM (ed), *Management of Endocrine Disorders,* Philadelphia, Lea & Febiger, Philadelphia, 1980, p 10. Copyright Lea & Febiger.

desired. Radiotherapy delivered as supervoltage photons from either ^{60}Co or linear accelerator devices, or as heavy particles (protons in Boston, Massachusetts, and alpha particles in Berkeley, California), has a slower onset of effect than surgery, generally taking 6–24 months for initial benefit to be seen, with progressive improvement over 2–5 years. Both surgery and radiation may result in hypopituitarism or occasionally damage adjacent structures. Recently, dopamine agonists such as bromocriptine and lisuride have been shown to produce remarkable shrinkage of PRL-secreting adenomas, and this medical therapy may ultimately be recommended as the sole or adjunctive therapy for such tumors (see page 32).

Patients scheduled for pituitary-hypothalamic surgery should not be subjected to a detailed preoperative hormonal evaluation, since testing will only need to be repeated postoperatively. Instead, one should measure the serum free T_4 index (untreated hypothyroidism may increase the risks of general anesthesia) and serum GH and PRL levels (to detect occult hypersecretion of these hormones). Rather than assess the ACTH reserve preoperatively, most physicians merely provide supplemental glucocorticoid in the perioperative period and during stressful diagnostic procedures.

In postoperative patients and patients receiving medical or radiation therapy alone, the need for hormone replacement should be evaluated by measuring the serum testosterone level (in men) and the free T_4 index and performing a test of the pituitary-adrenal axis with insulin-induced hypoglycemia or metyrapone. The presence of regular menses in a premenopausal woman usually indicates relatively normal estrogen secretion, and further testing is not needed unless infertility is present. Children should have provocative tests of GH secretion. Basal PRL and GH levels should be measured in all patients to detect occult hypersecretion.

Following initial treatment, patients are seen every 3–4 months for 1 year, and then every 6–12 months. At each visit, signs and symptoms of hormone deficiency or excess should be sought. The ACTH reserve and the serum free T_4 index should be tested every 1–2 years. Pituitary tumor patients should have visual field testing and a lateral skull roentgenogram every 6–12 months for the first 2 or 3 years after treatment, and then every 2–3 years thereafter. A contrast-enhanced cerebral CT scan should probably also be performed every 2–3 years in these patients.

ACROMEGALY AND GIGANTISM

Hypersecretion of GH results in the typical appearance of acromegaly, with enlargement of the hands, feet, and facial features in most patients. The presence of GH excess prior to the closure of long bone epiphyses in late puberty leads to increases in stature; if the process begins in childhood, gigantism may result. Other common symptoms include excessive perspiration, perhaps due to enlarged sweat glands or to hypermetabolism; the carpal tunnel syndrome, due to compression of the median nerve by hypertrophied fibrocartilaginous tissue in the wrist; degenerative arthritis, secondary to bony overgrowth and deformity around large weight-bearing joints; hypertension, perhaps related to the salt-retaining effects of GH; glucose intolerance or frank diabetes mellitus, due to the insulin-antagonistic properties of GH; hypercalciuria, perhaps secondary to stimulation of 1,25-dihydroxyvitamin D_3 production by GH; and galactorrhea, due either to the intrinsic lactogenic properties of GH or to the presence of a "mixed" adenoma secreting both GH and PRL. Increased mortality in acromegaly is attributed to cardiovascular, cerebrovascular, and pulmonary diseases.

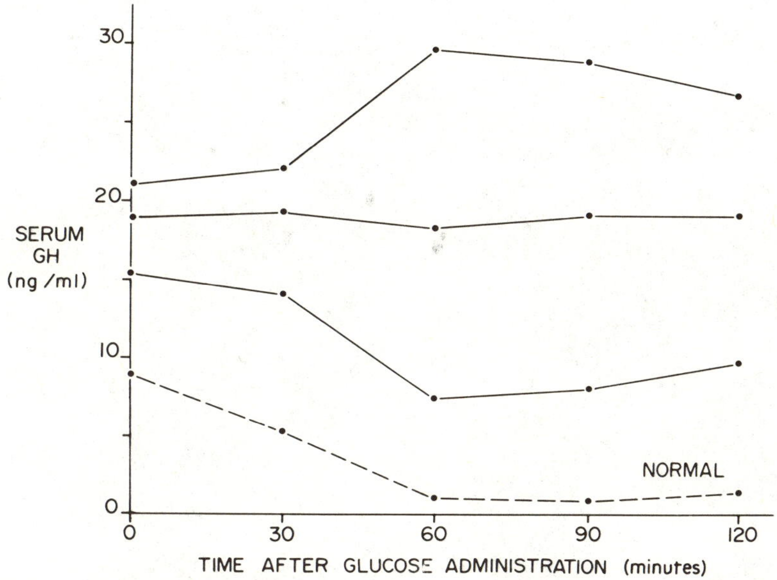

Figure 4. Lack of suppression of the serum GH level by glucose ingestion in acromegaly. In contrast to normal subjects (dashed line), patients with acromegaly may show partial suppression, no change, or a rise in the serum GH level after glucose ingestion (solid lines). Reprinted by permission of Carlson, HE, Functioning pituitary tumors, in Hershman JM (ed), *Practical Endocrinology.* John Wiley & Sons, New York, 1981, p 57. Copyright John Wiley & Sons.

Diagnosis of Acromegaly

When suspected in a patient with a compatible clinical history and appearance, the diagnosis of acromegaly is usually easy to confirm. The simplest and most reliable test involves the assessment of GH responses to oral glucose. In normal subjects, serum GH is suppressed to low levels (<5 ng/ml, often undetectable) 60–90 minutes after the oral administration of 50–100 g of glucose in solution. Nearly all acromegalics fail to show such suppression and may show a rise in GH levels instead (Fig. 4). Patients with borderline GH suppression by glucose may be studied with a TRH test; although TRH has little or no effect on GH in normal individuals, patients with acromegaly usually show a substantial transient rise in GH levels in response to TRH (Fig. 5). Two or three random measurements of the serum GH level should also be obtained, to serve as the average pretreatment baseline value. Baseline serum PRL levels should also be measured in all patients with acromegaly, since up to 40% of acromegalics have a mixed pituitary adenoma secreting both GH and PRL from two cell types in the same tumor.

After a hormonal diagnosis has been made, patients with acromegaly should also undergo an anatomic evaluation of their sellar contents with radiologic examinations (lateral skull film, sellar tomography, and contrast-enhanced CT scan) and a formal visual field examination.

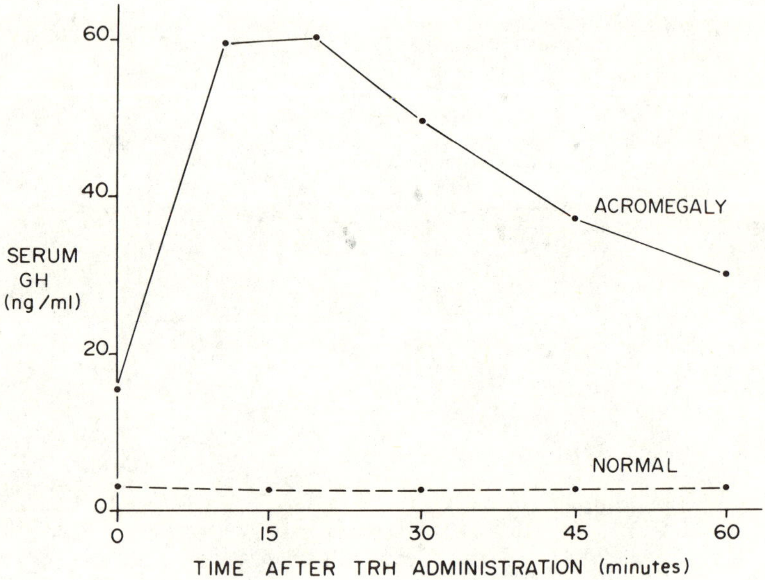

Figure 5. Normal subjects (dashed line) usually show no change in serum GH level in response to intravenous administration of TRH. Acromegalic patients (solid line) often demonstrate a marked rise in the serum GH level following TRH injection. Reprinted by permission of Carlson HE, Functioning pituitary tumors, in Hershman JM (ed), *Practical Endocrinology.* John Wiley & Sons, New York, 1981, p 58. Copyright John Wiley & Sons.

Treatment of Acromegaly

Radiotherapy and pituitary surgery both yield equivalent long-term results, with approximately 70–80% of patients achieving serum GH values <10 ng/ml. Surgery, however, offers the advantage of an immediate rather than a gradual lowering of GH; additionally, patients with very high pretreatment serum GH values (>50 ng/ml) are often left with residual GH hypersecretion after radiotherapy and are probably best treated with surgery as the initial therapy. As outlined above, factors such as visual field defects and large suprasellar extensions will also influence the choice of treatment (Table 4).

Although a variety of medical treatments for acromegaly have been proposed, the only practical therapy to date is the chronic oral administration of bromocriptine in doses of 15–30 mg/day. This ergot derivative with dopamine-like properties significantly lowers serum GH levels in a minority of acromegalics (10–40%). Some studies also report clinical improvement in patients who experience no fall in serum GH levels, although the validity of these uncontrolled observations has recently been questioned. Additionally, there are a few reports of pituitary tumor shrinkage in acromegalic patients given bromocriptine. At present, bromocriptine is used primarily as adjunctive treatment in acromegaly after surgery or radiation. The major side effects of bromocriptine consist of nausea and orthostatic hypotension; these are minimized by giving the drug in split doses with meals and by slowly increasing the daily dose to desired levels.

Successful treatment of acromegaly restores the serum GH level to normal and often results in regression of soft-tissue enlargement, improvement in carpal tunnel syndrome and glucose tolerance, increased pep and energy, and disappearance of excessive sweating. Bony changes and their sequelae (osteoarthritis) usually do not improve but at least stabilize.

Treated acromegalics should have serum GH levels measured in a random blood specimen every 6 months for 2 or 3 years after treatment, and then at yearly intervals. Radiologic assessment of sellar size, visual field examination, and measurement of serum PRL levels (if previously elevated) should be performed at similar time points. The serum free T_4 index and ACTH reserve should be evaluated every 1–2 years. The use of serum somatomedin measurements in the follow-up of treated acromegaly is still controversial.

PRL-SECRETING TUMORS

Adenomas secreting PRL (prolactinomas) are the most common functioning pituitary tumors. Hyperprolactinemia in women commonly leads to amenorrhea, with or without galactorrhea. Men usually manifest decreased libido and potency or symptoms of an intrasellar mass lesion; galactorrhea is uncommon in men, probably because the male breast has not been "primed" with endogenous estrogen. Menstruating women with prolactinomas may show infertility or a short luteal phase of the menstrual cycle. These manifestations of hypogonadism in both sexes appear to be due primarily to the inhibition of GnRH release from the hypothalamus by PRL, with resultant decreased LH and FSH secretion; a direct inhibitory action of PRL on the gonad may also contribute. Some women with PRL-secreting tumors also manifest hirsutism and elevated levels of serum androgens; the evidence for PRL stimulation of adrenal androgen production is still controversial.

Diagnosis

In addition to pituitary tumors, hyperprolactinemia may occur in a wide variety of other circumstances (Table 5). A careful history is of great importance in the investigation of medication-induced hyperprolactinemia. Pregnancy, hypothyroidism, and renal failure can be excluded by examination and simple laboratory tests. Radiologic examination and special endocrine testing then play a role in separating patients with pituitary or hypothalamic lesions from those with presumed "functional" hyperprolactinemia. Polytomography of the sella turcica may show generalized or focal bulging or thinning of the sellar floor in tumor patients, and computed tomography may reveal intrasellar or suprasellar mass lesions. Negative radiologic studies, of course, never rule out a small tumor; indeed, many patients initially believed to have functional hyperprolactinemia have been found in later follow-up, using more sensitive techniques, to have small pituitary neoplasms. It is helpful to obtain three separate or pooled determinations of the serum PRL level to account for spontaneous or stress-induced fluctuations. A serum PRL level persistently over 200 ng/ml is almost always associated with a pituitary tumor (normal male levels <15 ng/ml, normal female levels <20 ng/ml). However, since the elevation of the serum PRL level is roughly proportional to tumor mass, small tumors may cause smaller elevations of serum PRL levels to values commonly seen with hyperprolactinemia due to other causes (e.g., 30–50 ng/ml). Since there is currently no suppression test available to separate tumorous from nontumorous hyperprolactinemia, we must make do with a variety of stimulation tests. The best studied of these is the TRH test. In normal subjects, intravenous TRH results in a brisk rise in the serum PRL level in 15–30 minutes, with peak values exceeding 12 ng/ml and being at least twice baseline levels. In contrast, patients with PRL-secreting tumors usually show little or no increment (expressed as multiples of baseline values) in response to TRH,

Table 5 **Causes of Hyperprolactinemia**

Altered physiologic states
Sleep
Stress
Postprandial, especially in women
Coitus
Pregnancy, including pseudocyesis
Nursing or nipple stimulation
Chest wall or spinal cord lesions
Hypoglycemia
Hypothyroidism
Chronic renal failure
Medications
Phenothiazines
Butyrophenones (e.g., haloperidol)
Thioxanthenes (e.g., thiothixene)
Amoxapine
Reserpine
α-Methyldopa
Metoclopramide
Intravenous cimetidine
Estrogens
Opiates
PRL-secreting pituitary tumors
Decreased delivery of PRL-inhibiting factor to pituitary
Stalk section
Hypothalamic destruction

rarely exceeding a 100% rise (Fig. 6). Patients with elevated serum PRL levels due to other causes often (but not always) show a more normal response, with a TRH-induced rise in PRL levels of at least 100%.

Treatment

Ablative therapy, either surgical or radiologic, has been the traditional approach to the treatment of prolactinomas. Since the beneficial effects of radiotherapy are gradual and may require years for their full expression, this modality has not been favored for the typical patient with a prolactinoma, a young woman desiring fertility. Recent advances in transsphenoidal pituitary surgery have made selective adenomectomy an achievable alternative, and this is preferred at many centers where appropriate neurosurgical expertise is available. The best results are achieved with small tumors; 80–90% of patients with microadenomas are cured following surgery, but less than half of patients with larger tumors achieve normoprolactinemia. Within the last 5 years, however, medical therapy with dopamine agonists has emerged as a strong challenger to the primacy of surgical treatment of PRL-secreting tumors. Agents such as bromocriptine and lisuride are ergot derivatives with dopamine-like actions; as such, they are potent suppressors of PRL secretion and promptly restore normoprolactinemia, abolish galactorrhea, and restore normal gonadal function in patients with hyperprolactinemia of any cause. Although not yet officially approved for use in patients with PRL-secreting pituitary tumors, these drugs appear to be safe and effective in such subjects. Recent evidence indicates that they may also

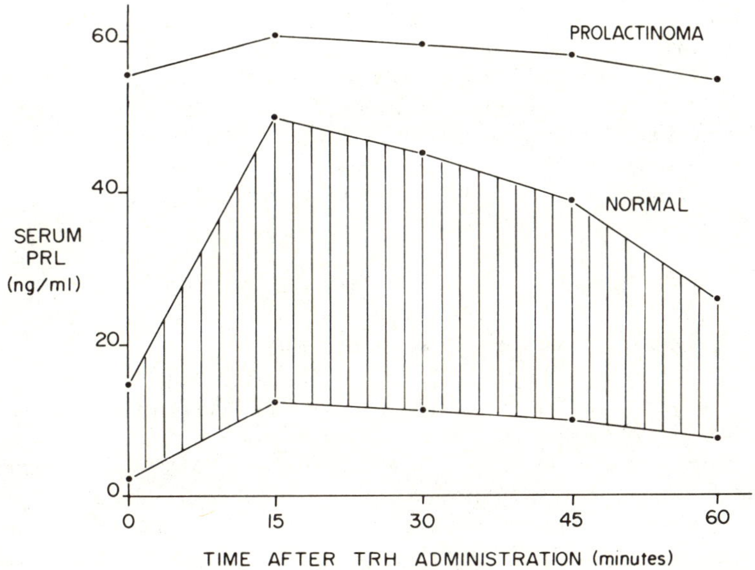

Figure 6. Normal subjects (hatched area) demonstrate at least a twofold rise in the serum PRL level after intravenous injection of TRH. In contrast, patients with PRL-secreting pituitary tumors (solid line) usually show little change in the serum PRL level after TRH administration. Reprinted by permission of Carlson HE, Functioning pituitary tumors, in Hershman JM (ed), *Practical Endocrinology.* John Wiley & Sons, New York, 1981, p 67. Copyright John Wiley & Sons.

cause a rapid shrinkage of prolactinomas in some patients. In general, these effects last only as long as the drug is taken, and tumor regrowth with recurrent hyperprolactinemia occurs once the medication is stopped. Nevertheless, it appears that we now have some most remarkable agents whose use may often obviate the need for surgery. Additionally, it has been suggested that preoperative treatment with bromocriptine or related drugs would, by shrinking large tumors, make surgery easier.

Ongoing concerns have been the effects of bromocriptine on pregnancy and the fetus, and the possible deleterious effects of resulting pregnancies on pituitary tumor growth. To date, there has been no evidence of an increase in spontaneous abortions, stillbirths, or fetal anomalies in patients given bromocriptine during pregnancy. Although the increased estrogen production during pregnancy does induce pituitary lactotroph hyperplasia, the incidence of clinically significant growth of small prolactinomas during pregnancy appears to be low—on the order of 3–5%. Patients with macroadenomas, however, have a 25–35% risk of complications. Such patients who do experience significant tumor growth during pregnancy with headaches and visual field problems can be treated with early delivery or with reinstitution of bromocriptine during gestation if necessary. Thus women with microprolactinomas who wish to become pregnant can be allowed to do so, with the patient having a clear understanding that there is a small but finite risk of significant tumor growth during the pregnancy. The routine use of pituitary radiotherapy prior to conception does not seem warranted in patients with microadenomas but may be useful in patients with larger tumors.

Bromocriptine is usually begun at a low dose (1.25–2.5 mg/day, usually at bedtime with a snack, to minimize nausea and orthostatic hypotension), with dose increments of 1.25 or 2.5

mg every 3–4 days until a total daily dose of 5–10 mg/day is reached (given in two or three divided doses, with meals). Some patients may require larger doses.

In men with prolactinomas or in women not desiring fertility, either radiotherapy or surgery may be the treatment of choice, as outlined in Table 4. In men, impotence and decreased libido resulting from hyperprolactinemia may not be fully reversed by testosterone administration and may additionally require lowering the PRL level to normal by medication or other modalities. Patients with PRL-secreting tumors should receive follow-up as outlined for acromegaly.

TSH-SECRETING TUMORS

Pituitary adenomas secreting TSH are rare, accounting for less than 1% of pituitary tumors. The clinical syndrome accompanying these tumors is characterized by hyperthyroidism with detectable or elevated serum TSH levels. Typically, serum TSH shows little response to TRH; serum levels of glycoprotein hormone alpha subunit are often elevated and also usually show no response to TRH. About one-third of TSH-secreting tumors also produce additional hormones, usually either GH or PRL. The greatest therapeutic benefit has been achieved with tumor ablation by either surgery or radiation; a few patients have responded to bromocriptine.

PITUITARY HYPERPLASIA

Patients with untreated primary endocrine end-organ failure (e.g., of the thyroid or gonads) manifest hypersecretion of the appropriate trophic hormone(s) (TSH, LH, and FSH). In some cases, hormonal hypersecretion of long standing is accompanied by sufficient hyperplasia of the pituitary to result in sellar enlargement. It is important to recognize this condition in order to avoid unneeded investigation and therapy for a supposed pituitary neoplasm. The elevated pituitary hormone level is readily suppressed to normal following replacement of end-organ hormones (T_4, gonadal steroids), and the sella may gradually return to a normal size.

EMPTY SELLA SYNDROME

When the pituitary gland does not fill the sella turcica, the remaining volume is often occupied by CSF, as an extension of the subarachnoid space. Such a situation has been called an *empty sella;* this is a bit of a misnomer, since the sella is not totally empty but is occupied in part by pituitary tissue and in part by CSF. The sella may also be enlarged.

An empty sella may arise in two ways. A *secondary* empty sella is found following infarction, shrinkage (e.g., by bromocriptine), or destruction (by surgery or radiation) of a hyperplastic or adenomatous pituitary. In this situation, the sellar enlargement was caused by initial expansion of the pituitary tumor. The remaining pituitary may function normally or may show residual impairment related to the primary pathologic process or its treatment.

More commonly, an empty sella is found without evidence of preexisting tumor. This situation, termed the *primary* empty sella, is also what is usually meant by the so-called empty sella syndrome. In such cases, it is believed that a congenitally incomplete diaphragma sellae (seen in 10–40% of normal persons) allows CSF to enter the sella. Normal pulsatile CSF pressures then compress the pituitary and gradually expand the sella turcica. If intracranial pressure is elevated (as in pseudotumor cerebri), sellar enlargement is more likely to occur.

The primary empty sella is most often found in obese, middle-aged women, perhaps because these individuals more commonly have increased CSF pressure. The primary empty sella may account for 20–30% of patients evaluated for radiologic sellar abnormality.

Pituitary function is usually normal in patients with a primary empty sella; a minority of patients show diminished GH or gonadotropin secretion, but this may be due to obesity rather than pituitary dysfunction. Occasional bona fide examples of hypopituitarism do occur with a primary empty sella; these likely result from compression of the pituitary stalk with resultant decreased delivery of hypothalamic releasing factors to the pituitary.

Diagnosis

Most patients with the primary empty sella come to medical attention when sellar enlargement is incidentally found on skull roentgenograms taken for unrelated purposes (head trauma, headaches, sinusitis). On lateral skull films or sellar tomograms, the sella is often smoothly and symmetrically ballooned; focal bulging and thinning of the sellar floor have been seen in some cases, however. A definitive diagnosis of an empty sella requires the demonstration of CSF within the sella. In the past, this usually required a limited pneumoencephalogram, an uncomfortable procedure. Nowadays, the diagnosis can usually be made with cerebral CT, especially if one of the newer high-resolution scanners can be utilized (Fig. 7).

Investigation of patients with a suspected primary empty sella should be kept to a minimum. In an *otherwise healthy* patient (i.e., with no endocrine signs or symptoms) referred for evaluation of a symmetrically enlarged sella, I believe a CT scan (with intravenous contrast) should be sufficient for an anatomic diagnosis; I would also measure serum PRL levels to exclude the possibility of a small occult prolactinoma. Patients with endocrine findings should receive a thorough evaluation of pituitary function, since they may have a secondary empty sella or may harbor a pituitary tumor in the empty sella.

Treatment

Usually, no treatment other than reassurance is required for patients with a primary empty sella. Hormone replacement may occasionally be required, but would more commonly be needed in patients with a secondary empty sella related to a pituitary tumor.

Rarely, the optic chiasm herniates downward into the gaping opening in the diaphragma sellae, putting pressure on the optic pathways and producing visual field defects. CSF rhinorrhea through openings in bony sutures of the sellar floor may also occur. These two rare complications are the only indications for surgery in patients with a primary empty sella. Removal of a residual pituitary tumor may be needed in patients with a secondary empty sella.

DISCUSSION CASES

Case 1

A 53-year-old man struck his head while diving into a swimming pool, receiving a scalp laceration; he did not lose consciousness. A skull x-ray series obtained at an emergency room showed an enlarged sella turcica. He denied headache, changes in vision, or any endocrine

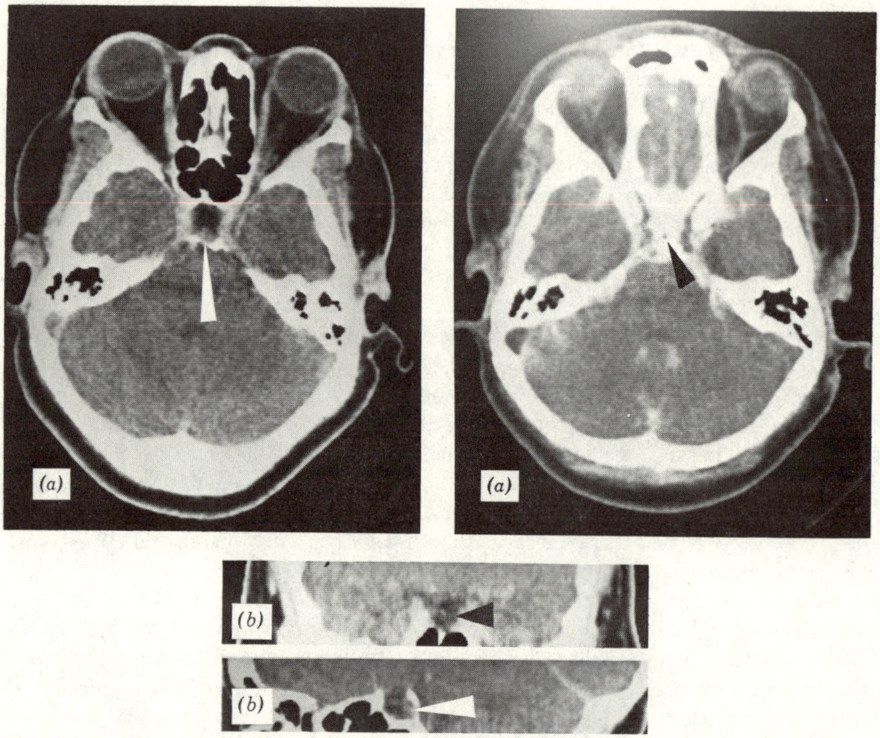

Figure 7. High-resolution computed tomography scans of a patient with an "empty sella." (*a*) Axial view of the sella following intravenous contrast agent (left) shows material of water density (CSF) filling most of the sella turcica; white arrowhead indicates the pituitary gland compressed against the posterior sellar wall. Following administration of intrathecal metrizamide (right), a water-soluble contrast agent, the sella is filled with contrast-density material; the pituitary stalk (arrowhead) can be seen entering the sella. (*b*) Reconstructed coronal (above) and sagittal (below) views of the same patient as in Figure 7*a*, demonstrating fluid within the sella. In the sagittal view, pituitary tissue can be seen against the posterior wall of the sella (white arrowhead). Scans courtesy of Huntington Memorial Hospital, Pasadena, California.

symptoms. The physical examination was entirely normal. Laboratory data were as follows: serum LH 10 mIU/ml, serum testosterone 677 ng/dl, free T_4 index 8.4, serum PRL 3.3 ng/ml. A high-resolution cerebral CT scan showed that most of the sella was occupied by material of the same density as CSF; there was no enhancement following intravenous injection of a contrast agent. A diagnosis of the empty sella syndrome was made, and the patient was reassured.

Discussion

This is a typical case of the empty sella syndrome in which a healthy patient is fortuitously found to have sellar enlargement. In most patients, a high-resolution CT scan is sufficient for anatomic diagnosis, replacing pneumoencephalography. Measurements of the serum LH level, testosterone concentration, and free T_4 index might have been omitted in view of the normal history and physical examination. It was wise to measure the serum PRL level, however, since a partially infarcted prolactinoma could have resulted in the same picture.

Case 2

A 27-year-old woman had an 8-year history of enlargement of her hands, feet, and facial features, along with excessive perspiration and oligomenorrhea; she denied galactorrhea or changes in vision. A lateral skull roentgenogram showed mild sellar enlargement. Visual field testing was normal, and a CT scan showed an intrasellar tumor. The basal serum GH level was 105 ng/ml and did not change following glucose ingestion. A diagnosis of acromegaly was made. She received ^{60}Co external radiotherapy (5,000 rads) to her pituitary gland.

Eighteen months after radiation therapy, there was no change in her acromegalic features, and she still perspired freely. Although her menses had become regular, she had been unable to become pregnant despite 2 years of unprotected intercourse. Her serum GH level was now 35 ng/ml, her serum PRL level was 16 ng/ml, and her free T_4 index was 8.5. After injection of TRH (500 μg i.v.), her serum GH level rose from 36 ng/ml to 61 ng/ml, her serum PRL level rose from 16 ng/ml to 26 ng/ml, and her serum TSH level rose from 1.1 μU/ml to 15 μU/ml.

She was given bromocriptine, 15 mg/day for 6 months. While taking the drug, she noted less perspiration and a subjective shrinkage of her extremities, manifested by looser rings. Although her serum GH level did not change appreciably during bromocriptine therapy, averaging about 29 ng/ml, her serum PRL level fell to <1 ng/ml. During the fifth month of bromocriptine treatment, she became pregnant. The drug was discontinued as soon as the pregnancy was confirmed. Gestation proceeded uneventfully, and she delivered a full-term healthy baby girl.

Two and one-half years later, with no further treatment, her basal serum GH level had fallen to 10 ng/ml and her serum PRL level to 9 ng/ml.

Comment

Although histologic confirmation was not obtained, this patient probably had a mixed pituitary adenoma secreting both GH and PRL. Her basal serum PRL level was in the high-normal range for women, and she clearly had a poor PRL response to TRH (normally, the serum PRL level should at least double after TRH administration). It is likely that her menstrual abnormality and infertility were both due to this borderline hyperprolactinemia. The TSH response to TRH was normal, while the dramatic rise in the GH level following TRH injection is typical of acromegaly.

She had an excellent GH response to radiotherapy. Because of her very high initial GH levels (>50 ng/ml), many physicians would have treated her with transsphenoidal surgery rather than radiation. Nevertheless, she had a typical slow fall in serum GH level over a period of 5 years after radiotherapy. It is hard to know if bromocriptine had any effect on her acromegaly. There was little change in her serum GH level, but, like many other patients, she noted subjective improvement while taking the drug. A recent study has suggested that these changes may be mostly placebo effects. More convincingly, bromocriptine suppressed her serum PRL to very low levels. This was probably responsible for her regaining fertility, as even mild hyperprolactinemia can interfere with ovulation and conception. Since her GH and PRL levels have continued to fall, she may not need bromocriptine again if she wishes to have a second child.

SUGGESTED READING

Alsever RN, Gotlin RW: *Handbook of endocrine tests in adults and children,* 2. Chicago, Year Book Medical Publishers, 1978.

Corenblum B: Successful outcome of ergocryptine-induced pregnancies in twenty-one women with prolactin-secreting pituitary adenomas. *Fertil Steril* 1979, 32:183–186.

Danziger J, Wallace S, Handel S, et al: The sella turcica in primary end organ failure. *Radiology* 1979, 131:111–115.

Ekblom M, Ketonen L, Kuuliala I, et al: Pituitary function in patients with enlarged sella turcica and primary empty sella syndrome. *Acta Med Scand* 1981, 209:31–35.

Foley KM, Posner JB: Does pseudotumor cerebri cause the empty sella syndrome? *Neurology* 1975, 25:565–569.

Gardeur D, Naidich TP, Metzger J: CT analysis of intrasellar pituitary adenomas with emphasis on patterns of contrast enhancement. *Neuroradiology* 1981, 20:241–247.

Lindholm J, Riishede J, Vestergaard S, et al: No effect of bromocriptine in acromegaly: A controlled trial. *N Engl J Med* 1981, 304:1450–1454.

Linfoot JA (ed): *Recent Advances in the Diagnosis and Treatment of Pituitary Tumors.* New York, Raven Press, 1979.

Marrs RP, Bertolli SJ, Kletzky OA: The use of thyrotropin-releasing hormone in distinguishing prolactin-secreting pituitary adenoma. *Am J Obstet Gynecol* 1980, 138:620–625.

Martin JB, Rechlin S, Brown GM: *Clinical Neuroendocrinology.* Philadelphia, FA Davis, 1977.

Molitch ME, Reichlin S: The amenorrhea, galactorrhea and hyperprolactinemia syndromes. *Adv Intern Med* 1980, 26:37–65.

Muhr C, Bergstrom K, Grimelius L, et al: A parallel study of the roentgen anatomy of the sella turcica and the histopathology of the pituitary gland in 205 autopsy specimens. *Neuroradiology* 1981, 21:55–65.

Rozario R, Hammerschlag SB, Post KD, et al: Diagnosis of empty sella with CT scan. *Neuroradiology* 1977, 13:85–88.

Salti IS, Nuha N-S, Bergman RA, et al: Thyrotropin secreting pituitary tumors: A cause of hyperthyroidism. *J Neurol Neurosurg Psychiatry* 1980, 43:1141–1145.

Schlechte J, Sherman B, Halmi N, et al: Prolactin-secreting pituitary tumors in amenorrheic women: A comprehensive study. *Endocrine Rev* 1980, 1:294–308.

Thorner MD, Martin WH, Rogol AD, et al: Rapid regression of pituitary prolactinomas during bromocriptine treatment. *J Clin Endocrinol Metab* 1980, 51:438–445.

Tucker HS, Grubb SR, Wigand JP, et al: Galactorrhea-amenorrhea syndrome: Follow-up of forty-five patients after pituitary tumor removal. *Ann Intern Med* 1981, 94:302–307.

Veldhuis JD, Hammond JM: Endocrine function after spontaneous infarction of the human pituitary: Report, review and reappraisal. *Endocrine Rev* 1980, 1:100–107.

Wass JAH, Thorner MD, Morris DV, et al: Long-term treatment of acromegaly with bromocriptine. *Br Med J* 1977, 1:875–878.

3 JAMES R. SOWERS

Disorders of Water Conservation

CONTROL OF AVP AND THIRST

Arginine vasopressin (AVP), the antidiuretic hormone (ADH), is an octapeptide synthesized by nerve cells located in the supraoptic and, to a lesser extent, in the paraventricular nuclei of the hypothalamus. It is transported along the neurohypophysial pathway attached to a large carrier protein (neurophysin) to be stored in the posterior lobe of the pituitary. It is released in response to many stimuli, the most important being increased plasma osmolality as seen in dehydration and hypovolemia as occurs with hemorrhage. The influence of plasma osmolality on AVP secretion is mediated by the osmosensitive centers of the anterior hypothalamus. Baroreceptors located in the aortic arch and carotid sinus and volume receptors in the left atrium also influence AVP secretion. Decreased arterial pressure or decreased blood volume results in increases in AVP secretion. Other factors that stimulate AVP secretion include stress, pain, noxious stimuli, retching and emesis, hypercapnea, hypoglycemia, angiotensin II, and numerous drugs.

Situated in close proximity to the sites of AVP synthesis is the ventromedial nucleus of the hypothalamus, which contains the thirst center. Neuronal input from the ventromedial nucleus either stimulates or inhibits the perception of thirst by the cerebral cortex, which in turn regulates drinking behavior. Thirst is also regulated by osmotic and volume stimuli and, in addition, is influenced by the renin–angiotensin system, other hormones, and hypokalemia. The anatomic and functional integration of the thirst system and the hypothalamoneurohypophyseal system allows close regulation of body fluid regulation. Water deprivation increases plasma osmolality, which stimulates both the thirst mechanism and the secretion of AVP. Subsequently, drinking increases total body water and dilutes plasma osmolality down to normal which, in turn, suppresses the thirst reflex and inhibits secretion of AVP. Thus orchestration of the thirst and AVP secretory mechanisms usually results in the maintenance of plasma osmolality within a narrow range of 285 mOsm $\pm$ 2%.

Because of the anatomic relationship between the thirst and AVP regulatory systems, clinical situations may occur that affect one or both of these systems. For example, large lesions of the hypothalamus resulting in destruction of both the sites of AVP synthesis and the thirst center permit polyuria and dehydration to occur without an appropriate increase in fluid intake. Such a situation can result in rapid dehydration, coma, and eventual death. Lesions involving only the thirst center can also occur, resulting in a condition called adipsic hypernatremia.

RELATIVE EFFECTS OF OSMOLALITY, BLOOD VOLUME, AND BLOOD PRESSURE ON AVP SECRETION

Under physiologic conditions the predominant controlling mechanism for secretion of AVP is plasma osmolality. At osmolalities below 280 mOsm/kg, AVP secretion is suppressed enough to permit excretion of maximally dilute urine. As osmolality then rises, increasing amounts of AVP are released until, at approximately 295 mOsm/kg, levels of AVP in the plasma are high enough to permit maximal concentration of the urine and water conservation. Activation of the thirst mechanism occurs at about the same osmolality, thus serving as an additional means of preventing further dehydration and any further increase in plasma osmolality. The change in plasma osmolality from 280 to 295 mOsm/kg and the associated changes in plasma AVP from 1 pg/ml to 5 pg/ml or greater are paralleled by changes in urinary osmolality from 100 to 900 mOsm/kg or greater. As basal plasma osmolality is normally located near the middle of the range at approximately 288 mOsm/kg, a small change in total body water of 2–3% in either direction is sufficient to produce a large change in plasma AVP concentration and in urinary osmolality. The sensitivity of AVP release in response to changes in blood volume or arterial pressure is not as great as for osmolality. Measurable increases in AVP secretion do not occur if blood volume is not altered by more than 2–3% throughout the day. Nevertheless, in clinical circumstances associated with hypovolemia or hypotension, plasma AVP levels may be 10 to 25 times higher than those required to produce maximal urinary concentration and may remain elevated even if plasma osmolality is very low. Thus, although osmolality under normal physiologic conditions is the major determinant of AVP secretion, in clinical states such as profound hypotension and hypovolemia AVP may be secreted in large amounts regardless of the osmolality.

AVP EFFECTS ON THE KIDNEY

Changes in plasma AVP concentration exert their effect on body water conservation by altering the rate of reabsorption of renal tubular fluid. The reabsorption of chloride and sodium without water in the ascending limb of the loop of Henle results in the formation of hypotonic tubular fluid and the generation of solute-free water. Thus glomerular filtrate is hypotonic to serum by the time it reaches the distal tubule of the nephron where the tubular fluid osmolality may be as low as 50 mOsm/kg. The eventual concentration of the urine is dependent upon the amount of AVP acting on the distal tubules and the collecting ducts. In the absence of AVP, the distal tubules and collecting ducts are impermeable to water, and maximally dilute urine with an osmolality approaching 50 mOsm/kg is excreted. With increasing AVP levels the renal tubular permeability to water progressively increases. The osmolality of the interstitial fluid surrounding the collecting ducts reaches levels as high as 1200 mOsm/kg. Thus, when sufficient AVP is secreted to permit maximum tubular permeability to water, complete osmotic equilibrium occurs between the interstitial and tubular fluid, resulting in maximally concentrated urine.

CLASSIFICATION AND ETIOLOGY OF DIABETES INSIPIDUS

Diabetes insipidus (DI) is characterized by polyuria (urine volumes in excess of 2.5–3 liters/day) and by the patient having a water diuresis with low ratios of urine to plasma osmolality (0.7 or less), with urine osmolality frequently less than 100 mOsm/kg. There are three possible defects in such patients: decreased secretion of AVP due to a disorder of the hypothalamoneurohypophyseal system (central or vasopressin-sensitive DI), renal resistance to AVP (nephrogenic DI), or decreased release of AVP due to hypo-osmolality of body fluids after greatly increased water intake (psychogenic polydipsia). In the first two groups, renal water losses result in elevations of plasma osmolality, which in turn stimulate thirst and water ingestion which then further enhance polyuria.

CENTRAL (NEUROGENIC) DI

Central DI can be further subdivided into the following four types:

1. Classical severe DI, characterized by failure to synthesize or release AVP.
2. Defective osmoreceptor DI, resulting in failure to secrete AVP in response to extremely high osmolality but normal release in response to hypovolemia.
3. Reset-osmoreceptor DI, in which AVP release is not initiated until plasma osmolality is higher than the usual threshold for stimulation of AVP secretion.
4. Partial DI, in which AVP release is initiated at the usual threshold but in subnormal amounts.

The causes of central DI are listed in Table 1. Central DI occurs rarely as an inherited disorder with either autosomal dominant or sex-linked inheritance and is associated with a marked reduction in the number of AVP neurosecretory cells in the supraoptic and paraventricular nuclei. As many as 40–50% of cases are idiopathic. In all other instances central disturbances of AVP secretion are acquired in association with other intracranial diseases. Intracranial neoplasms are an important cause of DI in children where polyuria may be a manifestation of craniopharyngiomas. An increasingly common cause of DI is damage to the pituitary stalk and posterior lobe of the pituitary associated with head trauma or a neurosurgical procedure. After these events a triphasic pattern of diuresis may be observed. There is an initial period of polyuria due to localized edema of neurosecretory pathways, an interphase lasting up to 5 days when previously synthesized AVP is released from the necrotic posterior lobe, and a final period of permanent polyuria when the stores of previously synthesized AVP are exhausted. Sarcoidosis, histiocytosis, and central nervous system infections, particularly tuberculosis and coccidioidal meningitis, are relatively common causes of central DI; alcohol and diphenylhydantoin transiently inhibit AVP secretion, causing temporary polyuria.

NEPHROGENIC DI

Various types of renal concentrating defects associated with unresponsiveness to maximum endogenous or exogenous AVP may result in impaired ability to concentrate urine maximally. In some cases there is a normal increase in water permeability of the collecting duct in response

Table 1 **Causes of Central DI**

Primary causes
Familial
Idiopathic
Secondary or acquired causes
Traumatic
Accidental (e.g., head trauma)
Iatrogenic (e.g., surgery)
Tumors
Craniopharyngioma
Primary pituitary tumors
Metastatic carcinoma—breast, lung
Acute leukemia
Granulomatous diseases
Sarcoidosis
Histiocytosis
Tuberculosis
Infections
Meningitis
Encephalitis
Vascular
Aneurysms
Sheehan's syndrome
Drugs
Alcohol
Diphenylhydantoin

to AVP, but the urine cannot be concentrated because of a defective osmotic gradient at the renal medullary tip. In other cases, the cellular response to AVP is impaired either by interference with renal medullary adenylate cyclase or by a more distal lesion such as impaired cellular response to cyclic AMP (CAMP) (Table 2). In familial DI severe, unremitting polyuria of up to 10 liters/day may occur, resulting in extreme thirst and making normal activity and sleep impossible. Polyuria in nephrogenic DI is usually much less severe, with a urine output of 2–3 liters daily, levels rarely approaching those seen with neurogenic DI. Because many of the causes of nephrogenic DI are easily correctable, their presence should always be excluded in patients with polyuria.

DIAGNOSIS

DI, both neurogenic and nephrogenic, must be distinguished from other causes of polyuria and polydipsia. One condition difficult to differentiate from DI is the polyuria seen in patients having a primary disturbance in thirst regulation, psychogenic polydipsia. In these patients, excessive water intake leads to body fluid dilution, physiologic suppression of AVP release, and polyuria. When this disorder persists over a long time, the renal medullary osmotic gradient is "washed out" and the maximal concentrating ability impaired. Historically, patients with neurogenic DI can often precisely date the onset of their polyuria and from that point on have unremitting symptoms, including nocturia. Polyuria in patients with psychogenic polydipsia is

Table 2 **Causes of Nephrogenic DI**

Breakdown of renal medullary osmotic gradient	
	Psychogenic polydipsia
	Low-protein diet
	Furosemide therapy
Disruption of the countercurrent system	
	Sickle-cell nephropathy
	Medullary cystic disease
	Chronic pyelonephritis
	Sjögren's syndrome
	Light-chain nephropathy
	Papillary necrosis
Interference with the adenylate cyclase–cAMP system	
	Lithium
	Demeclocycline
	Methoxyflurane
	Prostaglandin excess
	Familial nephrogenic diabetes insipidus
	Hypercalcemia–hypercalciuria
Impaired back-diffusion of water across the distal nephron	
	Amyloidosis

solely dependent on excessive fluid intake and usually is not associated with nocturia. This cause should be suspected when plasma osmolalities are slightly depressed or low-normal in the face of large urine volumes and almost maximally dilute urine. Unfortunately the overlap between osmolalities in this disorder and DI is considerable and limits the use of plasma osmolality measurements in distinguishing between these polyuric states.

Methods have been devised to differentiate between psychogenic polydipsia and neurogenic and nephrogenic DI. The simplest method involves fluid restriction combined with exogenous vasopressin administration. Patients are deprived of water (6–18 hours) until the osmolality of three consecutive urine specimens obtained at hourly intervals varies by less than 30 mOsm/kg In patients with a urine output exceeding 10 liters/day the test should begin at 6 AM to allow careful supervision during the period of water deprivation. The test should be terminated if weight loss exceeds 3% of the body weight. In severe polyuric states urine osmolality usually plateaus within 6–8 hours. In subjects with lesser degrees of polyuria, 12–18 hours of fluid restriction may be required for the stabilization of urine osmolality. Fluid deprivation begins at 6 PM or midnight in this group. Once urine osmolality has plateaued, 5 units of aqueous vasopressin is injected subcutaneously and urine osmolality measured 1 hour later. Plasma osmolality should be measured before water deprivation and again before administering vasopressin.

Normal individuals, patients with psychogenic polydipsia, and patients with partial neurogenic DI all have urine osmolalities greater than plasma osmolalities following fluid restriction. Only those with neurogenic DI will have an increase in urine osmolality greater than 9% after vasopressin. Urine osmolality in severe neurogenic and nephrogenic DI will remain hypotonic to plasma osmolality after dehydration. These two disorders can be distinguished from one another by the administration of vasopressin, which causes an increase in urine osmolality of greater than 50% in neurogenic but not nephrogenic DI. A normal increase in urine osmolality can also occur during fluid restriction in patients with reset osmoreceptors, but measurement of the plasma osmolality at the end of water restriction reveals hyperosmolarity which presumably is required to trigger AVP release in these patients. In institutions where measurements are available, plasma AVP levels are high in nephrogenic DI and low in neurogenic DI after dehydration.

Other diagnostic maneuvers include the infusion of hypertonic saline to determine the osmotic threshold for ADH release and the use of drugs such as nicotine and apomorphine, which stimulate AVP release. These tests may be of help in unusual or difficult cases, but their lack of simplicity and interpretability is a drawback to their wider clinical application.

TREATMENT

Management of polyuric states depends on the etiology and clinical setting. After head trauma and neurosurgical procedures patients should be followed closely for the possible development of neurogenic DI. Body weight, serum electrolyte levels, BUN levels, and urinary specific gravity should be measured before surgery and daily postoperatively. Fluid intake and urine output should also be monitored closely. When the patient is alert, the thirst mechanism is usually a satisfactory way of determining fluid intake. If polyuria occurs with urine output in excess of 250 ml/hr for two consecutive hours and exceeds 6–7 liters/day, or if adequate intake cannot be maintained, vasopressin administration is indicated.

Treatment of neurogenic DI revolves around the use of various forms of vasopressin and of other drugs that either enhance vasopressin secretion (carbamazepine, clofibrate) or augment its action on the kidney, such as chlorpropramide. Because of its short duration of action, thus minimizing the risk of water intoxication, aqueous vasopressin, 5–10 units s.c., is the treatment of choice after head trauma or neurosurgery. Pitressin tannate in oil in doses of 2.5–5 units has a duration of action of 24–72 hours but must be given intramuscularly. Lysine vasopressin (Diapid), a nasal spray, can be absorbed through the mucosa but must be administered every 4–6 hours. A synthetic analog of AVP, 1-desamino-8-D-arginine vasopressin (DDAVP, desmopressin), is available as a nasal spray, as well as for parenteral use, and has a duration of action of 18–22 hours. Administration of 10–20 μg of DDAVP twice daily is the current treatment of choice for patients with an absolute vasopressin deficiency. Dosages should be adjusted downward in children, but they often require administration twice daily. DDAVP appears effective even in the presence of nasal congestion or blockage. For patients in whom some AVP secretion remains, either carbamazepine (400–600 mg daily), clofibrate (500 mg four times daily), or chlorpropamide (200–500 mg daily) can be given singly or in combination. However, these oral medications may all involve serious side effects. Given the effectiveness and lack of side effects of DDAVP, there is little need to utilize oral antidiuretic agents. Thiazide diuretics are the most effective form of treatment in nephrogenic DI where they may reduce urine output by one-third to one-half. They appear to act through a reduction in the glomerular filtration rate and an increased proximal tubular reabsorption of sodium.

DISCUSSION CASE

Case 1

An 18-year-old boy developed excessive thirst and polyuria over a 2-day period approximately 1 year before being seen. He now drinks an estimated 7 qt of water daily and has a distinct preference for ice water. He has no family history of polyuria and is taking no medication for acne or otherwise. He denies orthostatic dizziness, heat or cold intolerance, and nausea or vomiting. He does note that his voice is rather high-pitched, that he shaves only once every 2 weeks, and that recently his vision has been somewhat blurred.

On physical examination he is a eunuchoidal appearing young man who has almost no facial hair. His vital signs are normal. He has sparse pubic and axillary hair, his testes measure 2.0 cm in their long diameter, and his penis is small. The remainder of the physical examination is normal except for a question of bitemporal hemianopsia on visual field examination.

His laboratory data included the following: Hematocrit 43%; WBC, 7,500/mm^3; sodium 144 mEq/liter; potassium 4.2 mEq/liter; bicarbonate 25 mEq/liter; chloride 105 mEq/liter; BUN 13 mg/100 ml; total protein 7.5 g/100 ml; glucose 86 mg/100 ml. Urinalysis: specific gravity 1.002; pH 6.7; protein, glucose, and microscopic negative; urine sodium 7 mEq/liter and urine potassium 5 mEq/liter; urine osmolality 70 mOsm/kg with a simultaneous serum osmolality of 292 mOsm/kg. Other laboratory data include an 8:00 AM serum cortisol level of 24 μg/100 ml and a serum TSH level of 2.8 μunits/ml with a serum free T_4 index of 4.2. Plasma gonadotropins are undetectable in the face of a plasma testosterone level of 60 ng/100 ml (normal male 400–1200 ng/100 ml). Lateral roentgenograms of the skull show suprasellar calcification.

Comment:

The data in this case are consistent with central DI, particularly in light of the rapid onset of polydipsia and polyuria. In this patient, evidence of hypogonadotropic hypogonadism, possible bitemporal hemianopsia, and suprasellar calcification all weigh against a diagnosis of idiopathic DI and suggest an intracranial lesion at or above the median eminence.

A carefully performed (in the hospital) water deprivation test followed by a test dose of aqueous Pitressin, 5 units s.c., should demonstrate an inability to concentrate urine spontaneously under conditions of high plasma osmolality but an appropriate renal concentrating response to exogenous AVP. Computed tomography would be very helpful in demonstrating the cause of the suprasellar calcifications.

The treatment for his neurogenic DI should be intranasal DDAVP given twice daily.

SYNDROME OF INAPPROPRIATE SECRETION OF ADH

Hyponatremia with hypo-osmolality is a common clinical disorder seen with circulatory insufficiency and a depleted extracellular fluid volume, circulatory insufficiency and an over-expanded extracellular fluid volume such as that seen in edematous patients, and adequate circulation and expanded extracellular fluid volume. The latter pathophysiologic mechanism is seen in the syndrome of inappropriate secretion of antidiuretic hormone (SIADH), first described in 1957 by Schwartz and associates in two patients with bronchogenic carcinoma. Careful metabolic studies on these patients revealed the following characteristics: hyponatremia and hypo-osmolality of the serum, urine less than maximally dilute, continued renal excretion of sodium, no clinical evidence of fluid volume depletion, and normal renal and adrenal function.

The causes of SIADH are listed in Table 3. About 75% of reported cases of SIADH are the result of tumors of which bronchogenic carcinoma, particularly the small-cell or oat cell type, is foremost. Although SIADH may not be clinically evident, many patients with bronchogenic carcinoma have impaired free water excretion, suggesting an excessive AVP effect.

Table 3 **Causes of SIADH**

Neurohypophyseal ADH

Central nervous system disorders: head trauma, subarachnoid hemmorrhage, brain tumors, encephalitis, meningitis, Guillain–Barre syndrome, lupus erythematosus, acute intermittent porphyria

Accentuated or abnormal physiologic states: physical or emotional stress, pain (surgical procedures), positive pressure breathing, postmitral commissurotomy

Pharmacologic agents: nicotine, narcotics, chlorpropamide (renal action), carbamazepine, clofibrate, vincristine, cyclophosphamide, thiazides (indirectly), psychotrophic agents

Ectopic ADH

Tumors: bronchogenic carcinoma (mostly oat cell), carcinoma of pancreas or duodenum, lymphosarcoma, thymoma

Nonmalignant pulmonary tissue (postulated): empyema, lung abscess, pneumonia, pulmonary tuberculosis

Production by these tumors of a substance having immunologic and biologic identity with neurohypophyseal AVP probably represents a derepression of the genes for synthesis of the hormone within the tumor.

SIADH has also been associated with tuberculosis, bacterial pneumonia, lung abscess, and other pulmonary disease. It has been speculated that some pulmonary diseases may alter pulmonary compliance and in turn influence the firing rate of intrathoracic baroreceptors. However, one patient who died of tuberculosis had a large quantity of AVP in the tuberculous granulomas.

SIADH has been associated with a wide spectrum of intracranial diseases, including meningitis, brain abscess, tumors, and head injuries. It is likely that the sustained production of AVP in these illnesses results from increased intracranial pressure.

Drugs are a relatively common cause of water retention and hyponatremia. Many of these drugs, including chlorpropramide, opiates, tricylclics, clofibrate, barbiturates, nicotine, vincristine, and cyclophosphamide, presumably cause hyponatremia by promoting secretion of AVP. In some cases, AVP release may not be the result of a direct effect on the hypothalamoneurohypophysial system but rather may be mediated via effects on other systems. For example, AVP secretion following systemic administration of nicotine can be markedly decreased by either baroreceptor denervation or pretreatment with antihistamines, suggesting mediation by vasomotor or emetic centers. Chlorpropamide production of SIADH is mediated through the drug's potentiation of AVP action at the collecting tubule level as well as through enhancement of AVP release. Some drugs, such as oxytocin, may bind to renal AVP receptors and initiate an antidiuretic response. Thus, with the increased use of oxytocin in obstetric cases, SIADH is being reported with increased frequency. Prostaglandins, which are also being used with increasing frequency in obstetrics and gynecology, may cause release of AVP, producing SIADH.

DIAGNOSIS OF SIADH

The following are characteristic of SIADH: no clinical evidence of intravascular volume depletion or edema; normal adrenal function, normal renal function, simultaneous hyponatremia, and hypo-osmolality of the serum; inappropriate hyperosmolality of the urine for the concomitant tonicity of the serum; inappropriately high urinary sodium excretion concomitant with the depressed serum sodium concentration.

The clinical symptoms and signs of SIADH are those of water intoxication. Although patients generally are asymptomatic when the serum sodium concentration is 120 mEq/liter or above, the clinical consequences of SIADH probably are as dependent on the rapidity of development of hyponatremia as the absolute serum sodium concentration. Headache, loss of appetite, nausea, vomiting, and abdominal cramps are frequent symptoms when serum sodium concentrations reach the 120–115 mEq/liter range. Personality changes, such as confusion, irritability, withdrawal, and hostility, are seen. At a serum sodium concentration of less than 110 mEq/liter neurologic disturbances may appear, such as muscle weakness, loss of reflexes, a positive Babinski response, and seizures. Psychotic states have been associated with SIADH; thus any personality changes in a psychiatric patient should be recognized as a potential manifestation of SIADH. Stupor may progress to convulsions, coma, and death. These events are almost uniformly seen in patients with serum sodium concentrations in the 100–90 mEq/liter range.

Making the diagnosis of SIADH depends primarily on ruling out other conditions that may manifest similar features. With its characteristic clinical background, hyperglycemia-induced hyponatremia can usually be easily eliminated. Because of an osmotically induced movement of water from the intracellular to the extracellular space, for every 100 mg/dl elevation of plasma glucose above 100 mg/dl, the serum sodium concentration will decrease approximately 1.6 mEq/liter. Marked hyperlipidemia may produce spurious hyponatremia because of the resulting occupation by lipids of a significant portion of the total plasma volume.

Dilutional hyponatremia may be observed in congestive heart failure, renal failure, and cirrhosis with ascites. Hyponatremia from sodium depletion states may be seen in diarrhea, renal disease, and diabetes mellitus. In these salt-losing states, however, evidence of dehydration, an elevated BUN level and hematocrit, and a concentration of urinary sodium <20 mEq/liter are usually observed. In contrast, in SIADH a BUN level of 10 mg/dl or less is often seen and the concentration of urinary sodium is usually >20 mEq/liter. Psychogenic polydipsia may present as hyponatremia, but a history of extremely large water intake, psychiatric disease, and a maximally dilute urine (specific gravity 1.000–1.004) all suggest the diagnosis of compulsive water drinking.

Patients with severe hypothyroidism may have an impaired ability of the kidney to excrete a free water load, have excessive urinary sodium loss, and develop hyponatremia without evidence of adrenal insufficiency. In most cases it appears that the hypothyroidism may alter the renal handling of water independent of AVP secretion. In a minority of hypothyroid patients, circulating AVP levels may be elevated, probably secondary to a decrease in cardiac output. Primary adrenal insufficiency can result in water retention, hyponatremia, and urinary sodium loss, primarily because of the associated aldosterone deficiency. Furthermore, in the absence of cortisol, it has been demonstrated that AVP effects at the renal tubule level may be potentiated, leading to a relative inability to excrete free water. Last, it has been reported that AVP levels are inappropriately high for the state of dehydration in hypoadrenalism.

TREATMENT

The selection of a particular modality of treatment of SIADH is determined in part by the degree of water intoxication and by the underlying cause as related to the expected duration of the syndrome. The recognized forms of therapy for SIADH are as follows: fluid restriction, infusion of hypertonic saline, diuretics, lithium, demeclocycline, removal of the underlying cause. In mild cases, fluid restriction usually is sufficient. A general guideline is that, until the serum sodium concentration normalizes and symptoms abate, water intake should not exceed urinary output; after normalization, intake should equal urinary output plus insensible fluid loss.

In a clinical setting of symptomatic hyponatremia ($<$110–115 mEq/liter), judicious intravenous administration of hypertonic saline in the form of 3% (514 mEq/liter) or 5% (855 mEq/liter) solutions over several hours may temporarily raise the serum sodium concentration. Two major disadvantages of using hypertonic saline alone are related to the already overhydrated state of the patient. Infused hypertonic saline draws large quantities of water from the cells into the intracellular space and potentially causes vascular congestion and pulmonary edema. Also, the renal sodium loss seen with fluid volume expansion, which is one of the hallmarks of SIADH, is accentuated by hypertonic saline infusion. Most of the administered saline is rapidly excreted, and hyponatremia returns. Furosemide can be administered in large doses along with hypertonic saline in order to promote renal excretion of water in excess of sodium. Furosemide blocks chloride reabsorption from the ascending limb of the loop of Henle and also increases renal prostaglandin production, resulting in elaboration of dilute urine and diuresis of free water. The enhanced free water clearance produced by furosemide results in a dehydrating effect with a consequent increase in serum sodium concentration. Also, by correcting the fluid overload in SIADH, furosemide helps prevent pulmonary edema as well as rapid excretion of the administered saline. Furosemide is administered as a single dose of 1 mg/kg body weight i.v. The need for subsequent doses of furosemide depends on the patient's clinical and laboratory response. If urinary loss of Na^+, K^+, and Mg^{2+} is replaced every 4 hours, the net effect will be a progressive loss of free water. An alternative approach is the use of peritoneal dialysis with a hypertonic dialysate, which removes large quantities of free water with little risk of pulmonary edema.

Both lithium carbonate and demeclocycline have been shown to be effective in treating chronic SIADH. Both drugs probably act by interfering with the normal effect of AVP to increase generation of cyclic AMP in the renal tubule. Demeclocycline appears to be more effective than lithium in the treatment of protracted SIADH. However, the delay of several days before onset of the effect of demeclocycline renders this agent ineffective for acute management. The demeclocycline dosage should not exceed 240 mg/day. Nephrotoxicity has been reported, necessitating the monitoring of renal function with use of this agent. Diphenylhydantoin has been demonstrated to be effective on a continuing basis in a patient with a basal skull fracture and persistent SIADH. Removal or suppression of the cause of SIADH should be attempted whenever possible. Treatment of benign pulmonary diseases, resection of tumors, or palliation with irradiation or chemotherapy may effectively control the SIADH.

DISCUSSION CASE

Case 2

A 65-year-old lawyer was brought to his internist because of confusion and disorientation. For about 4 months before admission his wife noted that he had complained of easy fatigability, weight loss, weakness, and a chronic, nonproductive cough. About 1 week before presentation he was noted to be irritable, and on the day before seeing his physician he became confused, irrational, and disoriented. Other than 60 pack-years of smoking, his history was unremarkable.

Physical examination revealed an irritable man, disoriented with respect to time and place. He was thin and had significant muscle wasting. His blood pressure was 152/84 mm Hg, supine, and did not change significantly with standing. Extremities showed early clubbing of the fingernails, but no edema was detectable. Bilaterally decreased deep tendon reflexes and extensor toe responses were present.

The following laboratory data were recorded: Hematocrit 28%; WBC 15,600/mm^3; Urinalysis: specific gravity 1.024; pH 6.7; glucose and protein, negative; serum was not lipemic; fasting serum glucose 105 mg/dl; BUN 8 mg/dl; creatinine 1.0 mg/dl; sodium 113 mEq/liter; potassium 4.0 mEq/liter; chloride 80 mEq/liter; CO_2 25 mEq/liter; calcium 9.0 mg/dl; phosphate 3.4 mg/dl; total protein 6.1 gm/dl; plasma cortisol 8:00 AM 24 μg/dl, 8:00 PM 14 μg/dl; chest x-ray film revealed a mass in the left upper lung field; skull roentgenograms, normal. Serum osmolality 234 mOsm/kg; concomitant urine osmolality 210 mOsm/kg.

Discussion

The tentative diganosis in this patient is brochogenic (likely oat cell) carcinoma, which has resulted in the SIADH. The marked hyponatremia (in the face of normal renal and adrenal function) is most likely due to decreased renal free water clearance and increased excretion of sodium resulting in hyponatremia and hypo-osmolality of the serum and extracellular fluid. In this man, who has marked plasma hypotonicity, the urine osmolality of 210 mOsm/kg, which is only slightly lower than the plasma osmolality of 233 mOsm/kg, clearly represents inappropriately concentrated urine. Thus the clinical and laboratory data in this patient are most consistent with the SIADH.

The initial treatment of this patient should be restriction of fluids to approximately 500–600 ml/day. A more aggressive approach to acute therapy would be to use a combination of hypertonic saline infusion and furosemide administration. Because of the infrequency with which oat cell carcinoma can be cured, this man will likely need chronic treatment for his SIADH, the preferable agent being demeclocycline.

SUGGESTED READING

Ahmed ABJ, Clark EH, Jacobs, HS: Water intoxication associated with oxytocin infusion. *Postgrad Med J* 51:249, 1975.

Andreoli TE, Grantham JJ, Rector F: Disturbances in body fluid osmolality. Bethesda, American Physiological Society, 1977.

Cobb WE, Spare S, Reichlin S: Neurogenic diabetes insipidus: Management with dDAVP (1-desamino-8-D-arginine vasopressin). *Ann Intern Med* 88:183, 1978.

De Fronzo RA, Thier SO: Pathophysiologic approach to hyponatremia. *Arch Intern Med* 140:897, 1980.

Forrest JN, Cox M, Hong C, et al: Superiority of demeclocycline over lithium in the treatment of chronic syndrome of inappropriate secretion of antidiuretic hormone. *N Engl J Med* 298:173, 1978.

Halter, J, Goldberg AP, Robertson GL, Porte D: Selective osmo-receptor dysfunction in the syndrome of chronic hypernatremia. *J Clin Endocrinol Metab* 44:609, 1977.

Hantman D, Rossier B, Zohlman R, et al: Rapid correction of hyponatremia in the syndrome of inappropriate secretion of antidiuretic hormone—An alternative treatment to hypertonic saline. *Ann Intern Med* 78:870, 1973.

Kleeman CR, Berl T: The neurophypophysial hormones: Vasopressin, in De Groot LJ, Cahill GF, Odell WD, et al (eds): *Endocrinology*, New York, Grune & Stratton, 1979, vol 1, pp 253–275.

Matuk F, Kalyanaraman K: Syndrome of inappropriate secretion of antidiuretic hormone in patients treated with psychotherapeutic drugs. *Arch Neurol* 34:374, 1977.

Moses AM: Diabetes insipidus and ADH regulation. *Hosp Pract* 12:37, 1977.

Moses AM, Miller M, Streeten DHP: Pathophysiologic and pharmacologic alterations in the release and action of ADH. *Metabolism* 25:697, 1976.

Newsome HH: Vasopressin: Deficiency, excess and the syndrome of inappropriate antidiuretic hormone secretion. *Nephron* 23:125, 1979.

Rado JP: Combination of carbamazepine and chlorpropramide in the treatment of "hyporesponder" pituitary diabetes insipidus. *J Clin Endocrinol Metab* 38:1, 1974.

Robertson GL: Vasopressin function in health and disease. *Recent Prog Horm Res* 33:333, 1977.

Schwartz W, Bennett N, Curelop S, et al: A syndrome of renal sodium loss and hyponatremia probably resulting from inappropriate secretion of antidiuretic hormone. *Am J Med* 23:529, 1957.

Shucart WA, Jackson I: Management of diabetes insipidus in neurosurgical patients. *J Neurosurg* 44:65, 1976.

Tanay A, Yust I, Peresecenschi G, et al: Long term treatment of the syndrome of inappropriate antidiuretic hormone secretion with phenytoin. *Ann Intern Med* 90:50, 1979.

Weissman PN, Shenkman L, Gregerman RI: Chlorpropamide hyponatremia. Drug-induced inappropriate antidiuretic hormone activity. *N Engl J Med* 284:65, 1971.

4 JEROME M. HERSHMAN

Hyperthyroidism and Hypothyroidism

HYPERTHYROIDISM

Hyperthyroidism is a disorder resulting from the effects of excessive amounts of thyroid hormones on body tissues. It is fairly common, with a lifetime prevalence estimated at 0.2–0.5% of the population.

Causes

Graves' Disease

Graves' disease is the most common cause of hyperthyroidism (Robert Graves, an English physician, described the condition in 1835). In addition to hyperthyroidism, about one-half of patients with Graves' disease have ophthalmopathy, and less than 1% have pretibial dermopathy. Graves' disease is an autoimmune disorder (see Chapter 18) that is four times more common in women than in men. Patients with Graves' disease have a significantly greater prevalence of the histocompatibility antigens HLA-B8 and DRw3. The patients' serum contains an immunoglobulin (IgG) thyroid stimulator that can be detected in several assay systems, giving rise to a variety of names. The IgG of patients with Graves' disease binds to the thyrotropin (TSH) receptor on the thyroid cell plasma membrane. It also activates thyroid adenylate cyclase and increases cyclic AMP levels. Thus the general term thyroid-stimulating immunoglobulin seems most appropriate. This IgG is synthesized by B lymphocytes, possibly because of a defect in suppressor T lymphocytes. The true etiology of this disorder of the immune system is still unknown.

Nodular Goiter

Multinodular goiter may cause hyperthyroidism, although most patients with multinodular goiter are euthyroid. In some of these patients, Graves' disease appears to be superimposed on nodular goiter, and thyroid-stimulating immunoglobulins may be detectable. In other patients, there is evidence of multiple autonomous thyroid follicles, presumed to develop over a long period of time. Radioiodine thyroid scans show intense diffuse or patchy uptake.

In some patients, there is a single large autonomous nodule, which on radioiodine thyroid scan concentrates all the radioiodine. The rest of the gland is suppressed because of the excessive secretion of thyroid hormone by the nodule. Administration of bovine TSH increases the uptake in the extranodular tissue. The autonomous hyperfunctioning nodule must exceed 3.5 cm to be large enough to cause hyperthyroidism and is usually the dominant nodule in a multinodular goiter. Solitary ''hot'' nodules on thyroid scans do not always cause hyperthyroidism; follow-up of some patients over many years shows that nodules may involute and that the patients remain euthyroid.

Spontaneously Resolving Lymphocytic Thyroiditis

In the past decade, short bouts of hyperthyroidism have been associated with lymphocytic thyroiditis, which appears to be very similar to Hashimoto's thyroiditis histologically. This disorder accounts for 10% of newly hyperthyroid patients. These patients have nontender thyroids, normal in size or slightly enlarged. Exophthalmos is absent. Tests of thyroid antibodies are often positive using both microsomal and thyroglobulin antigens. Thyroid uptake of radioiodine is very low. The hyperthyroidism is attributable to a ''leakage'' of thyroid hormone from the inflamed gland. Serum TSH and IgG thyroid stimulators are not detectable. Clinical features of hyperthyroidism tend to be mild and subside over a few months, with spontaneous recovery to normal. Long-term follow-up has revealed recurrent episodes of transient hyperthyroidism in about 10% of patients. Antithyroid antibodies persist; these patients should be followed regularly, because they may be predisposed to develop hypothyroidism.

Subacute Granulomatous Thyroiditis

This disorder may follow a viral infection. The thyroid becomes enlarged, tender, and quite firm; only one lobe may be involved at first, and then the other. Rarely the thyroid is nontender (''silent''). Patients appear febrile and hypermetabolic, in part because of the inflammatory process and in part because of the leakage of thyroid hormone which causes hyperthyroidism. Thyroid radioiodine uptake is very low in the acute phase which lasts for several weeks, often followed by a transient phase of hypothyroidism and then complete recovery. Table 1 compares the features of lymphocytic and granulomatous thyroiditis with hyperthyroidism.

Thyrotropin-Induced Hyperthyroidism

TSH-secreting pituitary tumors have been reported to cause hyperthyroidism in about 25 patients. The tumors may also produce growth hormone, causing acromegaly, or prolactin, causing galactorrhea. In general, these pituitary tumors tend to be large. The TSH secretion is autonomous and usually cannot be stimulated by thyrotropin-releasing hormone (TRH). TSH levels in different patients may be very high (25–50 μU/ml) or within the normal range but still inappropriately high for a hyperthyroid patient. This rare disorder should be suspected in a patient with other features of a pituitary tumor (see Chapter 2).

Excessive thyrotropin secretion also causes hyperthyroidism in patients without pituitary tumors. This is a very rare hereditary disorder in which there is resistance to the suppressive

Table 1 **Hyperthyroidism in Lymphocytic Thyroiditis and Subacute Granulomatous Thyroiditis**

	Lymphocytic	*Subacute Granulomatous*
Thyroid size	Normal to twice enlarged	Enlarged
Thyroid palpation	Smooth or finely nodular	Firm to hard
Fever	No	Yes
Sedimentation rate	Normal	High
Duration of hyperthyroidism	4–20 weeks	1–4 weeks
Severity of hyperthyroidism	Usually mild	Variable
Thyroid uptake	Low	Low
Thyroid biopsy	Lymphocytic	Granulomatous
Serum thyroglobulin level	Increased	Increased
Antithyroid antibodies	Positive	Negative

effect of thyroid hormone on pituitary TSH secretion, but there is no resistance in other tissues, so that the patient is hyperthyroid. Some patients have a resistance to the effect of thyroid hormone on peripheral tissues as well, so they appear euthyroid despite increased levels of circulating thyroid hormones. If the peripheral resistance is severe, the patients may be cretinous.

Other Causes

Excessive ingestion of thyroid hormone (thyrotoxicosis medicamentosa) is fairly common in patients, particularly medical personnel, who do this to control their weight. In some cases, the patients deny taking the thyroid medication. In these patients, the thyroid gland is usually not palpable, and the radioiodine uptake is suppressed to a low value; serum thyroglobulin levels are not elevated, in contrast to the situation in patients with silent thyroiditis (Table 1). Serum thyroid hormone levels reflect the exogenous thyroid hormone intake. In the past, excessive amounts of thyroid hormone were prescribed to suppress TSH secretion in patients with thyroid cancer. However, effective suppression of TSH secretion occurs with doses of thyroid hormone only 10–20% greater than replacement doses; these suppressive doses do not cause thyrotoxicosis medicamentosa.

Trophoblastic tumors, either the benign hydatidiform mole or the malignant choriocarcinoma, may cause hyperthyroidism by secretion of a thyroid stimulator. This stimulator is human chorionic gonadotropin (hCG) which has weak TSH-like activity. When serum hCG concentrations exceed 300 units/ml in some of these patients (levels severalfold greater than the peak concentrations of normal pregnancy), hyperthyroidism develops. It can be cured by surgical removal of the mole or effective chemotherapy of the choriocarcinoma, which eliminates the hCG.

Rarely, hyperthyroidism occurs in patients with metastatic follicular thyroid carcinoma; even though hormone secretion per unit mass is low, the large mass of tumor may be sufficient to cause hyperthyroidism. Another rare cause of hyperthyroidism is the ovarian teratoma with thyroid elements, ovarian struma. This may be associated with cervical goiter and Graves' disease. Most likely the ovarian thyroid tissue also responds to thyroid-stimulating immunoglobulins.

Iodine-induced hyperthyroidism may develop when a patient with euthyroid multinodular goiter is treated with large amounts of iodine. Many of the follicles in these glands are autonomous and incorporate the iodine into thyroid hormones. Excess substrate leads to excessive secretion of thyroid hormones.

Clinical Features

A typical patient with Graves' hyperthyroidism is a young woman who enjoys moderate weight loss despite a hearty appetite but complains of nervousness, palpitation, tremor, and weakness. In contrast, hyperthyroidism in the elderly may be heralded by poor appetite with weight loss, muscle wasting, atrial fibrillation, and heart failure. Hyperthyroidism affects nearly every body system, but few patients have all the clinical features.

Cardiovascular and Respiratory Systems

Cardiac symptoms are often prominent, because the conductive system is sensitive to thyroid hormone. An increase in heart rate is typical. Rapid tachycardia and atrial fibrillation occur, even in patients with otherwise normal hearts, but atrial fibrillation is usually superimposed on underlying coronary or rheumatic heart disease, and severe heart failure may develop.

The cardiac manifestations resemble increased adrenergic activity. Although circulating catecholamine concentrations are not increased, cardiac β-adrenergic receptor levels are increased, which may explain the tachycardia.

Excessive metabolic demands also lead to increased cardiac output. Brisk arterial pulsations, a forceful cardiac impulse, flow murmurs, and an extracardiac systolic scratch are sometimes heard.

Exertional dyspnea without heart failure is frequent and is probably due to respiratory muscle fatigue. Vital capacity and pulmonary compliance may be reduced.

Gastrointestinal, Hepatic, and Hemopoietic Systems

Increased gastrointestinal motility leads to more frequent bowel movements, but diarrhea rarely occurs. In the elderly, constipation occurs, possibly as a result of dehydration. Abnormal liver function tests correlate with the severity of hyperthyroidism and may be related to weight loss and malnutrition.

Anemia is infrequent in a previously healthy person but may develop on a nutritional basis because of increased demands for hemopoietic factors. It is usually normochromic but may be megaloblastic if the patient with Graves' disease has coexistent pernicious anemia (which occurs in about 3% of patients). Moderate granulocytopenia and lymphocytosis are common.

Neurologic, Muscular, and Skeletal Systems

Nervousness is a common complaint. Concentration is reduced, leading to reduced performance at work and in school. Some patients feel exhilarated and claim to work faster and sleep less. Others attribute fatigue to sleeplessness. Hyperthyroidism may precipitate psychosis or seizures in predisposed individuals. Tendon reflexes are brisk. Finger tremor is common; patients complain of shaking when handling cups.

Muscle strength is reduced, and athletic performance declines precipitously. Prolonged hyperthyroidism leads to severe muscle atrophy. In Orientals with Graves' disease there is an increased prevalence of hypokalemic periodic paralysis.

Thyroid hormone has a catabolic effect on bone leading to hypercalciuria and, in some patients, hypercalcemia. Serum levels of bone-derived alkaline phosphatase are increased and may increase further as the bones heal.

Skin and Water Metabolism

Hyperthyroid patients have smooth, moist, velvety skin. In older patients, the skin may feel like a baby's skin. To provide cooling of the body, there is increased perspiration. Pruritus is also fairly common.

Intolerance to heat is common, as is kicking off the blankets at night. The increased insensible loss causes mild polydypsia. Polyuria and nocturia should alert one to consideration of hypercalcemia as well as hyperglycemia.

Some patients, even blacks, note darkening of the skin. Vitiligo is associated with Graves' disease, as is premature graying of the hair. Onycholysis (retraction of the nail beds) causes dirt to get under the nails. The rare pretibial dermopathy (myxedema) of Graves' disease is a knobby or orange peel thickening of this area due to infiltration with mucopolysaccharide. In severe instances, the hands are also affected.

Reproductive System

Severe hyperthyroidism causes oligomenorrhea and relative infertility, but it is not a reliable form of birth control. In men, there may be gynecomastia or impotence, and recent studies show oligospermia. The gynecomastia is attributed to increased conversion of androgens to estrogens.

Graves' Ophthalmopathy

Increased sympathetic tone of Müller's levator palpebrae muscle causes a "stare" and lid lag. Proptosis (quantitated on an exophthalmometer: greater than 20 mm in caucasians, 22 mm in blacks) is attributed to swelling of retroorbital contents. The extraocular muscles are thickened from edema and inflammation, leading to eventual scarring which causes dysconjugate vision. Reduced upward gaze is most common and attributed to tightening of the inferior rectus muscles. Chemosis, tearing, and photophobia are common. Papilledema, reduced visual acuity, and corneal abrasions from the proptosis are ominous signs of malignant exophthalmos, a rare disorder affecting only 1% of Graves' patients. The pathogenesis is unclear. There may be a circulating immunoglobulin causing exophthalmos or deposition of immune complexes on the membranes of retroorbital muscles and other structures.

Diagnostic Tests

The diagnosis of hyperthyroidism is established by measurement of serum thyroid hormone concentrations. This involves the assumption that increased metabolic effect of thyroid hormone is caused by increased secretion of thyroid hormone and that serum concentrations are proportional to the secretion rates. The simplest and most direct test is the serum thyroxine (T_4) concentration determined by radioimmunoassay (RIA); normal levels are about 4.5–11 μg/dl. Because T_4 is strongly bound to binding proteins and only 0.03% is unbound or free, an increase in the binding proteins (principally T_4-binding globulin, TBG) may raise the total serum T_4

concentration into the hyperthyroid range. To compensate or correct for this, the free T_4 concentration can be measured directly or estimated as a free T_4 index. An elevated free T_4 index or free T_4 concentration confirms the diagnosis.

The serum triiodothyronine (T_3) concentration, measured by RIA (normal ~80–180 ng/dl), is also high in hyperthyroidism, usually even higher in relation to normal than the serum T_4 level. In addition, some patients have an elevated serum T_3 level and a normal serum T_4 concentration, giving rise to the name T_3 thyrotoxicosis. For this reason, the serum T_3 level should be measured to consider this possibility in a hyperthyroid patient with a normal serum T_4 level and free T_4 index. On the other hand, the serum T_3 concentration may be lowered into the normal range in a hyperthyroid patient because of systemic illness or malnutrition. This occurs because about one-half of the T_3 production in hyperthyroidism arises from peripheral monodeiodination of T_4 to T_3, mainly in the liver. This process may be substantially reduced by liver disease, severe systemic illness, or starvation.

Measurement of the thyroid uptake of radioiodine is useful in distinguishing thyroiditis (an inflamed gland leaking thyroid hormone) from a hyperfunctioning thyroid with a high thyroid uptake (>30% at 24 hours). Because of the frequency of silent thyroiditis, the uptake should be carried out in nearly all patients without exophthalmos, since exophthalmos has been associated only with Graves' disease and not with thyroiditis with hyperthyroidism.

In patients with borderline elevations of serum T_4 and T_3 values, testing with TRH (protirelin) may be useful in diagnosis. The normal response to TRH, 500 μg i.v., is an increment in the serum TSH level so that the peak level at 30 minutes exceeds 5 μU/ml in men and 7 μU/ml in women. Failure of the TSH to rise after TRH indicates suppression of the pituitary by excessive circulating levels of T_4 and T_3. However, a euthyroid subject may have a diminished TSH response to TRH on one occasion that is normal on repeated testing. In addition, some depressed patients have subnormal TSH increments after administration of TRH.

Administration of T_3 (75 μg daily for 8 days) or of T_4 (3 mg at a single dose) will suppress the thyroid uptake measured 7 days later to less than 50% of the baseline level in a normal subject. Hyperthyroid patients with Graves' disease do not suppress their thyroid uptake normally. Because this is a cumbersome test and the exogenous T_3 may exacerbate cardiac symptoms, I prefer the TRH test for borderline cases.

At the present time, tests for thyroid-stimulating antibodies are not of practical utility.

Table 2 summarizes the diagnostic tests for hyperthyroidism.

Therapy

Therapy depends on the etiology of the hyperthyroidism. Because Graves' disease is responsible for almost 90% of cases of hyperthyroidism and there is no specific therapy aimed at its etiology, this section will focus on the modes of treatment of the hyperthyroidism of Graves' disease.

Drugs

Propylthiouracil and Methimazole. Medical therapy with antithyroid drugs of the thionamide series has been used for 35 years. The two drugs used in the United States are propylthiouracil and methimazole (Tapazole). Both are concentrated in the thyroid cells and block the peroxidase enzyme system; coupling of iodotyrosines to form T_4 and T_3 is inhibited more than organic binding and formation of iodotyrosines. Thus complete blockage of organic binding of iodine is not essential for beneficial effects.

Table 2 **Diagnostic Tests for Hyperthyroidism**[a]

Step 1:	Serum T_4 level, free T_4 index. High value indicates hyperthyroidism. Go to step 3.
Step 2:	Serum T_3 concentration if serum T_4 level and free T_4 index are normal. High value indicates T_3 thyrotoxicosis. Step 3 unnecessary.
Step 3:	Thyroid radioiodine uptake. Low value indicates thyroiditis, thyroid hormone ingestion, iodine contamination. High value indicates hyperthyroidism.
Step 4:	TRH test if serum T_4 and T_3 levels are normal. Failure of TSH to respond suggests hyperthyroidism.

[a]This sequence should be followed in evaluating a patient.

With the usual daily starting dose of 300 mg propylthiouracil or 30 mg methimazole, serum T_4 and T_3 levels fall in 2 weeks and clinical improvement occurs in 2–4 weeks. Because propylthiouracil is rapidly degraded (plasma $t_{1/2}$ is 1–2 hours), I prescribe it in divided doses every 8 hours. Methimazole is metabolized more slowly and can be given once or twice daily; it is preferable for the forgetful patient.

Propylthiouracil also blocks the peripheral monodeiodination of T_4 to T_3, but methimazole does not have this action. Both drugs have an immunosuppressive effect which may in part be responsible for their long-term beneficial effects.

When the patient has become euthyroid, the dose can be reduced by one-third. Successive adjustments of the dose are based on clinical evaluations every 2 months and measurements of serum T_4 and T_3 concentrations which should be maintained in the normal range.

For optimal results, therapy is continued for 12–24 months. With this approach, nearly one-half of patients have a long-term remission after the drugs are stopped. Recurrence is usually apparent within 6–12 months, and a second course of antithyroid drugs may be given. Antithyroid drugs are more likely to cause a prolonged remission in patients with small goiters and symptoms for less than a year. Patients with chronic hyperthyroidism or large goiters are much less likely to experience a long-term remission.

The main problem in deciding how long to continue the antithyroid drug is the lack of a sensitive and precise marker for the activity of the disease. Measurement of thyroid suppression by making short thyroid uptake measurements (20 minutes to 1 hour) and suppression tests (75 μg T_3 daily) during therapy is difficult. It is simpler merely to follow the activity of the hyperthyroidism clinically and with blood tests.

Some have advocated stopping therapy as soon as the patient becomes euthyroid, rather than continuing the drug at a reduced dose. However, many groups have shown that the incidence of long-term remission seems related to the duration of treatment. As therapy is continued, an increasing proportion of patients regain normal thyroid suppressibility.

Side effects of the thionamide drugs include skin rash, serum sickness, arthralgia, hepatic toxicity, and rarely agranulocytosis. Most clinicians do not follow white cell counts routinely, because this alarms the patients and does not predict the onset of the agranulocytosis with precision, since it can develop suddenly. These side effects usually occur within the first few months of treatment. For minor reactions, the patient can be switched from propylthiouracil to methimazole (or vice versa).

Iodine and Lithium. Iodine was the first effective drug for treatment of hyperthyroidism. A saturated solution of potassium iodide or Lugol's solution, 5 drops two or three times daily, will slow release of hormone from the gland. In addition, it may block biosynthesis. Serum T_4

and T_3 levels fall rapidly, sometimes to normal, but most patients escape from the beneficial effects in 10–14 days.

Lithium, in doses of 900–1,200 mg of lithium carbonate daily, also slows the release of hormone from the gland, but has gastrointestinal side effects.

β-Adrenergic Blockers. Many of the clinical features of hyperthyroidism resemble β-adrenergic effects. These features (tachycardia, palpitation, tremor, sweating, and nervousness) are blocked by β-adrenergic antagonists. Propranolol has been widely used for this purpose. Doses of 20–40 mg every 4–6 hours usually result in rapid symptomatic relief. The main indication for propranolol administration is resting tachycardia. The dose may be increased to slow the resting heart rate to less than 90. Although propranolol does not affect thyroid secretion, it reduces monodeiodination of T_4 to T_3 peripherally and may lower the serum T_3 concentration by 30%. The drug may be useful while awaiting the results of diagnostic tests or waiting for the response to antithyroid drugs or radioiodine. Propranolol is the best agent for treating hyperthyroidism due to thyroiditis. Propranolol is contraindicated in obstructive pulmonary disease and congestive cardiac failure; however, it is beneficial in hyperthyroid patients when the cardiac failure results from rapid tachycardia.

Biliary Tract Contrast Agents. The iodinated contrast agents for cholecystography, sodium ipodate (Oragrafin) and iopanoic acid (Telepaque), potently inhibit peripheral conversion of T_4 to T_3. In hyperthyroid patients a 1- to 3-g dose of sodium ipodate may lower the serum T_3 level by 50–80%. Because of the iodine in these drugs, there is also a reduction in thyroid secretion, which lowers the serum T_4 concentration. Therapy for 1–3 weeks is associated with significant improvement. These drugs are still experimental in the treatment of hyperthyroidism. Short-term administration appears to be free of any significant side effects.

Subtotal Thyroidectomy

Surgical thyroidectomy is dramatically effective for the eradication of hyperthyroidism. For optimal results, the patient should be prepared with antithyroid drugs to reverse the catabolic state and cardiovascular effects. Administration of iodine for 7–10 days preoperatively reduces the vascularity of the thyroid and is reputed to make surgery easier. In recent years, many patients have been prepared for surgery with propranolol as the sole agent for controlling tachycardia. Proponents say the surgery is simple and the results are excellent, but postoperative thyroid storm is still hazardous and can be avoided completely if the patient is euthyroid preoperatively.

Surgeons usually aim to leave about 5 g of residual thyroid to preserve normal thyroid function. Unfortunately, about 10% of patients develop a recurrence of hyperthyroidism, and 30% become permanently hypothyroid. Permanent hypoparathyroidism is a bad complication in 1–4% of patients, and recurrent laryngeal nerve palsy occurs in about 1%. These complications, as well as the trauma and expense of surgery, make it less appealing than medical therapy or radioiodine.

Iodine-131

Radioiodine-131 has been used for the treatment of hyperthyroidism for over 30 years. The hyperactive thyroid follicular cells concentrate the ^{131}I, and the radiation exerts a destructive effect on the tissue. Oral administration is simple. The usual doses are calculated to deliver 5,000–7,000 rads to the thyroid and are about 2–10 mCi. Each microcurie taken up by a gram of thyroid produces about 90 rads. The dose in microcuries can be calculated from the following formula for a therapeutic dose of 5,000 rads:

$$\text{Microcuries } (\mu\text{Ci}) = \frac{5{,}000 \text{ rads}}{90 \text{ rads-g}/\mu\text{Ci}} \times \frac{\text{thyroid weight (g)}}{\text{24-hr uptake (fractional)}}$$

For a 50-g thyroid gland with a 24-hour uptake of 50%, the dose would be 5,600 μCi (5.6 mCi). This dose is relatively small. A high proportion of patients receiving it, perhaps 50%, require a second dose of ^{131}I at a later date to control the hyperthyroidism. However, if larger initial doses are given, there will be a higher incidence of hypothyroidism, the main undesirable consequence of ^{131}I therapy. With conventional ^{131}I doses (5,000–7,000 rads), the long-term incidence of hypothyroidism is about 30–50%. Depending on the dose of ^{131}I, the incidence of hypothyroidism is 5–20% after 1 year, and then it increases more slowly at a rate of 1–3% per year. Because of this, some clinicians prefer to give a large dose of ^{131}I to cure the hyperthyroidism with certainty and to induce definite hypothyroidism. This approach may be justified in older patients for whom recurrent hyperthyroidism may be dangerous. In younger patients, I prefer to give a dose of ^{131}I to deliver 5,000 rads in the hope that hypothyroidism will be avoided or delayed. Because the effect of this dose is uncertain, antithyroid drugs are continued afterward for 1 year before stopping them to assess the effect of the radioiodine. If hyperthyroidism recurs, a second treatment with ^{131}I is given.

Hypoparathyroidism after ^{131}I is extremely rare. The parathyroids, which lie posterior to the thyroid, are apparently protected and also quite radioresistant.

Fear of carcinogenesis from the radiation is unjustified. There is no increase in the incidence of leukemia, which has been studied very carefully. Thyroid cancers after this treatment are also rare and occur in a lower incidence than in the general population. Thyroid neoplasia increases progressively with radiation doses from 50 to 2,000 rads but does not occur in the hyperthyroid gland treated with doses larger than 2,000 rads. This may be attributable to damage to the genetic apparatus, which impairs replication. Radiation to the gonads of women has been calculated carefully and is no greater with ^{131}I therapy for hyperthyroidism than that with diagnostic pelvic roentgenograms such as pyelography. Studies of offspring of men and women who received ^{131}I for treatment of hyperthyroidism as children have shown no increase in congenital anomalies. These points should be explained carefully to patients to relieve anxiety about radiation hazards. Unfortunately, there are an increasing number of patients, often well educated, who express grave concern about radioiodine therapy because of a totally unfounded fear of radiation hazards. These patients require additional education. If ^{131}I is the best therapy for such a patient, then the patient's unfounded anxiety seems to be a poor basis for choosing other treatment.

Specialists in nuclear medicine often administer the radioiodine and follow these patients. A generation ago, when nuclear medicine was less complex, these specialists were well trained in clinical thyroidology. This is often not the case nowadays. Hyperthyroid patients should be followed by an internist or endocrinologist. This physician, rather than the nuclear medicine specialist, should determine the dose of ^{131}I (the number of rads), additional medicine, and when the next dose should be given.

For severely hyperthyroid patients, it is important to control the hyperthyroidism with drug therapy before administering ^{131}I. To avoid delay of ^{131}I treatment, drugs containing iodine should not be used. Propylthiouracil or methimazole can be stopped 2–3 days before giving the ^{131}I and will not interfere with the treatment. These drugs may be used again 2–3 days after the ^{131}I has been given.

Table 3 summarizes the therapeutic recommendations.

Table 3 **Recommendations for the Treatment of Hyperthyroidism**

Propylthiouracil or methimazole	
	Children
	Young and middle-aged adults
	Preparation for ^{131}I therapy or surgery
	Pregnant women
Beta blockers (propranolol)	
	Control of tachycardia
	Waiting for diagnostic tests
	Before and after ^{131}I therapy
Radioiodine-131	
	Recurrence after drug treatment
	Recurrence after surgery
	Older patients
	Coexistent cardiac disease
	Autonomous hyperfunctioning nodule
	Multinodular goiter
Surgical thyroidectomy	
	Severe reactions to thionamides
	Recurrence after drugs; patients refuse ^{131}I therapy
	Pregnancy (drug treatment preferable)
	Coexistent thyroid carcinoma (rare)

Thyroid Storm

Thyroid storm or thyrotoxic crisis is a dangerous worsening of hyperthyroidism with fever, rapid tachycardia, agitation or delirium, nausea, vomiting, diarrhea, and volume depletion. It is usually precipitated by stress, such as an infection or surgery, but sometimes the fever is due to the thyrotoxic state itself. Gastrointestinal symptoms are ominous as harbingers of storm because they reduce the caloric and fluid intake of a severely hypermetabolic patient.

Serum T_4 and T_3 levels are no higher than in other patients with hyperthyroidism. The condition has a high mortality if it is not treated vigorously.

Treatment consists of multiple modalities: 200–300 mg of propylthiouracil (by gavage if necessary) or 20–30 mg methimazole (given as a rectal solution), sodium ipodate (1 g by mouth) or sodium iodide (1 g i.v. over 8 hours). Iodine should be given 1 hour after the thionamide, so that blockage of organic binding will prevent the iodine from being made into thyroid hormone. Propranolol is given to reduce the tachycardia: It may be administered intravenously, 1 mg every 2 minutes up to 10 mg, with the patient on a cardiac monitor to reduce the heart rate to 100/minute. Repeated doses of propranolol intravenously are given every 2–4 hours based on heart rate. Corticosteroids have beneficial effects in hyperthyroidism by blocking conversion of T_4 to T_3. Plasmapheresis may be used to reduce circulating thyroid hormones as a desperate measure in an otherwise unresponsive patient.

Treatment of the underlying disorder with antibiotics for infections, vigorous fluid and electrolyte replacement, administration of oxygen, and other supportive measures are equal in importance to therapy directed at the thyroid. These supportive measures must not be overlooked.

Hyperthyroidism in Pregnancy

Hyperthyroidism complicates pregnancy in about 1 per 1,000 pregnancies. Because hyperthyroidism impairs fertility, pregnancy is more likely to develop after the hyperthyroidism has been controlled by treatment. To avoid this complication, some form of birth control should be prescribed in hyperthyroid women of child-bearing age until the hyperthyroidism has been resolved.

Estrogen increases the level of TBG, the protein that binds 70% of T_4 and 50% of T_3. Therefore, total T_4 and T_3 levels rise during pregnancy, but the free hormone levels and indexes generally remain normal. Thus the free hormone levels or indexes are useful for diagnosis of hyperthyroidism.

Therapy for hyperthyroidism during pregnancy is controversial. Radioiodine is not used because the fetal thyroid concentrates iodine after the tenth week of gestation. Giving ^{131}I after this time has caused fetal hypothyroidism. Antithyroid drugs are effective and safe when used judiciously in the lowest possible dose to control the hyperthyroidism. Both propylthiouracil and methimazole cross the placenta and can impair fetal thyroid hormone production and cause fetal goiter. Thyroid hormones and TSH do not cross the placenta. The fetal thyroid gland operates independently. IgG crosses the placenta, so that thyroid-stimulating antibody could cause fetal hyperthyroidism. In theory, fetal hyperthyroidism could be prevented by an antithyroid drug. During pregnancy, antithyroid drugs should be given in doses sufficient to control hyperthyroidism. The dose is tapered as quickly as possible, and the serum free T_4 index is maintained in the upper portion of the normal range. Most pregnant women tolerate mild hyperthyroidism very well. Patients are seen at monthly intervals or more frequently if necessary to evaluate the therapy.

To control severe symptoms and rapid tachycardia, propranolol may be useful, but it should not be continued throughout pregnancy because of potential deleterious effects on the fetus. Stable iodine in therapeutic doses is contraindicated, because the fetal thyroid concentrates it avidly; the resulting high intrathyroidal iodine concentration blocks biosynthesis of hormone, and large obstructing goiters have resulted.

Surgical thyroidectomy has also been effective for curing hyperthyroidism in pregnancy. If it is to be done, it is preferable to perform it during the second trimester after the hyperthyroidism has been controlled with medical treatment. General surgery in the first trimester may precipitate a spontaneous abortion, and during the third trimester it may induce premature delivery. Postsurgical hypothyroidism should be anticipated and treated early to avoid prolonged maternal hypothyroidism.

Comparisons of the results of medical and surgical treatment of hyperthyroidism in pregnancy show similar results: 80–90% of the pregnancies yield a successful outcome with a healthy infant, no fetal goiter, and no neonatal thyrotoxicosis. I prefer medical treatment because it eliminates the possibility of surgical complications and because patients may go into a prolonged remission after completing the pregnancy.

HYPOTHYROIDISM

Hypothyroidism is the condition resulting from a deficiency of thyroid hormone.

Causes

Congenital hypothyroidism has been carefully studied by screening over a million newborns. Its frequency is about 1 in 4,000 births, and the most common cause is thyroid hypoplasia or aplasia or a lingual thyroid remnant. Hereditary defects in the biosynthesis or action of thyroid hormone are much rarer than thyroid hypoplasia.

Endemic cretinism occurs only in relatively primitive societies that suffer severe iodine deficiency, often coupled with ingestion of goitrogenic foods, such as cassava. Cassava increases plasma thiocyanate concentration which displaces or washes out the little iodine that is available to the thyroid.

Chronic lymphocytic (Hashimoto's) thyroiditis is the most common cause of spontaneous hypothyroidism in adolescents and adults. It is four times more common in women than in men. Its prevalence rises with age, reaching about 12% in middle-aged women, based on detection of thyroid microsomal antibodies; about one-tenth of patients have overt hypothyroidism, and some, but not all, will become hypothyroid later.

Treatment of hyperthyroidism with surgery or radioiodine may result in hypothyroidism; hypothyroidism occurs uniformly after surgery for thyroid cancer. Radiation therapy for Hodgkin's disease or for laryngeal cancer often damages the thyroid. The main drugs causing reversible hypothyroidism are thionamides, iodine, and lithium. Nearly one-twentieth of patients taking lithium for depression will have reversible mild hypothyroidism.

Hypopituitarism or hypothalamic disease may be caused by a large variety of lesions. Reduced secretion of TSH causes thyroid atrophy and results in *central* hypothyroidism.

Clinical Features

Mild hypothyroidism is much more common than severe myxedema in our population. This may be attributed to earlier diagnosis and therapy. A common pattern of symptoms is mild fatigue, slight cold intolerance, weight gain of only a few pounds, and dry skin. Although these symptoms are nonspecific, they should suggest a diagnostic evaluation for hypothyroidism. Anyone with goiter who is not hyperthyroid should be suspected of hypothyroidism. All patients with hyperlipidemia should be screened for hypothyroidism.

Myxedema causes a characteristic appearance. The face is puffy, especially around the eyes, the features are slightly coarsened, the eyelids are droopy, and the forehead is wrinkled in an effort to keep the eyes open. The voice may be hoarse; speech and movement are slow. The hair is coarse and the lateral eyebrows are thin. The skin is dry and thickened as a result of the deposition of mucoprotein (which is the basis of the term myxedema), and it has a yellowish cast from the deposition of carotene. Rarely, there is pitting edema of the ankles and feet without another overt cause.

Patients complain of exertional dyspnea but have few other cardiac symptoms. Myocardial contractions are feeble because the myocardium is also myxedematous. The heart rate is slow. Small pericardial effusions, detected by echocardiography, are common and enlarge the cardiac silhouette. The ECG shows low-voltage and flat T waves. The hypercholesterolemia and hypertriglyceridemia of hypothyroidism may accelerate atherosclerosis. Ventilatory responses to hypoxia and hypercapnea are reduced. With severe myxedema respiratory acidosis may develop.

Reduced gastrointestinal motility causes constipation. Ascites is rare and is usually superimposed on another etiology such as portal hypertension.

Muscle weakness and cramps may be prominent. The muscles may be hypertrophied, especially in children, but contraction is slow and weak. The levels of muscle enzymes, especially creatine phosphokinase (CPK), are elevated in the serum. Neurologic syndromes include peripheral neuropathy, carpal tunnel syndrome, cerebellar ataxia, dementia, and functional psychiatric disorders, particularly depression.

Hypothyroidism causes primary amenorrhea or precocious puberty in children, possibly because of the luteotropic activity of TSH. In adult women, secondary amenorrhea and galactorrhea can occur with increased prolactin secretion attributed to the prolactin-releasing effect of TRH. With milder hypothyroidism, menses may be prolonged and anovulatory cycles may occur. Men sometimes complain of a decrease in libido.

Hypothyroidism causes anemia, usually normocytic, which may be an adaptive response to a decreased oxygen need. About 8% of patients with hypothyroidism and Hashimoto's thyroiditis have coexistent pernicious anemia, reflecting a more generalized autoimmune diathesis (see Chapter 18).

Primary hypothyroidism causes pituitary enlargement as a result of hyperplasia of the thyrotrophs. The sella turcia is enlarged on lateral skull roentgenograms, especially in children, and this raises suspicion of a pituitary tumor causing hypothyroidism. The lack of thyroid hormone reduces growth hormone secretion. It was believed that the pituitary enlargement of primary hypothyroidism was a benign process, but recently several hypothyroid patients were reported who had visual field abnormalities from chiasmal compression. These features improved as the thyrotrophs involuted with treatment of the hypothyroidism.

Hypothyroid patients have reduced oxygen consumption and hypothermia. Excretion of a water load is delayed. Hyponatremia may occur, partly as a result of inappropriate secretion of vasopressin.

Diagnostic Tests

Diagnosis of primary hypothyroidism is relatively simple using the combination of serum T_4 concentration, free T_4 index, and serum TSH concentration. The free T_4 index will "adjust" a low serum T_4 level into the normal range if the low serum T_4 level is due to reduction in the serum protein-binding capacity for T_4. This occurs in the following conditions: cirrhosis, severe malnutrition, nephrotic syndrome, congenital deficiency of TBG, and therapy with large doses of corticosteroids, testosterone, or salicylates. On the other hand, in hypothyroidism, the protein-binding capacity is relatively increased, so that the free T_4 index is even less than the total serum T_4 concentration. TSH secretion is very sensitive to mild changes in levels of circulating thyroid hormones. Serum TSH levels are clearly increased above the normal range in patients with mild hypothyroidism; however, serum TSH levels may also be increased in euthyroid patients who have a normal serum T_4 concentration but slightly compromised thyroid function. This may occur in some patients with Hasimoto's thyroiditis and after ^{131}I therapy for hyperthyroidism.

For screening patients who do not have clinical features of hypothyroidism, measurement of the serum T_4 level is probably sufficient and cost-effective. This is as important in the geriatric population as in the newborn, because the prevalence of hypothyroidism in the aged is about 2-4%.

Measurement of the serum T_3 concentration is not a sensitive test for hypothyroidism. Many patients with mild hypothyroidism have a normal serum T_3 concentration. A low T_3 level is found with more severe hypothyroidism. In systemic illness, monodeiodination of T_4 to T_3 is reduced, and the serum T_3 level may be low in a euthyroid patient with a normal serum T_4 concentration.

To differentiate primary from central hypothyroidism, the serum TSH level and the TSH response to TRH may be helpful. In patients with central hypothyroidism due to pituitary lesions, the serum TSH level is low or undetectable. In patients with central hypothyroidism due to

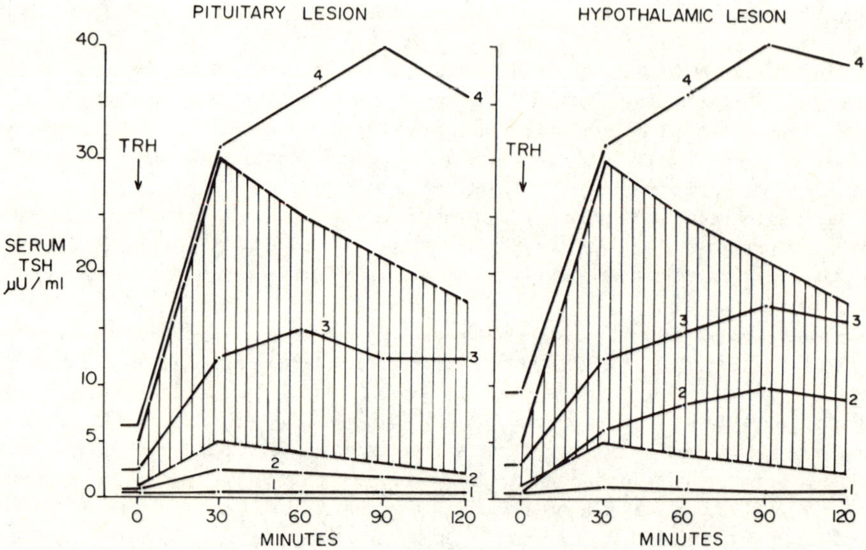

Figure 1. Patterns of TSH response to 500 μg of TRH (protirelin) given intravenously. Hatched area shows the normal range of responses. Pituitary lesions (left) usually cause a subnormal response (patients 1 and 2), sometimes a normal response (patient 3), and rarely an exaggerated response (patient 4). Hypothalamic lesions (right) usually cause a normal response with a delayed peak (patients 2 and 3) or sometimes high baseline TSH with an exaggerated response (patient 4).

hypothalamic lesions, such as craniopharyngioma, the serum TSH level is low, normal, or even slightly elevated. The TSH in these patients with elevated serum TSH levels has been shown by RIA to have reduced biologic activity, but the reason for the lack of biologic potency is unknown. Figure 1 shows the various patterns of TSH response to TRH in patients with central hypothyroidism. In patients with pituitary lesions, the TSH response is usually blunted. In patients with hypothalamic lesions, the TSH response is delayed, so that the peak TSH level may occur at 60–90 minutes after TRH administration rather than at 30 minutes, and the height of the response may be exaggerated. Unfortunately, a common cause of a ''hypothalamic'' pattern is suprasellar extension of a pituitary tumor. Because of the variability of the TSH response to TRH in patients with central hypothyroidism, the test has limited diagnostic utility.

Other Tests

A variety of tests have been used to assess the metabolic action of thyroid hormone, but these tests are not very sensitive or specific for diagnosis of hypothyroidism. They include measurement of the serum cholesterol level, creatine phosphokinase (CPK) level, speed of Achilles reflex contraction, basal metabolic rate, and systolic time interval.

Antibodies to thyroid microsomes and thyroglobulin are useful in diagnosing Hashimoto's thyroiditis as the cause of hypothyroidism. Approximately 70–80% of patients with Hashimoto's disease will have diagnostically abnormal titers of one or both antibodies.

Patients Taking Thyroid Hormone

A common problem is the diagnosis of hypothyroidism in a patient who takes thyroid hormone for indications that are relatively flimsy, based on the patient's history. Measurements of thyroid hormone levels reflect the patient's present dose of thyroid hormone. One approach in establishing the diagnosis is to stop the thyroid therapy. Because it has suppressed the pituitary-thyroid axis, the patient will experience mild physiologic hypothyroidism about 1–2 weeks after the preparation is stopped. The axis usually recovers from this suppression in 3–4 weeks in patients with normal thyroids, whereas hypothyroid patients become progressively more hypothyroid. Serum T_4 and TSH concentrations should be measured 5 weeks after stopping the thyroid medication. At this time, the levels should reflect the true diagnosis. Figure 2 diagrams this situation.

Therapy

Treatment of hypothyroidism is simple and effective. Synthetic sodium L-thyroxine is the preparation of choice. The usual replacement dose for adults is 2–2.5 μg/kg. In young and middle-aged adults, it is safe to begin treatment with a T_4 replacement dose of about 100–150 μg as a single daily dose. The dose is increased by 25 μg each month until the serum T_4 level and free T_4 index are in the normal range *and* the serum TSH level is suppressed to the normal range *or* the serum T_3 level is normal. Patients on T_4 replacement therapy may have a normal serum T_4 concentration on a suboptimal dose, which is associated with an elevated serum TSH level and a subnormal serum T_3 concentration. Of course the serum T_3 levels arise from conversion of T_4 to T_3.

In older patients who may have cardiovascular disease and in those with known heart disease, it is better to start with a low dose of thyroid hormone such as 25–50 μg of thyroxine and to increase by 25 μg monthly until the desired clinical effect is obtained. This concept of "low and slow" thyroid dosage in the cardiac patient has been exaggerated, leading to prolonged symptomatic hypothyroidism due to inadequate therapy. In some patients, treatment actually alleviates cardiac symptoms, because the myxedematous myocardium works poorly. Another

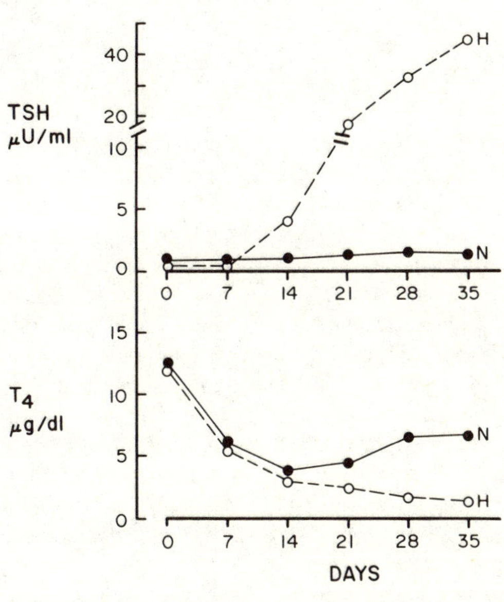

Figure 2. Patterns of serum T_4 and TSH levels after stopping a 0.2-mg daily dose of T_4 in a normal euthyroid patient (N) compared to a patient with primary hypothyroidism (H).

possibility is to block the cardiac effects of thyroid hormone and prevent severe arrhythmias by concomitant use of propranolol.

In a hypothyroid patient with severe coronary heart disease who is a candidate for coronary revascularization surgery, surgery may be carried out without replacement therapy with T_4. Instead, T_4 is given in the postoperative period.

Many patients continue to take biologic thyroid preparations, desiccated thyroid, or partially purified thyroglobulin. The ratio of T_4 to T_3 in these preparations is about 3.3 : 1. Each microgram of L-thyroxine is equivalent to 1 mg of desiccated thyroid. Within a few hours after ingestion of preparations containing T_3, the serum T_3 concentration may rise to supranormal levels. USP standardization of desiccated thyroid requires only that the iodine content be about 0.2% rather than that there be an assessment of hormonal activity. For these reasons, synthetic L-thyroxine is the better preparation for therapy. Many patients prefer to take desiccated thyroid, perhaps because the supraphysiologic T_3 levels provide some stimulation they do not feel while taking an equivalent amount of T_4.

The Patient in a Myxedema Coma Versus the Sick Euthyroid Patient

Myxedema coma is a life-threatening emergency that is the end stage of myxedema. Often the coma has been precipitated by a sedative given to a querulous elderly patient who then cannot be aroused. Other precipitating factors include severe cold exposure, surgery, infections, and other intercurrent illnesses. Factors contributing to the obtundation or coma are respiratory acidosis, severe hyponatremia, and cerebral edema. These patients are often severely hypothermic. Host response to infection is poor, and the temperature may not rise above normal. Rewarming such patients may cause peripheral vasodilation and precipitate shock because of diminished plasma volume.

A patient with myxedema coma must be differentiated from a severely sick euthyroid patient with low serum levels of thyroid hormone due to systemic illness. Severe systemic illness, liver disease, and advanced renal failure may impair conversion of T_4 to T_3 and cause a low serum T_3 concentration. In addition, severe systemic illness lowers the serum T_4 concentration; the mechanism is not really understood. The free T_4 index, rapid measurements of free T_4 by kits, and even free T_4 measured by equilibrium dialysis are often subnormal in these patients, but the values are usually less depressed (in relation to normal) than the total serum T_4 level. The serum TSH level is generally normal, but the clinician must be aware that large doses of corticosteroids and dopamine infusion can lower the serum TSH concentration in hypothyroid patients. Although the bandages, indwelling tubes, and lines attached to patients in the medical intensive care unit make clinical evaluation difficult, these sick patients generally do not have the obvious clinical features of myxedema. Table 4 summarizes the guidelines for evaluation of patients with nonthyroidal illness and a low serum T_4 concentration.

In addition to supportive measures for underlying disorders, therapy for myxedema coma consists of the administration of a large dose of thyroxine intravenously to restore the extrathyroidal T_4 pool to one-half normal. The usual dose of T_4 is 500 μg. The patient may be observed afterward for 2 or 3 days before additional doses are necessary. With this large dose, serum T_4 may rise from virtually undetectable levels to 3–5 μg/dl. Subsequent daily doses are 50–100 μg i.v. T_4. Since only one-half of T_4 given by mouth is absorbed, the intravenous doses are equivalent to larger oral doses.

With this vigorous therapy, the majority of patients survive and their prognosis is related to their general health otherwise. One should not hesitate to treat myxedema coma promptly; euthyroid patients are not harmed by a single 500-μg dose of T_4.

Table 4 **Guidelines for Evaluation of Thyroid Function in Patients with Low Serum T_4 Concentration and Nonthyroid Illness**

Clinical evaluation must serve as the basis for the decision about treatment.

Initial thyroid laboratory data: If free T_4 index $\gg T_4$ (or if free $T_4 \gg T_4$), patient is probably not hypothyroid. Do not treat with T_4.

Measure TSH and free T_4.

Treat for hypothyroidism if free T_4 is low and TSH >10 μU/ml *or* if free T_4 is low, TSH is low or normal, and patient has definite evidence of organic pituitary-hypothalamic disease.

DISCUSSION CASES

Case 1:

Description

A 29-year-old secretary developed poor appetite and a weight loss of 8 lb in 2 months attributed to job stress. She also complained of nervousness, shaking, weakness, heat intolerance, and palpitation. She had been married 3 months earlier and recalled that her eyes bulged out slightly in her wedding pictures. Her menstrual periods had been slightly shorter and lighter for the past 2 months. Her mother had hypothyroidism.

She was 64 in. tall and weighed 120 lb. Her pulse was 96/minute, blood pressure 130/60, temperature 36.6°C. She had a prominent stare and normal ocular motility; her eyes measured 20 mm bilaterally on the exophthalmometer (normal <20 mm). Her thyroid was diffusely enlarged to 50 g with a prominent isthmus and was not tender. She had a forceful cardiac pulsation, a faint systolic ejection murmur, and a "scratch" at the left sternal border. She had smooth, moist skin, a faint fine tremor, and brisk tendon reflexes.

Thyroid function tests showed a serum T_4 level of 13.7 μg/dl, a free T_4 index of 15 (normal 4.5–11), a serum T_3 level of 450 ng/dl, and a free T_3 index of 490 (normal 90–180).

Treatment with propylthiouracil, 100 mg every 8 hours, was started, and she returned in 6 weeks. Her symptoms had improved, she had gained 6 lb, and she reported that she had missed her last menstrual period.

Her serum T_4 level was 6.7 μg/dl, her free T_4 index 4.9, her serum T_3 level 240 ng/dl, and her free T_3 index 180. A pregnancy test was positive. After the alternatives were explained to her and her husband, they decided to think about pregnancy versus elective abortion for a few days. She called back the next week to say she wished to continue her pregnancy. The dose of propylthiouracil was reduced to 200 mg daily and 1 month later to 150 mg/day in three divided doses. When seen at monthly intervals, she was euthyroid; her serum T_4 level ranged between 13 and 19, her free T_4 index between 10 and 15, and her T_3 level between 210 and 300 ng/dl.

Her labor was uncomplicated, and the baby was born 1 week after the expected date. He was euthyroid (cord T_4 level 9.5 μg/dl) and did not have a goiter. Because she wanted to nurse, propylthiouracil therapy was stopped after the delivery. One month later, she felt well but was nervous; her thyroid was estimated to be 40 g, her serum T_4 level was 6.4 μg/dl, her free T_4 index 6.4, and her T_3 level 130 ng/dl.

Question

1. Why is there a discrepancy between the T_4 and free T_4 index values during pregnancy? What is the free T_3 index?

Answer

The increased estrogen of pregnancy raises the TBG level and thus raises the total T_4 concentration. The free T_4 index corrects for this alteration in TBG. The T_3 in the serum is also bound to TBG (but to a smaller extent than T_4), so the total T_3 concentration is raised in pregnancy. The free T_3 index adjusts for the changes in the total T_3 level in the same way as the free T_4 index.

Question

2. What was the cause of her hyperthyroidism? Should a radioiodine uptake have been performed?

Answer

She had Graves' disease as indicated by the diffuse enlargement of her thyroid and the mild ophthalmopathy. The proptosis, even though minimal, made it unlikely that lymphocytic thyroiditis was the cause of her hyperthyroidism. Although she subsequently developed amenorrhea and a positive pregnancy test, hydatidiform mole as the cause of her hyperthyroidism was not a viable diagnostic consideration because she had significant thyromegaly without evidence of pregnancy initially and the proptosis. These features have not been reported in molar pregnancy with thyrotoxicosis, because the moles and the abdomen are large and there is only slight thyromegaly.

Question

3. Was it necessary that propylthiouracil therapy be stopped in order for her to nurse her baby?

Answer

This has been standard dogma because early studies showed concentration of propylthiouracil in the milk. However, a recent report claimed that less than 0.1% of propylthiouracil is excreted in the milk, so this concept may need revision.

Question

4. What are her chances for long-term remission?

Answer

The subsidence of her hyperthyroidism after delivery was surprising, because 150 mg propylthiouracil was required to maintain her in a borderline hyperthyroid-euthyroid condition during the pregnancy. Many hyperthyroid women improve during pregnancy, possibly because of the immunosuppression of the gravid state. She has about a 50% chance of maintaining the remission and needs close follow-up in the next year. A substantial decrease in the size of her thyroid would have suggested regression of the disease.

Case 2

Description

A 31-year-old woman noted discomfort high in her neck which felt like "a popcorn husk stuck in her throat." This was accompanied by mild dysphagia which persisted for 1 month. She had felt "exhausted all the time" for several months and was crabby. She had gained 5 pounds during this time. She also felt unusually cold, and her pattern of bowel movements had changed to one every 2 days rather than daily. She had noted slight menorrhagia for the past 3 months. She denied taking medicine or food with a high iodine content.

She consulted an otolaryngologist who noted a swelling in her pharynx at the base of her tongue.

She was a pleasant, attractive woman, 67 in. tall and 136 lb, with a pulse of 72 and a blood pressure of 110/76. Her voice was low. There was no periorbital puffiness. The thyroid was not palpable. Her skin was dry. A biceps jerk showed a slightly delayed return phase, but her ankle jerk appeared normal.

Her serum T_4 level was 1.1 μg/dl, and her free T_4 index was 0.9. Her TSH level was 290 μU/ml. Antithyroid antibodies showed positive antithyroglobulin at 1:160 and antimicrosomal at 1:25,600. A thyroid scan showed a small focus of uptake high in the neck and no uptake in the usual thyroid area.

She was given 100 μg T_4 daily. She noted a loss of the discomfort in her neck 3 weeks later; her serum T_4 level was 7.4 μg/dl, her free T_4 index 6.4, and her serum TSH level 150 μU/ml at this time. The dose of T_4 was increased to 125 μg daily (serum T_4 level 8.6 μg/dl, serum TSH level 18 μU/ml after 1 month) and then to 150 μg with loss of all symptoms. Her serum T_4 level on this dose was 9.8 μg/dl, and her TSH level was <0.5 μU/ml.

Question

1. What is the pathogenesis of her symptoms?

Answer

This woman had a mass in her neck at the base of the tongue that was shown on scan to be lingual thyroid tissue. This tissue had hypertrophied under stimulation by her very high levels of thyrotropin. Obviously this thyroid tissue was incapable of secreting sufficient thyroid hormone to keep her euthyroid. In embryologic development, a small remnant of thyroid tissue may remain at the base of the tongue. A lingual thyroid is much more common in young children with hypothyroidism who have failed to develop normal thyroid tissue. Screening of newborns for hypothyroidism has yielded an incidence of about 1 in 4,000 births. About one-fourth of these hypothyroid infants have lingual thyroid tissue which shows up on a thyroid scan.

This patient also had typical symptoms of hypothyroidism including fatigue, feeling cold, and a slight weight gain. Her menorrhagia was also typical. Hypothyroidism of long standing causes amenorrhea and occasionally galactorrhea, but mild menorrhagia is the most common menstrual disorder caused by hypothyroidism. Her constipation was also minimal and is the main gastrointestinal symptom of hypothyroidism.

Hashimoto's chronic lymphocytic thyroiditis is the most common cause of spontaneous hypothyroidism in adults. The antithyroid antibodies were elevated to titers diagnostic of this disorder: antithyroglobulin $>1:25$ and antimicrosomal $>1:100$. Usually, the antimicrosomal antibody level is more elevated than the antithyroglobulin antibody level, as in this patient, but sometimes only one value may be abnormal. In patients with Hashimoto's thyroiditis, ingestion of large amounts of iodine, as in a saturated solution of potassium iodide, may cause hypothyroidism. The diseased thyroid, which is stimulated by TSH, is particularly susceptible to the blocking effect of iodine on the biosynthesis of T_4. Iodine could not be incriminated as a contributory factor in this instance.

In her case, therapy with T_4 suppressed the serum TSH level and caused involution of the lingual thyroid tissue and loss of her symptoms.

Question

2. Why was the dose of L-thyroxine increased beyond 100 μg daily?

Answer

The 100-μg dose elevated the serum T_4 level to 7.4 μg/dl, a normal value, but her serum TSH level was still elevated, indicating an incomplete therapeutic and suppressive effect. Although the serum TSH concentration might have continued to fall over the next few weeks, it probably would have remained supranormal because even 125 μg did not lower the TSH level to the normal range. The 150-μg dose was necessary to suppress the TSH completely.

SUGGESTED READING

Astwood EB: The use of antithyroid drugs during pregnancy. *J Clin Endocrinol* 11:1045–1053, 1951.

Davis PJ, Davis EB: Hyperthyroidism in patients over the age of 60 years, *Medicine* 53:161–181, 1974.

Fisher DA, Dussault JH, Foley TP Jr, et al: Screening for congenital hypothyroidism: Results of screening one million North American infants. *J Pediatr* 94:700–705, 1979.

Gordin A, Lamberg B-A: Natural course of symptomless autoimmune thyroiditis. *Lancet* ii:1234–1238, 1975.

Hamburger JI: Evolution of toxicity in solitary autonomously functioning thyroid lesions. *J Clin Endocrinol Metab* 50:1089–1093, 1980.

Hershman JM, Bray GA: *The Thyroid: Physiology and Treatment of Disease*. Oxford, Pergamon, 1979.

Higgins HP, Hershman JM, Kenimer JG, et al: The thyrotoxicosis of hydatidiform mole. *Ann Intern Med* 83:307–311, 1975.

Hollander CS, Mitsuma T, Nihei N, et al: Clinical and laboratory observations in cases of triiodothyronine toxicosis confirmed by radioimmunoassay. *Lancet*, i:609–611, 1972.

Kampman JP, Johansen K, Hansen JM: Propylthiouracil in human milk. *Lancet* i:736–738, 1980.

Krugman LG, Hershman JM, Chopra IJ, et al: Patterns of recovery of the hypothalamic-pituitary-thyroid axis in patients taken off chronic thyroid therapy. *J Clin Endocrinol Metab* 41:70–80, 1975.

Sawin CT, Hershman JM, Fernandez-Garcia R, et al: Comparison of thyroxine and desiccated thyroid in patients with primary hypothyroidism. *Metabolism* 27:1518–1525, 1978.

Stock JM, Surks MI, Oppenheimer JH: Replacement dosage of L-thyroxine in hypothyroidism: A reevaluation. *N Engl J Med* 290:529–533, 1974.

Volpé R: Thyrotoxicosis. *Clin Endocrinol Metab* 7:1–243, 1978.

Werner SC, Ingbar SH: *The Thyroid*, ed 4. Hagerstown, Harper & Row, 1978.

Woolf PD: Transient painless thyroiditis with hyperthyroidism: A variant of lymphocytic thyroiditis? *Endocr Rev* 1:411–420, 1980.

Yamada T, Tsukei T, Ikejin K, et al: Volume of sella turcica in normal subjects and in patients with primary hypothyroidism and hyperthyroidism. *J Clin Endocrinol Metab* 42:817–822, 1976.

Yamamoto M, Igarashi T, Kimura S, et al: Thyroid suppression test and outcome of hyperthyroidism treated with antithyroid drugs and triiodothyronine. *J Clin Endocrinol Metab* 48:72–77, 1979.

Zakarija M, McKenzie TM, Banovac K: Clinical significance of assay of thyroid-stimulating antibody in Graves' disease. *Ann Intern Med* 93:28–32, 1980.

5

ANDRE J. VAN HERLE

Thyroid Nodules and Thyroid Cancer

The thyroid nodule is one of the most common endocrine problems encountered in clinical practice. The Framingham study indicated that the overall incidence of thyroid nodules in the population under study was 4.2%, with an annual increase in new nodule detection of 0.09% per year. These values are concordant with data recently reported by Tunbridge and co-workers who described an increase in nodularity from ~1% in the second decade of life to ~5% in the seventh decade; this increase is especially noticeable in the female population (Fig. 1). In addition, thyroid nodules as well as thyroid cancer are more common in women all over the world, except for anaplastic carcinomas of the thyroid gland. These facts indicate that thyroid nodules will become more common as the age of a given population increases. We are consequently dealing with a large population that potentially can develop thyroid nodules, and in addition a wide differential diagnosis should be considered. Indeed, varying pathologies can manifest themselves as a thyroid nodule or neck mass; these include inflammatory processes, developmental abnormalities, traumatic events, intrinsic metabolic defects, and, last but not least, the occurrence of neoplasms (benign and malignant). The exact incidence of thyroid carcinoma in a given population is difficult to establish. Although clinically apparent thyroid nodules are common, thyroid cancer among them is rare. The third National Cancer Survey indicates that the overall adjusted incidence of thyroid cancer for both sexes is 3.9/100,000 per year. The prevalence of occult thyroid cancer is more common, ranging from 0.45 to 28.4% in autopsy studies. The clinical significance of occult thyroid cancer, however, is questionable to say the least, since the tumor in these cases represents an incidental autopsy finding and is never the cause of death. Although the mortality and morbidity of thyroid cancer are relatively low when compared to cancers of other organs, they nevertheless cannot be ignored. Pathology departments of large institutions have reported a number of subjects who died from thyroid cancer despite the generally favorable prognosis of differentiated thyroid tumors. Therefore, correct selection by the internist of patients with thyroid nodules who are in need of surgical exploration because of the presence of a malignancy is an important and challenging task. The histologic types of tumors under consideration will, to a certain extent, determine the therapy chosen (Table 1). The present discussion will primarily deal with strategy and selection of patients with thyroid nodules who need surgical therapy. The prognosis of various malignancies will also be discussed.

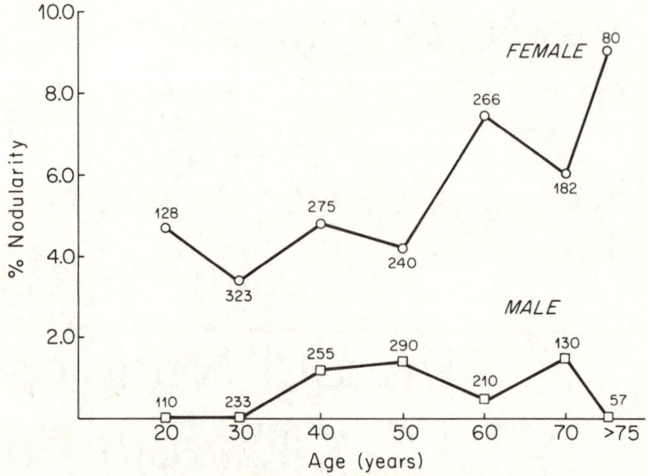

Figure 1. Prevalence of thyroid nodules in a community. The Whickham study. A clear increment in the prevalence of thyroid nodularity is seen in the female population with increasing age. A similar increment was not clearly demonstrated in the male population. Reproduced with permission of Tunbridge WMG, The spectrum of thyroid disease in a community: The Whickham survey. *Clin Endocrinol* 7:481–493, 1977. Copyright Blackwell Scientific Publications, Ltd.

ETIOLOGY

The cause of many thyroid conditions that can lead to thyroid nodule (single or multiple) or goiter formation is essentially unknown. In subacute thyroiditis a viral agent has been isolated, and in chronic lymphocytic thyroiditis the exact cause of the breakdown of normal immune mechanisms remains to be determined. Dietary iodine deficiency has been and still is a major cause of goiter formation in many areas of the world, but this factor can no longer be solely incriminated in the pathogenesis of goiter and nodule formation in the United States since the introduction of iodized salt. The pathogenic mechanism responsible for goiter formation in iodine-deficient areas is presumably mediated via excessive thyrotropin release, which in turn causes hyperplasia of the thyroid gland in an effort to ensure a normal thyroid hormone economy. The presence of goitrogens in the diet as well as in the water supply has been incriminated in goiter formation in certain areas of the world. As far as the etiopathogenesis of thyroid cancer is concerned two factors have come into focus in the last decade:

1. The relationship between external irradiation of the thyroid gland and carcinogenesis of the thyroid gland.
2. The recognition of the familial occurrence of medullary carcinoma of the thyroid gland and in rare instances of papillary carcinoma of the thyroid gland.

Irradiation-Induced Thyroid Cancer

This is a topic that has received wide attention in the medical literature as well as in the lay press. From the 1920s through the 1950s a large number of infants and children and a

Table 1 **Histologic Classification of Thyroid Tumors**

Epithelial tumors
Benign
Follicular adenoma
Others[a]
Malignant
Follicular carcinoma
Papillary carcinoma
Squamous cell carcinoma
Undifferentiated (anaplastic) carcinoma
Spindle cell type
Giant-cell type
Small-cell type
Medullary carcinoma
Nonepithelial tumors
Benign
Malignant
Fibrosarcoma
Others
Miscellaneous tumors
Carcinosarcoma
Malignant hemangioendothelioma
Malignant lymphoma
Teratoma
Secondary tumors[b]
Unclassified tumors
Tumor-like lesions[c]

Reprinted with permission of the World Health Organization.
[a]Papillary adenoma.
[b]Metastatic carcinoma.
[c]Adenomatous (nodular) goiter.

smaller number of adults underwent therapeutic irradiation for various medical conditions including an enlarged thymus, tonsils and adenoids, cervical adenitis, impetigo, sinusitis, pertussis, acne, hemangioma or keloid formation after a burn, Bell's palsy, eosinophilic granulomas, Hodgkins' disease, and other medical conditions.

The exposure to environmental irradiation occurring in nuclear plants and exposure to atomic weaponry should also be considered. The use of ^{131}I as a therapeutic tool in Graves' disease has also been mentioned, but this appears to not alter the risk of thyroid cancer. It is clear that the above-mentioned exposure to external irradiation leads to benign as well as malignant tumors of the thyroid gland in a certain percentage of the population. A recent survey carried out in the Chicago area revealed 27.3% of irradiated patients had abnormalities of the thyroid gland; of the subjects who were operated upon one-third had a malignancy of the thyroid gland and two-thirds had a benign lesion of the thyroid gland. Most of the malignant tumors were of the well-differentiated type (papillary, follicular, or mixed papillary-follicular cancer). However, a small number of anaplastic tumors developing after external irradiation have independently been reported by another group of investigators. The time interval between irradiation and tumor development extends beyond 25 years, and the patients who are exposed may in fact be at risk for the rest of their lives. There appears to be a good correlation between the total irradiation exposure and the incidence of nodule formation. At higher doses of irradiation exposure however, the incidence of thyroid tumors appears to fall off but does not disappear.

It should be stated that not only tumors of the thyroid gland develop after radiation exposure to the neck area, but also tumors of the parathyroid gland and of the parotid gland. A careful review of the patient's history with respect to radiation exposure is thus of paramount importance in the evaluation of all patients with thyroid nodules.

Genetic Inheritance of Thyroid Tumors

Medullary carcinoma of the thyroid gland is a rare tumor (5–10% of all thyroid malignancies) of the C cell of the thyroid gland, which characteristically produces thyrocalcitonin (TCT) and occasionally is responsible for the production of other hormones as well, such as ACTH and vasoactive intestinal peptide (VIP). The patients can be clustered in families (20%), or the tumors can occur sporadically (80%). The familial cases are part of the so-called multiple endocrine neoplasia syndrome (MEN). In the Sipple syndrome (MEN-IIa) medullary carcinoma of the thyroid gland is frequently (50%) associated with bilateral pheochromocytoma, parathyroid adenoma, or hyperplasia. In the MEN-IIb (or MEN-III) syndrome the presence of mucosal neuromas on the tongue, lips, and eyelids, as well as the Marfanoid habitus of the patient, allows one to suspect the diagnosis of medullary cancer and pheochromocytoma. Recognition of this familial occurring tumor is important, since total thyroidectomy in subjects with such tumors is indicated. Both these syndromes are inherited in an autosomal dominant pattern.

More recently a familial occurrence of papillary carcinoma of the thyroid gland has been reported in two kindreds in Norway. The frequency and mode of inheritance of the latter syndrome has not been clearly defined.

CLINICAL FEATURES

It is generally believed that certain clinical characteristics of a thyroid nodule are indications of a malignant process, namely, rapid expansion of an existing nodule, a firm and bulging texture of a lesion, pressure on adjacent structures, fixation of a nodule, obstructive symptoms, dysphagia, paralysis of the vocal cords, and Horner's syndrome. All the above symptoms, however, have been associated with benign lesions of the thyroid gland as well and are consequently only of relative value in the distinction between benign and malignant tumor of the thyroid gland. To illustrate this further, vocal cord paralysis has been invoked as the hallmark of a malignancy; however, in one study describing 10 cases of a thyroid nodule with vocal cord paralysis, 4 cases were due to a benign adenoma and in 6 cases a carcinoma was present.

In constrast to the clinical characteristics of the lesions present in the thyroid gland, the presence of enlarged lymph nodes is a very important indicator of malignancy. Delphian node involvement and involvement of the deep jugular lymph nodes are reliable signs of the presence of a malignancy. These phenomena may be even more important in children, in whom lymph node enlargement is frequently (75%) the first sign of a thyroid malignancy. The lymph nodes are described as having a firm feel on palpation and are usually movable, nontender, and mostly ~2 cm in size. The Delphian lymph node can also be enlarged in other thyroidal disorders such as Hashimoto's thyroiditis, Graves' disease, infections, and rarely amyloidosis.

The presence of a thyroid lesion combined with palpable lymph node enlargement is suggestive of a thyroid malignancy on a purely clinical basis. Since the clinical findings surrounding a thyroidal nodule are frequently not reliable in the distinction between a benign and a malignant lesion, a battery of tests have been developed to aid the internist in the differential diagnosis of a thyroid nodule.

DIAGNOSIS

Blood Tests

There is little doubt that thyroid function studies play a certain role in the evaluation of patients with a thyroid nodule. Indeed an elevated serum thyroxine (T_4) or triiodothyronine (T_3) level in a patient with a nodule of the thyroid gland could reflect the presence of a toxic adenoma, and as such the thyroidal lesion is not indicative of a malignancy. If such elevated serum T_4 and T_3 levels occurred in a patient with clear-cut Graves' disease and a coexisting solitary cold nodule in the gland, the benign nature of the lesion would still be in doubt. Except for toxic adenomas and the occurrence of hyperthyroidism in patients with a nodular goiter, thyroid function studies are of limited value in the distinction between a benign and a malignant nodule in the thyroid gland. The determination of serum thyroglobulin (Tg) itself has not played a role in distinguishing benign lesions from malignant lesions of the thyroid gland either. Indeed, a number of other benign conditions of the thyroid gland summarized in Table 2 are associated with elevated serum Tg levels. The use of Tg, however, has revolutionized the follow-up of patients with a differentiated thyroid gland in the postoperative period. The determination of anti-Tg antibodies or antimicrosomal antibodies levels has been of limited use in the distinction between benign and malignant lesions.

Serum thyrocalcitonin (TCT) was considered until recently an excellent marker in the diagnosis of medullary carcinoma of the thyroid, especially when measured during a stimulatory test (i.e., calcium infusion or pentagastrin stimulation) (Fig. 2). This initial enthusiasm has been somewhat

Table 2 **Serum Tg Levels in Normal Subjects and in Patients with Various Benign Pathologic Conditions of the Thyroid Gland**

Condition	*Serum Tg Level, Mean ± SEM (ng/ml)*	*No. of Subjects*
Control subjects (blood donors)	5.1 ± 0.49	95
Active Graves' disease	176.0 ± 30.0	33
Non-Graves' disease thyrotoxicosis[a]	145.0 ± 27.0	7
Subacute thyroiditis (acute phase)	136.8 ± 74.5	12
Thyroid adenoma	424.6 ± 189.4	27
Endemic goiter	208.1 ± 19.8	77

[a]Multinodular toxic goiter and toxic adenomas.

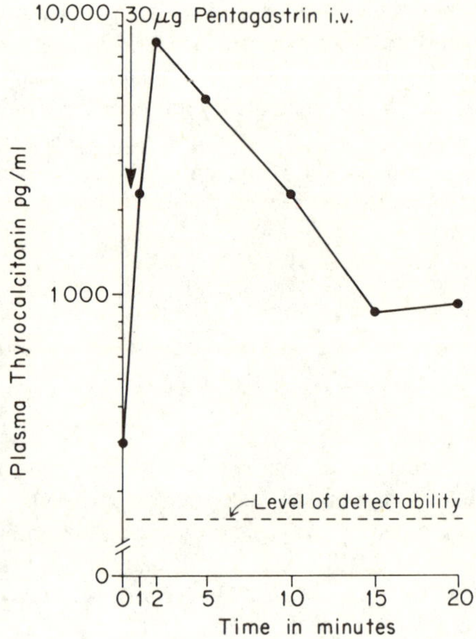

Figure 2. H.F. ♀ Medullary CA of the thyroid and pheochromocytoma. TCT stimulation. Injection of pentagastrin is responsible for the rise in TCT in the serum in this subject with multiple endocrine neoplasia type II.

dampened, since recent studies indicate that the TCT level can be elevated in subjects with nonthyroidal disorders. Indeed, Schwartz and co-workers recently indicated that elevated immunoreactive calcitonin was found in a number of patients with tumors other than medullary thyroid malignancies: lung (38%), colon (24%), breast (38%), pancreas (42%), and gastric carcinoma (30%). These findings indicate that calcitonin can no longer be regarded as an organ-specific tumor marker. Furthermore, of equal importance is the fact that an elevated calcitonin level is also observed in subjects with nontumor disorders, such as chronic obstructive pulmonary disease, renal failure, acute gastrointestinal bleeding, and granulomatous lung disease. Notwithstanding, TCT remains an excellent tumor marker in patients with medullary thyroid cancer, analogous to serum Tg measurements in patients with papillary and follicular tumors of the thyroid gland.

Roentgenogram Studies

Roentgenogram studies have been used to delineate the presence of calcifications within the thyroid gland. Shell-like calcifications usually reflect the presence of a benign lesion, and stippled calcifications caused by an aggregate of psammoma bodies usually reflect the presence of a malignancy. These findings, however, are not entirely specific, since exceptions occur for both roentgenogram findings. Angiography and lymphangiography have no place in the diagnosis of thyroid cancer. The use of a computerized axial tomography (CAT) scan for evaluation of the thyroid gland has not been explored but may be useful in assessing the relationship of a large goiter to the surrounding structures (Fig. 3).

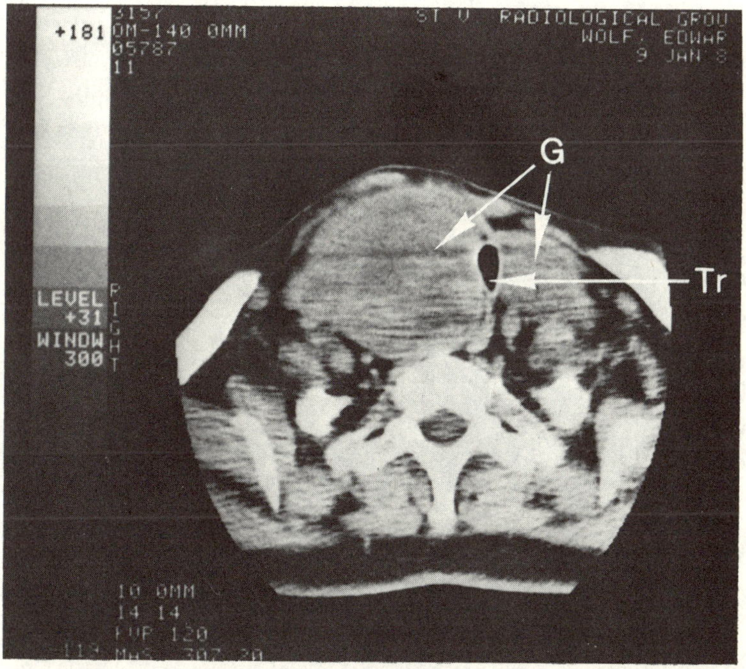

Figure 3. CAT scan of a multinodular thyroid gland. The study was performed with a third-generation scanner. The goiter leads to severe "drop"-like compression of the trachea. The usefulness of CAT scans in the evaluation of thyroid nodules has not been firmly established. G, Goiter; Tr, trachea.

Ultrasonography

Gray scale ultrasonography is now commonly used in the evaluation of thyroid nodules. The technique allows not only a precise measurement of the size of a lesion but also the distinction among cystic, solid, and mixed cystic-solid lesions. This factor is of some importance in the differential diagnosis of benign versus malignant lesions (Table 3). The data in Table 3 represent a review of 16 studies culled from the world literature, which analyzes the ultrasound results in a total of 1,166 subjects with thyroid nodules. About 20% of nodules are pure cysts. The data indicate that the incidence of malignancies in solid lesions was 21% and only 7% in cystic lesions. In mixed solid-cystic lesions the incidence of malignancy was 12%. The overall incidence of thyroid cancer in all the studies compiled was 17%.

Although the ultrasound technique can be used to reveal gross anatomy of the thyroid gland, it does not provide histopathologic information. There is no typical pattern for benign or malignant lesions. It is generally believed that cystic lesions are benign; however, if the lesion is >4 cm in diameter, a higher incidence of a malignancy can be expected. The information provided by ultrasonography is usually useful, for example, during pregnancy where additional testing by other techniques (isotopic scans) may not be desirable. Ultrasonography can also provide the multinodular characteristics of a thyroid lesion that is not always obvious on clinical examination alone. In multinodular goiters the incidence of thyroid malignancy has been reported

Table 3 **Ultrasonography of Thyroid Nodules: Comparison of Preoperative Ultrasonographic and Surgical Pathologic Findings**

Solid			*Mixed*			*Cystic*			*Total*		
No. of Cases	*No. Operated On*	*No. Malignant*	*No. of Cases*	*No. Operated On*	*No. Malignant*	*No. of Cases*	*No. Operated On*	*No. Malignant*	*No. of Cases*	*No. Operated On*	*No. Malignant*
807	734	151 (21%)[a]	138	124	15 (12%)[a]	221	151	10 (7%)[a]	1166	1009	176 (17%)[a]

Reprinted with permission of Ashcraft MW and Van Herle AJ, *Head Neck Surg* 3:216–230, 1981, and John Wiley & Sons, Inc.

[a]Represents percentages of malignancy found in operated cases only within this subcategory.

by some investigators to be lower than in cases with a single nodule, however, this has been seriously questioned.

Thyroid-Scanning Techniques

Various radioactive isotopes have been used to analyze thyroidal nodules. The development of different isotopes reflects the lack of satisfaction provided by the existing techniques. The visualization of nodules by various nuclides is based on trapping and/or organification of isotopes of iodine or technetium or the increased replication rate characteristic of tumors (^{131}I, cesium, and ^{67}Ga). Unfortunately, most of these techniques are nonspecific and consequently unreliable in the differentiation of benign and malignant nodules. The results of radioiodine scans and technetium scans of thyroid nodules are summarized in Table 4, which represents a compilation of a number of studies gathered from the world literature. It is clear from this table that the criteria presently used to refer patients to surgery (cold nodule with isotopes of iodine or hyperfunctioning lesions with ^{99m}Tc) are poor, since about 90% of nodules are cold. Indeed, based on these criteria roughly 70–80% of patients are referred to surgery for a benign lesion. In terms of morbidity and medical economics this is a high price to pay. Of note is the observation that hyperfunctioning lesions when visualized with ^{99m}Tc are more frequently malignant than cold lesions using the same isotope.

The question can now be raised whether or not other techniques have been developed with higher specificity and sensitivity. Recently ^{241}Am fluorescent scanning has been used for diagnostic purposes on a limited experimental basis (Table 5).

The technique is based on the characteristic roentgenogram recorded when gamma rays from ^{241}Am are directed at a given area of the thyroid gland, where they excite iodine. The intensity of the x-ray emission is directly proportional to the amount of stable iodine present in the gland or lesion. A lesion with a low iodine content produces a "light" area and is more likely to be malignant, while a lesion with a high iodine content appears "dark" and is most likely benign.

The limitation of the technique presently used is the specialized and costly equipment required and the less sensitive resolution of small thyroidal lesions (<1.5 cm). Apart from this, the technique seems to be promising and further exploration in this area is certainly warranted.

Thyroid Hormone Suppression

As early as 1894, Burns and co-workers described the excellent response to thyroid extract feeding in patients with diffuse goiter and the rather poor response in subjects with nodular goiters. The basic assumption in these observations is that thyroid-stimulating hormone (TSH, thyrotropin) initiates and promotes growth of thyroid nodules. The goal of thyroid hormone administration is then to suppress TSH release by giving suppressive doses of T_4 (usually 150–200 μg/day) and to follow the size of the thyroid nodule during the ensuing 3–6 months. Total or partial regression of the lesion has been considered a favorable result, and further growth has been considered an ominous sign. Neither of these criteria with regard to suppression is absolute, since on the one hand a number of lesions may grow under suppressive therapy, are not necessarily malignant, and can be due, for example, to bleeding in a cystic lesion; regression under suppression on the other hand is not necessarily an indication of the benign nature of the lesion, since it may reflect a response of extratumoral tissue to suppressive therapy. It is consequently not surprising that the data in the literature are extremely confusing and that results of suppressive therapy are uninterpretable because of the lack of adequate control studies. It is,

Table 4 **Results of Radioiodine or Technetium-99m Scans in Patients with Thyroid Nodules Subsequently Referred for Surgery**

Nonfunctioning			*Hypofunctioning or Normofunctioning*[a]			*Hyperfunctioning*			*Total*		
No. of Cases	*No. Operated On*	*No. Malignant*	*No. of Cases*	*No. Operated On*	*No. Malignant*	*No. of Cases*	*No. Operated On*	*No. Malignant*	*No. of Cases*	*No. Operated On*	*No. Malignant*
Isotopes of iodine[b]											
4,457	4,457	708 (16%)[c]	554	554	49 (9%)[c]	283	283	10 (4%)[c]	5,294	5,294	767 (14%)[c]
Technetium-99m											
176	176	38 (22%)[c]	47	47	6 (13%)[c]	21	21	6(29%)[c]	244	244	50 (20.5%)[c]

Reprinted with permission for Ashcraft MW and Van Herle AJ, *Head Neck Surg* 3:297–322, 1981, and John Wiley & Sons, Inc.

[a]In this column, for isotopes of iodine hypo- and normofunctioning lesions were combined, and for ^{99m}Tc only normofunctioning lesions were categorized.
[b]Studies with various isotopes of iodine were combined.
[c]Represents percentage of malignancy found within this subcategory.

Table 5 **Results of Americium-241 Fluorescent Scans in Patients with Thyroid Nodules Subsequently Referred for Surgery**[a]

Light		*Normal of Irregular*		*Dark*		*Total*	
No. of Cases	*Number Malignant*	*No. of Cases*	*Number Malignant*	*No. of Cases*	*Number Malignant*	*No. of Cases*	*Number Malignant*
113	45 (40%)[b]	93	0 (0%)[b]	26	0 (0%)[b]	232	45 (19%)[b]

Reprinted with permission for Ashcraft MW and Van Herle AJ, *Head Neck Surg.* 3:297–322, 1981, and John Wiley & Sons, Inc.

[a]This represents a summary of five studies.

[b]Percentage of malignancies within subcategory.

however, advisable to use suppressive therapy in subjects where surgery is for other reasons contraindicated. This therapy should be considered merely as a therapeutic trial and not as a functional test. One conclusion seems inescapable: The internist is left with a very poor armamentarium in sorting out the vast array of possible diagnostic possibilities.

Fine Needle Aspiration

This state of affairs changed, however, when in 1952 Söderstrom popularized the thyroid aspiration biopsy technique in Scandinavia. It is curious to observe that Martin and Ellis in the United States laid the groundwork for this technique in 1930. It was not until nearly a half-century after the latter publication and 25 years after the publication of Söderstrom that this technique was accepted on the North American continent. If one analyzes the data collected from the literature, the following conclusions are reached (see Table 6).

The incidence of false negative diagnoses obtained with fine needle aspiration (FNA) was 2.6%. The incidence of false positive diagnoses was only 1.5%. The total degree of reliability was consequently greater than 95%. In 51 of the subjects in which insufficient material was obtained for analysis no malignancies were found when all patients were operated upon. It is clear that this case finding method (FNA) is the only one with high specificity and sensitivity. The procedure has additional advantages—its lack of side effects and its cost-effectiveness. The procedure can be easily carried out by a trained internist in his or her office (Fig. 4) and by sending the specimens to a cytologist trained in the evaluation of thyroid aspirates. A number of academic centers in the country, as well as community hospitals, have such expertise available. A flow diagram integrating the various techniques utilized in the diagnosis of thyroid nodules is provided in Table 7.

TREATMENT

Surgical Approach

The indications for removal of a thyroid nodule are fourfold: the malignant nature of a lesion, compression phenomena, associated thyrotoxicosis, and cosmesis. Surgery, however, is imperative when the thyroid nodule is malignant. The type of surgery performed for a thyroid nodule ranges from a simple nodulectomy (a procedure hardly recommended when a malignancy

Table 6 **Results of Needle Aspirations for Cytologic Processing**[a]

Benign			*Malignant or Suspicious*				*Insufficient Material*			*Total*		
No. of Cases	*No. Operated On*	*No. False Negative*[b]	*No. of Cases*	*No. Operated On*	*No. Found Malignant at Surgery*	*No. False Positive*	*No. of Cases*	*No. Operated On*	*No. Found Malignant at Surgery*	*No. of Cases*	*No. Operated On*	*No. Found Malignant at Surgery*
848	848	22 (2.6%)[c]	482	482	246	7 (1.5%)[d]	51	51	0 (0%)	1381	1381	268 (19.4%)[c]

[a]Includes biopsy of solitary and multinodular goiters.
[b]Found to be malignant at surgery.
[c]Represents percentage of malignancy found in operated cases within this subcategory.
[d]Represents percentage of benign tumors found in operated cases within this subcategory.

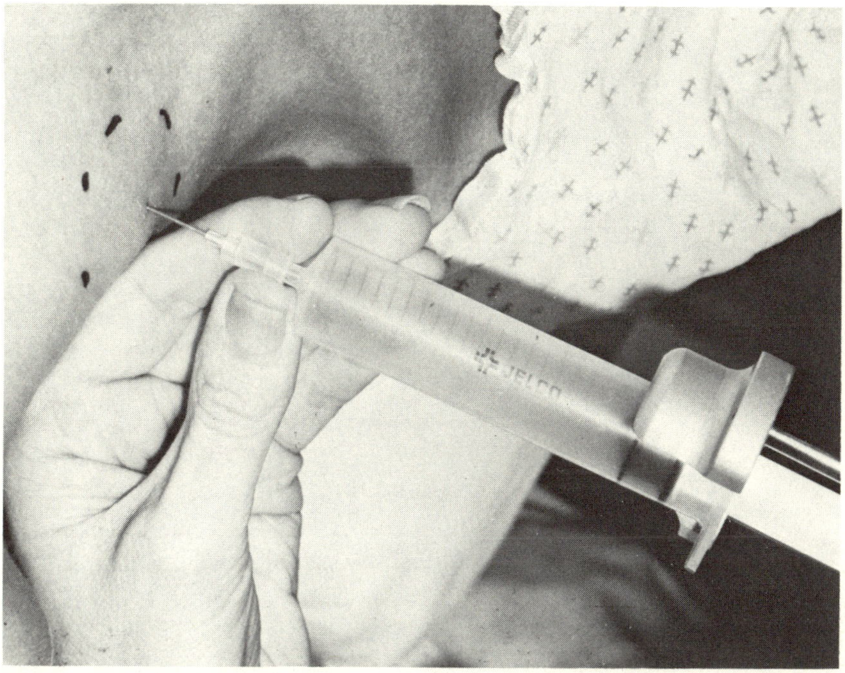

Figure 4. Thyroid aspiration biopsy. A 23-gauge needle is introduced into the nodule. The 20-ml syringe fits into a special holder, which permits fixation of the lesion with one hand and aspiration with the other. The procedure is carried out without anesthesia.

is present) to total thyroidectomy with radical neck dissection, a technique rarely applied these days. Several arguments can be brought forward in favor of near-total thyroidectomy when a malignancy is known to be present. These data are summarized in Table 8.

It is clear that only general guidelines can be provided in terms of the surgical approach, since the surgical modalities are sometimes tailored by the surgeon during the operation. A few guidelines can be summarized as follows:

1. If the nodule is located in a thyroid lobe, a thyroid lobectomy should be performed and an isthmectomy on the side of the nodule. If a frozen section is benign, no further resection is indicated; if it is malignant, near-total thyroidectomy or total thyroidectomy is indicated.
2. If the nodule is located in the isthmus, resection of the nodule and removal of the anterior one-third of each lobe are indicated. If the frozen section is benign, no further surgery is indicated; if it is malignant, a near-total thyroidectomy or total thyroidectomy is indicated.
3. Modified neck dissections are recommended for medullary carcinoma of the thyroid. Prophylactic modified neck dissections are not recommended for papillary or follicular cancer.

The complications of radical surgery should also be kept in mind, such as hypoparathyroidism, laryngeal nerve palsy, and the morbidity and mortality associated with all surgical procedures.

Table 7 **Flow Diagram for the Evaluation and Therapy of the Most Common Lesion Presenting as a Single Thyroid Nodule**

Result of FNA			*Therapy*
Malignant or suspicious →			Surgery[a]
Insufficient material for diagnosis →			Repeat FNA
Benign lesion →	Colloid goiter, Hashimoto's thyroiditis, Cyst →		T_4 administration[b]
	Subacute thyroiditis →		Observation
Follicular neoplasm →	Thyroid scan and ^{123}I uptake	Hot (patient thyrotoxic) →	^{131}I or surgery
		Hot (patient euthyroid) →	Observation
		Normo- or hypofunctioning →	Surgery

[a]Surgery may not be indicated in the case of an anaplastic carcinoma.
[b]The dose of T_4 given depends on the disease state. The purpose is usually to prevent further cysts, nodules, or goiter formation. If compressive symptoms have developed surgery may be indicated.

Table 8 **Factors Favoring a Total Thyroidectomy in a Recognized Case of Thyroid Malignancy**

In subjects with thyroid cancer more than 70% have intra- and/or extrathyroidal spread of the tumor at the time of surgery
Approximately 7–10% of the patients develop recurrent clinical cancer in the lobe left behind
The degeneration of differentiated tumors to undifferentiated anaplastic carcinoma has been documented and provides further impetus for advocating total removal of the thyroid gland
Follow-up studies with radioactive iodine scanning and serum Tg levels become feasible only after total thyroidectomy

POSTOPERATIVE MANAGEMENT

Benign Nodules

In the postoperative period, T_4 is frequently administered (150 μg/day). This therapy is given in the hope of preventing further nodule or goiter formation in the remainder of the thyroid gland. A yearly follow-up examination is usually recommended.

Cancer

In the postoperative period radioactive iodine is usually used to further ablate residual or metastatic disease. The rationale for such therapy in patients with differentiated thyroid tumors who concentrate ^{131}I has been more clearly defined by the studies of Varma and co-workers and more recently Mazzaferri and co-workers. These studies indicated that ^{131}I therapy, in addition to surgery, in patients with thyroid cancer over the age of 40 significantly lowered the death rate when compared with subjects undergoing surgery alone. Mazzaferri et al. confirmed these data recently by indicating that patients treated with ^{131}I for papillary carcinoma of the thyroid had a better survival rate than those not treated with this isotope. The procedure can be summarized as follows.

Following thyroidectomy for thyroid cancer of the papillary or follicular type, the patient is given L-triiodothyronine, 25 μg orally 3 times a day, for a period of up to 2 months, when there is full recovery from the surgical procedure. At that time the patient's T_3 administration is discontinued for 2 weeks and a tracer dose (100–250 μCi) of ^{123}I is then given. If residual thyroid tissue is found in the patient's neck area, an ablative dose of ^{131}I (range 30–100 mCi) is given, and thyroid hormone therapy is resumed with 0.15–0.2 mg L-thyroxine daily.

Serum Tg levels should be obtained at regular intervals, since this represents an extremely useful marker in the establishment of residual or metastatic disease, especially if total thyroid ablation as been performed. A recent study by Ashcraft and Van Herle provides the reader with a flow diagram (Fig. 5) representing a guide to ordering Tg levels as well as ^{131}I total body scans. If during physical examinations in the ensuing years lymph nodes enlarge and it can be established by FNA biopsy that these are indeed due to metastatic disease, that is, not due to infection, one should perform a modified radical neck dissection. If no lymph nodes are palpable but if an ^{131}I scan is positive, further treatment with ^{131}I is recommended. The recommended dose varies from 30 to 150 mCi. External radiation is less effective in treating metastatic disease

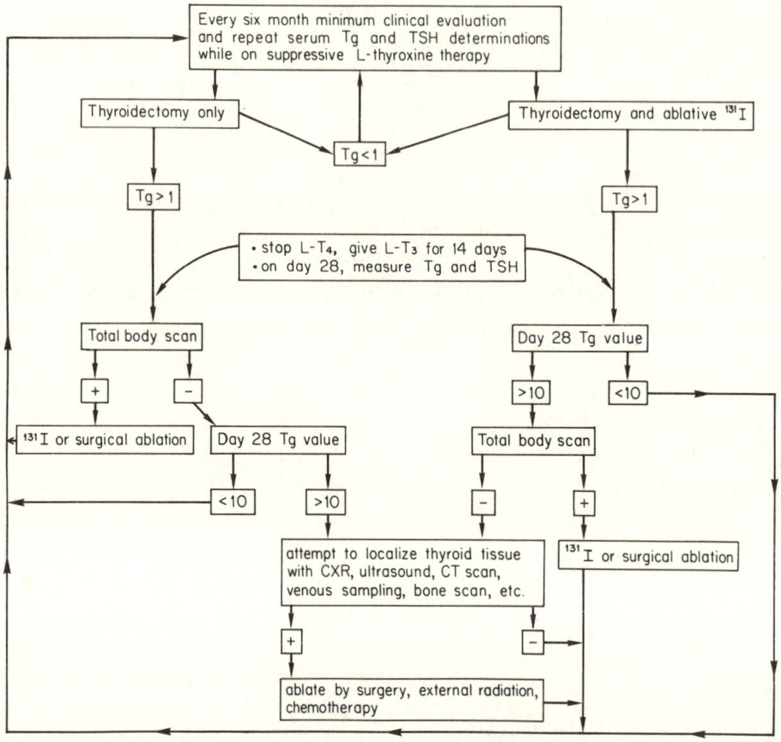

Figure 5. Clinical strategy for follow-up. Study of patients with treated, well-differentiated thyroid cancer, with no antithyroglobulin antibodies in serum. Tg values are expressed in nanograms per milliliter. Reproduced by permission of Ashcraft MW, Van Herle AJ, *Am J Med* 71:806–814, 1981. Copyright Technical Publishing Company.

of the lymph nodes. External supervoltage irradiation, however, can be used for treating invasive thyroid cancer left behind in the thyroid bed (4,500–5,000 rads given over 4.5–5 weeks) or to treat metastatic disease of bones (3,500–4,500 rads in 3–4.5 weeks).

Administration of thyroid hormone is needed in the postoperative care of all patients with thyroid cancer. First, because operative procedures intended to remove the thyroid gland leave the patient invariably athyreotic. Second, thyroid tumors have been shown to contain TSH receptors which may mediate growth; thyroid hormone should therefore be given to suppress endogenous TSH levels. In the follow-up of these patients serum TSH as well as Tg measurements should periodically be obtained to assess whether the thyroid hormone dose is sufficient to suppress TSH to undetectable levels (<1.0 μU/ml) and whether serum Tg levels are also undetectable (<1.0 ng/ml). The lowest dose of thyroid hormone that completely inhibits serum TSH levels in response to TRH administration should be used. A dose between 150 and 200 μg/day of L-thyroxine is usually sufficient to achieve this goal.

Chemotherapy has not gained a major place in the treatment of patients with thyroid cancer. Adriamycin has been used by Gottlieb and Hill. Patients selected for this study had recurrent disease and widespread metastases no longer responsive to radiotherapeutic or surgical approaches. Partial remissions were observed for all histologic types of tumor. The cumulative dose of the drug was limited to 550 mg/m^2 because of the cardiac toxicity associated with higher doses.

PROGNOSIS

Thyroid cancer is more lethal than is generally accepted. Indeed, 19% of 554 patients treated by Ibanez and co-workers died of their disease, and these data are consistent with the findings accumulated by Woolner and coinvestigators who found a mortality rate of 22.2% in a 10-year follow-up study of 333 patients with papillary, follicular, and medullary carcinoma. More recently Konrad and Canalis reported on data accumulated between 1955 and 1977 at UCLA. In this study 452 patients with benign thyroid neoplasms were identified, and 208 with malignant thyroid neoplasms (2 : 1). Of the latter, 43 patients died of their disease. When the anaplastic carcinomas were excluded, 15% died of differentiated thyroid cancer—a figure close to the previously mentioned 19% reported by Ibanez and co-workers and the 22.2% reported by Woolner and co-workers. Anaplastic carcinoma of the thyroid is a lethal disorder because of its extensive local invasion and dissemination.

As far as the influence of sex on survival is concerned, female patients in the study reported by Konrad and Canalis had an average survival of 12.3 years. Males, however, had a survival of only 6.4 years, the difference being of borderline significance. It is clear from studies carried out by Woolner et al. that in differentiated thyroid cancer survival is better if extrathyroidal spreading has not occurred. It is our hope that early detection of thyroid malignancies will influence the future death rate of patients harboring such tumors, especially in subjects 40 years or older, in whom papillary follicular tumors carry a poor prognosis.

DISCUSSION CASES

Case 1

Description

A 30-year-old man consults his internist because of possible exposure to viral hepatitis. His physican discovers on routine examination a 2 × 3 cm nodule in the lower part of the right lobe of the thyroid, which is nonfunctioning on ^{123}I scanning. No adenopathy is present. The patient has no history of previous irradiation to the neck, tonsils, or chest. The thyroid function studies are normal. A thyroid aspiration biopsy is performed which contained insufficient material for diagnosis. The patient is on a course of T_4 suppression (200 μg daily for 6 months), which results in partial regression of the lesion.

Question

1. What do you recommend now?
   (a) Repeat the ^{123}I scan.
   (b) Perform a TRH test.
   (c) Repeat the aspiration biopsy of the thyroid.

Answers

(a) Repetition of the ^{123}I scan would add nothing to the assessment of this nodule and should not be done.

(b) A TRH study while the patient is on T_4 would give an answer concerning the adequacy of the T_4 dose administered to the patient but diagnostically it would be fruitless.

(c) Since the first biopsy yielded insufficient material, a second FNA is indicated.

Description

At the end of 6 months of suppression an intravenous TRH test is performed and no TSH response following TRH is observed. Because of the partial regression of the lesion, a FNA biopsy is performed. The cytologist reports: "positive for malignant cells consistent with papillary carcinoma." A total thyroidectomy is performed. A well-differentiated papillary carcinoma of the thyroid is found on pathologic section. The left lobe of the thyroid reveals no changes, and a right paratracheal lymph node reveals metastatic disease.

Question

2. Which of the following statements are correct with respect to diagnosis and treatment of papillary thyroid carcinoma?

(a) Papillary cancers can easily be diagnosed by FNA biopsy.

(b) Serum Tg levels are useful in monitoring such patients after total thyroidectomy and ablation.

Answer

(a) This is correct.

(b) Tg levels are indeed useful in monitoring these patients.

Case 2

Description

A 19-year-old construction worker underwent a total thyroidectomy for papillary carcinoma of the thyroid which had metastasized to the cervical lymph nodes. Postoperatively, an ablative dose of ^{131}I (50 mCi) was administered, and the patient was placed on suppressive doses of thyroid hormone and lost for follow-up.

Three years after the intervention the patient noted the development of a few firm lymph nodes in the cervical area, which he attributed to a tooth infection. One year later, he consulted his physician who advised a tooth extraction, which did not lead to resolution of the lymph nodes. Thyroid hormone therapy was then discontinued for 6 weeks and a total body ^{131}I scan was performed. No tracer activity was observed in the neck area or, for that matter, elsewhere in the body.

Question

1. Which of the following test(s) would you now order to pursue his problem further?

(a) Serum calcitonin measurement.

(b) Ultrasound study of the neck area.

(c) Serum Tg level measurement.

Answer

1. (a) Serum TCT measurements are not useful in papillary cancer of the thyroid, since they are normal.

(b) An ultrasound examination of the neck could detect whether the deeper cervical lymph nodes were involved, which may represent tumor spread. Ultrasound would not yield a pathologic diagnosis.

(c) Serum Tg measurement is the test of choice, since Tg levels can be elevated in the absence of ^{131}I uptake. The elevated Tg levels usually reflect metastatic disease.

Question

2. If evidence for recurrence of the tumor was overwhelming, which one of the following therapeutic modalities would you now select?

(a) External radiation to the cervical area.
(b) ^{131}I therapy with ablative doses.
(c) Modified radical neck dissection.
(d) An increase in the T_4 dose from 0.2 mg q.d. to 0.3 mg q.d.

Answer

2. (a) External radiation to the neck area is not the first modality of therapy utilized.

(b) ^{131}I treatment is not in order, since no uptake of tracer occurred.

(c) Modified radical neck dissection is probably the treatment of choice in the presence of elevated Tg levels and enlarged lymph nodes.

(d) Increasing the dose of T_4 further would only lead to thyrotoxicosis and is not advisable.

SUGGESTED READING

Ashcraft MW, Van Herle AJ: Management of thyroid nodules. I and II. *Head Neck Surg* 3:216–277 and 298–325, 1981.

Ashcraft MW, Van Herle AJ: The comparative value of serum thyroglobulin measurements and iodine 131 total body scans in the follow-up study of patients with treated differentiated thyroid cancer. *AM J Med* 71:806–814, 1981.

Favus MH, Schneider AB, Stachura ME, et al: Thyroid cancer occurring as a later consequence of head-and-neck irradiation: Evaluation of 1056 patients. *N Engl J Med* 294:1019–1025, 1976.

Gottlieb JA, Hill CS Jr: Chemotherapy of thyroid cancer with adriamycin: Experience with 30 patients. *N Engl J Med* 290:193–197, 1974.

Hoffer PB, Gottschalk A: Fluorescent thyroid scanning: Scanning without radioisotopes. *Nucl Med* 99:117–123, 1971.

Ibanez ML, Russell WO, Albores-Savedra J, et al: Thyroid carcinoma, biological behavior and mortality. *Cancer* 19:1039–1053, 1966.

Young RL, Mazzaferri EL, Rahe AJ, Dorfman SG: Pure follicular thyroid carcinoma: Impact of therapy in 214 patients. *J Nucl Med* 21:733–737, 1980.

Konrad HR, Canalis RF: Lethal thyroid carcinoma. *Arch Otolaryngol* 104:454–455, 1978.

Martin HE, Ellis EB: Biopsy by needle puncture and aspiration. *Ann Surg* 92:169–181, 1930.

Mazzaferri EL, Young RL, Oertel JE, et al: Papillary thyroid carcinoma: The impact of therapy in 576 patients. *Medicine* 56:171–596, 1977.

Melvin KEW, Tashjian AJ Jr, Miller HH: Studies in familial (medullary) thyroid carcinoma. *Recent Prog Horm Res* 28:399, 1972. Astwood EG (ed): *Proceedings of the Laurentian Hormone Conference*. New York, Academic Press, 1971.

Schwartz KE, Wolfsen AR, Forster B, et al: Calcitonin in nonthyroidal cancer. *J Clin Endocrinol Metab* 49:438–444, 1979.

Söderstrom N: Puncture of goiters for aspiration biopsy. *Acta Med Scand* 144:237–244, 1952.

Tunbridge WMG, Evered DC, Hall R. et al. The spectrum of thyroid disease in a community: the Whickham survey. *Clin Endocrinol* 7:481–493, 1977.

Vander JB, Gaston EA, Dawber TR. The significance of nontoxic thyroid nodules. *Ann Intern Med* 69: 537–540, 1968.

Van Herle AJ, Uller RP: Thyroid cancer classification, clinical features, diagnosis and therapy. *Pharmacol Ther* 2:215–238, 1977.

Van Herle AJ: Pathophysiology of thyroid cancer, in Greenfield LD (ed): *Thyroid Cancer*. Boca Raton, Fla., CRC Press 1978, pp. 23–36.

Van Herle AJ, Vassart G, Dumont JE: Control of thyroglobulin synthesis and secretion. I. *N Engl J Med* 301:239–249, 1979.

Van Herle AJ, Vassart G, Dumont JE: Control of thyroglobulin synthesis and secretion. II. *N Engl J Med* 301:307–314, 1979.

Van Herle AJ, Rich P, Ljung B-ME, et al: The thyroid nodule. *Ann Intern Med* 96:221–232, 1982.

Varma VM, Beierwaltes WH, Nofal MM, et al: Treatment of thyroid cancer: Death rates after surgery and after surgery followed by sodium iodide I^{131}. *J Am Med Assoc* 214:1437–1442, 1970.

Woolner LB, Beahrs OH, Black BM, et al: Classification and prognosis of thyroid carcinoma: A study of 885 cases observed in a thirty year period. *Am J Surg* 102:354–378, 1961.

6

HAROLD E. CARLSON
ARNOLD S. BRICKMAN

Hypercalcemia and Hypocalcemia

HYPERCALCEMIA

Calcium ion is required for the normal functioning of many organs in the body, and the circulating concentration of calcium in the serum is therefore normally kept within rather narrow limits. In most laboratories, the normal range for total serum calcium is 9.0–10.5 mg/dl. Since this range is usually defined as including 95% of normal subjects, by definition 2.5% of determinations in normal subjects will exceed 10.5 mg/dl; however, on repeat testing, further measurements in these subjects will fall within the normal range. Serum calcium values *persistently* above 10.5 mg/dl are abnormal and require further consideration. (In some laboratories, careful analysis of normal subjects has narrowed the normal range to 9.0–10.2 mg/dl.)

About 35–40% of the total serum calcium is bound to serum proteins (mainly albumin), 5–15% is complexed with other anions (citrate, sulfate, phosphate), and 50% is free or ionized. It is this free or ionized fraction that is biologically active and is sensed and regulated by the body's homeostatic mechanisms. Major changes in serum albumin can therefore alter the total serum calcium level. For every 1-g/dl increase or decrease in serum albumin from the normal mean of 4.0 g/dl, the total serum calcium level should increase or decrease by about 0.8 mg/dl. In practice, this correction factor is useful primarily in evaluating serum calcium levels in patients with hypoalbuminemia and is usually not applied for patients with mildly increased serum albumin concentrations. Ionized calcium may be measured directly, using calcium-sensitive electrodes, in difficult situations; ultrafiltrable calcium, which includes both ionized and complexed calcium, may also be assessed.

When to Measure the Serum Calcium Level

Nowadays serum calcium is measured in many patients as part of a biochemical profile or panel of tests performed as part of a screening evaluation. In instances when the determination of serum calcium levels must be specifically requested, one should obtain a measurement in the following circumstances:

1. Known malignancy.
2. Signs or symptoms of hypercalcemia (see Table 1).
3. Other diseases that may *cause* hypercalcemia (see Table 2).
4. Other conditions known to be associated with or due to hyperparathyroidism (see Table 3).
5. Multiple endocrine neoplasia (see Chapter 17).

Signs and Symptoms of Hypercalcemia

Hypercalcemia per se may produce a variety of signs and symptoms, some of which are life threatening (Table 1). In general, greater elevations of the serum calcium level produce more severe features, although a rapid increase in the serum calcium level may evoke more symptoms than a slow, gradual rise. In addition, one of the common causes of hypercalcemia, primary hyperparathyroidism, may produce additional features which may be due to elevated serum parathyroid hormone (PTH) rather then hypercalcemia (Table 3).

Causes of Hypercalcemia

A rather large number of medical conditions may cause hypercalcemia; these are listed in Table 2, along with the postulated mechanism of development of hypercalcemia, if known. Three of the more common conditions are discussed in greater detail below.

Hyperparathyroidism

Primary hyperparathyroidism may occur in up to 0.1% of the general population. Although most cases are sporadic, familial hyperparathyroidism has been well described both as a separate entity and as part of multiple endocrine neoplasia syndromes (Chapter 17). Although it has been recognized for several years that radiation to the head and neck during childhood (for treatment of tonsillitis, acne, enlarged thymus) leads to a high incidence of thyroid nodules and cancer, it has recently been shown also to lead to an increased incidence of hyperparathyroidism.

The disorder is protean in its manifestations; some of the features of primary hyperparathyroidism are due to hypercalcemia (Table 1), while others may represent a more direct effect of PTH. Table 3 lists some of the features unique to hyperparathyroidism. In recent years, more

Table 1 **Symptoms and Signs of Hypercalcemia**

Neuropsychiatric	Headache, mood depression, psychosis, poor concentration, lethargy, confusion, obtundation, coma
Eyes	Gritty or sandy sensation, calcium deposition in cornea (band keratopathy) or conjunctivae
Musculoskeletal	Fatigue, weakness, hyporeflexia
Cardiovascular	Hypertension, arrhythmias
Gastrointestinal	Anorexia, nausea, vomiting, constipation, abdominal pain, peptic ulcer, pancreatitis
Urinary	Polyuria, nephrolithiasis, nephrocalcinosis, renal failure

Table 2 **Causes of Hypercalcemia**

Primary hyperparathyroidism—excessive PTH
- Adenoma (80–85%), hyperplasia (10–15%), or carcinoma (2–3%)

Familial hypocalciuric hypercalcemia

Cancer-related
- Skeletal metastases—local osteolysis
- Hematologic malignancies—production of osteoclast-activating factor
- Humorally-mediated—PTH, prostaglandins, other substances?

Endocrine disorders
- Hyperthyroidism—increased bone resorption
- Hypothyroidism—slow clearance of dietary calcium loads?
- Adrenal insufficiency—hemoconcentration, increased calcium binding to serum proteins and anions
- Pheochromocytoma—humoral substance secreted from tumor

Drugs
- Vitamin A intoxication—increased bone resorption?
- Vitamin D intoxication—increased absorption of dietary calcium
- Thiazide diuretics—enhanced effects of PTH on kidney and bone
- Lithium—unmasks primary hyperparathyroidism?
- Milk-alkali syndrome—increased absorption of calcium from gut

Granulomas—enhanced sensitivity to vitamin D
- Sarcoidosis
- Tuberculosis
- Coccidioidomycosis
- Histoplasmosis
- Berylliosis

Idiopathic infantile hypercalcemia—hypersensitivity to vitamin D?

Renal failure—dialysis, posttransplant, recovery phase of acute renal failure

Immobilization in states of rapid bone turnover (e.g., Paget's disease)—relative increase in bone resorption relative to bone formation.

Increased serum proteins—normal ionized calcium
- Hemoconcentration
- Calcium binding to myeloma paraprotein (rare)

Table 3 **Features of Primary Hyperparathyroidism**

Hypercalcemia and its effects (Table 1)

Hematologic—anemia, due to marrow fibrosis and/or possible toxic effects of PTH on erythropoiesis

Skeletal—bone pain, osteopenia, subperiosteal reabsorption, pathologic fractures, bone cysts, loose teeth, due to PTH-mediated bone resorption

Neuromuscular—paresthesias, neurogenic proximal muscle weakness and atrophy, possibly due to toxic effect of PTH

Rheumatologic—gout, pseudogout, chondrocalcinosis, arthralgias and more patients with essentially asymptomatic, mild disease have come to medical attention, largely as a result of routine screening measurements of the serum calcium level. Currently, 40–50% of patients operated on for primary hyperparathyroidism are asymptomatic. The disease is chronic, with apparently only slow progression in most patients. Indeed, documentation of hypercalcemia over a period of a year or more in a healthy subject almost guarantees a diagnosis of primary hyperparathyroidism.

Hypercalcemia in primary hyperparathyroidism is the consequence of a number of factors including enhanced gut absorption of dietary calcium (as a result of stimulation of 1,25-dihydroxyvitamin D_3 production by PTH), enhanced renal tubular reabsorption of filtered calcium mediated by PTH, and liberation of calcium from bone by enhanced PTH-induced osteoclastic activity.

Familial Hypocalciuric Hypercalcemia

A small fraction (1%) of patients with suspected primary hyperparathyroidism have been found to have instead a disorder known as familial hypocalciuric hypocalcemia. This condition is characterized by hypercalcemia, mild hypermagnesemia, and normal or slightly elevated serum PTH levels (as in primary hyperparathyroidism) but is distinguished from the latter condition by the presence of hypocalciuria rather than hypercalciuria and by the general absence of the renal complications of hypercalcemia (stones, renal failure), hence its alternate name of familial benign hypercalcemia. Urinary cyclic AMP (cAMP) levels tend to parallel those of PTH and are normal or only slightly elevated. In most families, the condition is inherited in an autosomal dominant pattern. The importance of recognizing this condition lies in its relatively benign course and the lack of response to subtotal ($3\frac{1}{2}$ gland) parathyroidectomy.

Hypercalcemia of Malignancy

Several mechanisms underlie the development of hypercalcemia in patients with cancer. First, metastatic deposits in bone have a direct osteolytic effect, partly as a result of tumor-secreted prostaglandins which activate osteoclasts. Second, occasional tumors may produce hypercalcemic hormones; this is most often seen with hypernephroma, hepatoma, and squamous cell tumors originating in the lung, head, neck, esophagus, or urogenital tract. Contrary to initial reports, it now appears that only a few of these instances represent true "ectopic" PTH secretion; rather, other as yet unidentified substances with some PTH-like actions are produced. In some cases hypercalcemia has developed in patients with tumors that produce excessive amounts of specific prostaglandins. The latter appear to stimulate bone resorption by activation of osteoclastic activity. Finally, hematologic malignancies involving the bone marrow (myeloma, leukemias, lymphomas) may produce a substance called osteoclast-activating factor which acts locally to promote bone resorption.

Differential Diagnosis

In a given patient with newly discovered, persistent hypercalcemia, many of the entities listed in Table 2 may be excluded from further consideration on the basis of history and physical examination (e.g., vitamin A or D intoxication, thiazide use, hyperthyroidism, postrenal transplant). In most instances, the ultimate differentiation is between primary hyperparathyroidism and malignancy. Several surveys have shown that, among generally healthy outpatients, the vast majority of hypercalcemic subjects have primary hyperparathyroidism. Conversely, among hospital inpatients, true hypercalcemia is most often due to a malignancy, usually one that is readily diagnosed. Nevertheless, we are still faced with the problem of diagnosis in each individual patient. Several tests have been proposed to more clearly distinguish hyperparathyroid patients from those with cancer.

1. Serum chloride, phosphorus, and the chloride/phosphorus ratio: In general, patients with primary hyperparathyroidism manifest mild hypophosphatemia due to urinary phosphate loss and mild hyperchloremia, reflecting a metabolic acidosis due to PTH-induced bicarbonaturia; together these lead to an elevated serum chloride/phosphorus ratio (>33). However, there is some overlap between the two groups with each of these parameters, and the measurement is not useful in the differential diagnosis.
2. Serum PTH levels: Depending on the laboratory, the serum PTH level is elevated in 30–80% of patients with primary hyperparathyroidism and in 0–95% of those with hypercalcemia due to malignancy. These differences probably reflect the interaction of different radioimmunoassay antibodies with the multiple, heterogeneous forms of circulating PTH. To interpret the results of PTH assays meaningfully, it is essential that the practitioner be familiar with the detection characteristics of the assay used.
3. Nephrogenous cAMP: Initial reports claimed that all patients with elevated urinary nephrogenous cAMP had PTH-mediated hypercalcemia, presumably due to primary hyperparathyroidism. Subsequent series, however, demonstrate that many patients with hypercalcemia of malignancy have elevated nephrogenous cAMP levels, apparently because of stimulation of renal adenylate cyclase by factors other than PTH. Thus this test is apparently of little use in distinguishing primary hyperparathyroidism from cancer.

Recommendations for Investigation of Hypercalcemia

Patients with signs or symptoms suggestive of cancer or other diseases should, of course, receive appropriate investigations directed at the likely sites of pathology. In apparently healthy patients, it is useful to perform a limited screening examination to exclude common occult malignancies and familial hypocaliuric hypercalcemia; one such protocol includes:

1. Determination of serum PTH and serum calcium levels simultaneously.
2. Determination of serum phosphorus and alkaline phosphatase levels.
3. Serum protein electrophoresis.
4. Chest roentgenogram.
5. Abdominal roentgenogram or intravenous pyelogram.
6. Complete blood count.
7. Urinalysis.
8. Twenty-four-hour urine collection for calcium and creatinine levels.

A patient with hypercalcemia, a high-normal or elevated serum PTH, a urinary calcium level of over 200 mg/day, and normal results on the other tests probably has hyperparathyroidism and can be considered for surgery or other therapy. Routine radiographs of the hands and skull are usually positive only in rather advanced, obvious cases of hyperparathyroidism (<5–10% of cases) and thus add little useful information.

Treatment of Hypercalcemia

The treatment of hypercalcemia can be considered in two phases: acute management of severe hypercalcemia, and treatment of chronic, milder elevations in serum calcium levels.

Patients with signs and symptoms of severe hypercalcemia (obtundation, arrhythmia, dehydration, rapidly progressive renal failure) or any patient with a serum calcium level over 13 or 14 mg/dl should receive immediate therapy to lower the serum calcium level to a more nearly normal value.

1. In patients with normal renal function, the most useful measure is rehydration with intravenous saline followed by treatment with furosemide to induce a brisk diuresis (6–12 liters/day), replacing fluid and potassium intravenously. This usually results in a lowering of the serum calcium concentration within 12–24 hours. Unfortunately, the massive diuresis is uncomfortable for the patient; this treatment is therefore only a temporary measure until more definitive therapy can be applied. Moreover, careful monitoring of the fluid and electrolyte status and cardiovascular function is required when this therapy is carried out in a vigorous manner.

Certain other measures, alone or in combination, can be tried if diuresis fails; these may also be used for longer periods of time, if necessary:

2. Large doses of salmon calcitonin (4–8 MRC units/kg s.c., i.m., or i.v. one to four times a day) are beneficial in many subjects.
3. Mithramycin, an antitumor antibiotic, usually produces a fall in serum calcium levels within 24 hours, often lasting several days. In doses of 25 μg/kg, the drug reversibly poisons osteoclasts, diminishing bone resorption. Bone marrow (thrombocytopenia), renal, and hepatic toxicity may occur as a function of dose and duration of treatment as well as idiosyncratic reactions.
4. In pharmacologic doses (40–80 mg prednisone/day), glucocorticoids given in specific clinical settings have a beneficial effect on hypercalcemia. These disorders include multiple myeloma, sarcoidosis, vitamin D intoxication, and some cancers metastatic to bone. Corticosteroids appear to prolong the action of calcitonin in the treatment of hypercalcemia due to malignancy.
5. A 3-day trial of indomethacin, 50 mg orally three times a day, may be worthwhile if a prostaglandin-producing malignancy is a possible cause of the hypercalcemia.
6. With oral doses of 2–3 g of elemental phosphorus daily, serum calcium levels will be lowered 1–2 mg/dl. Because of the dangers of soft tissue calcification, parenteral administration of phosphate should be used only by those experienced in its effects. Neither oral nor parenteral phosphate therapy should be employed in individuals with significant renal insufficiency.
7. Propranolol (Inderal) 160–320 mg/day is sometimes useful in treating hypercalcemia due to primary hyperparathyroidism or hyperthyroidism; cimetidine has been used with some success in treating primary hyperparathyroidism, apparently by suppressing PTH secretion; intravenous dichlorodimethyl phosphonate has been used to lower the serum calcium level but the drug has recently been withdrawn because of toxicity. However, all three of these forms of therapy should currently be regarded as experimental.

Management of chronic hypercalcemia involves:

1. Control of underlying diseases (e.g., hyperthyroidism, cancer).
2. Avoidance of immobilization.
3. Withdrawal of offending or aggravating drugs (vitamin D, thiazides, etc.).
4. Surgical treatment of primary hyperparathyroidism.
5. Medical management with oral phosphate.
6. Observation with no specific therapy.

The question often arises, Should all patients with primary hyperparathyroidism be subjected to neck exploration? This question is still unanswered, since we do not yet know the complete natural history of untreated disease. An ongoing study at the Mayo Clinic has found that about 19% of 112 otherwise healthy patients with mild primary hyperparathyroidism (serum calcium level <11 mg/dl) required surgery during a 5-year follow-up; of these, 5% developed new complications of the hyperparathyroidism (renal failure, bone disease), 2% had a rise in the serum calcium level to over 11 mg/dl; 7% underwent surgery for unspecified reasons, and 5% were operated on at the patient's or physician's request. Thus it appears that patients with mild hyperparathyroidism may be followed without surgical intervention *if* they are willing to return for frequent follow-up examinations every 3–6 months. Chronic oral phosphate treatment is another option that needs further study; however, although the serum calcium level may be decreased, renal function theroretically may be worsened by phosphate therapy, suggesting that its use possibly should be restricted to patients for whom there is no other recourse.

Ancillary Diagnostic Measures in Primary Hyperparathyroidism

About 80–85% of patients with primary hyperparathyroidism have a single parathyroid adenoma as the cause of their hypercalcemia; a few have two adenomas, a few have parathyroid carcinoma, and 10–20% have diffuse hyperplasia. If possible, it would be useful to distinguish among these entities preoperatively and localize adenomas to guide the surgeon. Most parathyroid adenomas are small and consequently impalpable; some success has been claimed for ultrasound examinations and computerized axial tomography (CAT) scanning in detecting parathyroid adenomas, but the procedures are most accurate for the larger adenomas readily found by the surgeon. Selective catheterization of parathyroid venous drainage with measurement of the PTH level has been of use in localizing recurrent tissue or glands missed during an initial exploration; its hazard, expense, and sometimes misleading results lead to its use only in difficult cases, however.

In general, the best procedure is a careful and thorough exploration of the neck by an experienced surgeon. Attempts to find all four glands should be made. Patients with a single adenoma are likely to be cured by removal of the single enlarged gland. If diffuse hyperplasia is present, however, most authorities recommend removing three or three and one-half glands, marking the remaining gland or remnant with permanent surgical clips for easy retrieval later. Alternatively, some surgeons have recently removed all four glands, transplanting one whole or half gland subcutaneously or intramuscularly into the forearm; recurrent hypercalcemia can then be treated by a minor procedure on the arm, rather than by a more difficult reexploration of the neck. Parathyroid tissue may also be frozen and preserved in tissue banks for later reimplantation if hypocalcemia develops; treatment of hypocalcemia is discussed later in this chapter. Hypocalcemia and injury to the recurrent laryngeal nerves are the major complications of extensive parathyroid surgery and are inversely proportional to the experience of the surgeon.

HYPOCALCEMIA

Signs and Symptoms of Hypocalcemia

Hypocalcemia produces a variety of clinical findings, listed in Table 4. Acute decreases in the serum calcium level of relatively minor degree (e.g., 1–2 mg/dl) may provoke severe tetany; conversely, many patients with chronic hypocalcemia may tolerate serum calcium levels of 6–7 mg/dl with few or no complaints. Hypocalcemia increases neuromuscular irritability and is directly responsible for muscle cramps, paresthesias, and convulsions. Calcium deposition at extraskeletal sites reflects not so much the ambient calcium level (since hypocalcemia would be expected to retard tissue calcification) but rather the increase in the serum phosphorus level that typically accompanies hypoparathyroid states. This increase in the serum phosphorus concentration increases the calcium-phosphate ion product to levels above that required for solubility, leading to precipitation of calcium phosphate salts in tissues. There is some evidence that brain

Table 4 **Symptoms and Signs of Hypocalcemia**

Neuromuscular
Muscle cramps and tetany
Paresthesias
Seizures
Laryngeal stridor
Weakness and fatigue
Diminished intellectual functioning
Psychiatric disorders
Pseudotumor cerebri
Prolonged Q-T interval on electrocardiogram
Extraskeletal calcification
Brain (especially basal ganglia, cerebellum, sometimes with resultant Parkinsonism or choreoathetosis)
Soft-tissue ossification (primarily in pseudohypoparathyroidism)
Vascular (arterial media)
Renal?
Cataracts
Dermatologic
Dry, scaly skin
Brittle nails
Sparse, coarse, dry hair (scalp, axillae, pubic, eyebrows)
Dental (if hypocalcemic during tooth development)
Enamel pitting and defects
Short, blunted roots
Delayed or absent eruption of teeth
Prone to caries

Table 5 **Causes of Hypocalcemia**

Hypoparathyroidism
Congenital
Associated with thymic aplasia (DiGeorge's syndrome) or other branchial cleft anomalies
Unassociated with other anomalies—pure parathyroid hypoplasia
Acquired
Idiopathic—probably autoimmune; often associated endocrinopathies, monilia infections
Surgical
Following radioactive iodine therapy
Hemochromatosis
Resistance to parathyroid hormone
Congenital
Pseudohypoparathyroidism
Acquired
Osteomalacia
Renal failure
Combined hypoparathyroidism and resistance to PTH
Magnesium deficiency
Drugs
Colchicine
Actinomycin D, mithramycin
Ethanol
Citrated blood (lowers ionized calcium level)
Other
Acute pancreatitis
Medullary carcinoma (rare)
Osteoblastic metastases (rare)

calcification may impair function of the central nervous system. Cataracts occur frequently, since hypocalcemia interferes with ion and water transport in the lens.

Causes of Hypocalcemia

A variety of conditions may cause hypocalcemia; these are listed in Table 5. In general, these disorders produce hypocalcemia by one of three mechanisms: (a) deficient PTH secretion, (b) resistance to PTH action, or (c) a combination of these two mechanisms.

Deficient PTH Secretion (Hypoparathyroidism)

Most cases of hypoparathyroidism arise as a consequence of the inadvertent surgical removal of or damage to the bulk of functioning parathyroid tissue, usually in connection with either thyroid or parathyroid surgery.

A less common cause of hypoparathyroidism is so-called idiopathic hypoparathyroidism, thought to reflect autoimmune destruction of the parathyroid glands (see Chapter 18). Such patients often have evidence of autoimmune disease affecting other endocrine glands (thyroid, adrenal, gonad) or the skin (vitiligo, alopecia).

Finally, congenital maldevelopment of the parathyroids may occur, often accompanied by an immunologic deficiency (e.g., DiGeorge's syndrome), reflecting the common origin of the parathyroids and the thymus from the third and fourth pharyngeal pouches. In each of these disorders, hypocalcemia results from decreased mobilization of calcium from bone, diminished renal production of 1,25-dihydroxyvitamin D_3 with a resultant decrease in intestinal calcium absorption and, possibly, renal calcium wasting.

Resistance to PTH

Pseudohypoparathyroidism. In this disorder, PTH secretion is adequate but peripheral tissues (kidney, bone) are resistant to PTH action. This disorder is inherited, most often in an X-linked dominant fashion. Some patients (perhaps half) manifest a characteristic phenotype which may include short stature, round face, obesity, low intelligence, dental anomalies, and shortening of some of the bones of the hands and feet (most typically the metacarpals, metatarsals, and phalanges). Additional features may include hypertension, hypothyroidism (almost always primary), and prolactin deficiency.

Recent investigations have shown that about half of patients with pseudohypoparathyroidism have a defect in the protein that couples membrane hormone receptors to adenylate cyclase in the cell interior, thus leading to resistance to PTH action (see Chapter 1). Patients with this form of illness may also show resistance to other hormones acting via adenylate cyclase (e.g., glucagon, antidiuretic hormone, thyroid-stimulating hormone), although the clinical effects of this multihormonal resistance are unknown. The cause of PTH resistance in pseudohypoparathyroid patients with normal amounts of receptor–cyclase coupling protein is not known.

Rarely, patients secrete an abnormal, biologically inactive PTH, resulting in hypocalcemia in the presence of high serum levels of immunoreactive PTH. Such patients respond normally to the administration of exogenous PTH, however, thus differentiating their disease from more classic forms of pseudohypoparathyroidism.

Rickets and Osteomalacia. Dietary vitamin D deficiency still occasionally occurs but is uncommon. More often, vitamin D deficiency is seen with intestinal malabsorption or chronic renal insufficiency (due in the latter case to failure of the kidney to produce 1,25-dihydroxyvitamin D_3, the active metabolite of vitamin D). As the serum calcium level falls, the serum PTH level increases. If renal function is normal, the elevated serum PTH level will increase renal phosphate loss, leading to hypophosphatemia in classic osteomalacia. Renal phosphate retention with *hyper*phosphatemia is seen in renal failure. In malabsorption syndromes, diminished absorption of dietary calcium and vitamin D as well as hypomagnesmia (vide infra) may contribute to the genesis of hypocalcemia.

Combined Defects of PTH Secretion and Action.

Hypocalcemia due to magnesium depletion is the best example of this mechanism. As total body magnesium stores fall, PTH action on bone and kidney becomes progressively impaired, ultimately leading to hypocalcemia. Although PTH levels may initially rise transiently, when magnesium deficiency becomes more severe PTH secretion is diminished. Thus two defects occur: insufficient secretion of and peripheral resistance to PTH. Hypomagnesemia is commonly seen in chronic alcoholism, intestinal malabsorption, diabetes mellitus, and overuse of diuretics.

Table 6 **Serum Chemistries in Hypocalcemic Disorders**

Disorder	*Calcium*	*Phosphorus*	*Alkaline Phosphatase*	*PTH*
Hypoparathyroidism	↓[a]	↑[b]	NL[c]	↓ or NL
Pseudohypoparathyroidism	↓	↑	NL or ↑	↑
Osteomalacia	↓ or NL	↓	↑	↑
Renal failure	↓ or NL	↑	↑	↑
Magnesium deficiency	↓	NL	NL	↓ NL, or ↑

[a] ↓, decreased
[b] ↑, increased.
[c] NL, Normal level.

Differential Diagnosis of Hypocalcemia

A presumptive diagnosis may often be made on the basis of the patient's history and a physical examination. A history of neck surgery or the presence of a thyroidectomy scar should suggest surgical hypoparathyroidism. A history of endocrine autoimmunity in the patient or in his or her family raises the possibility of idiopathic hypoparathyroidism. The presence of the characteristic phenotype suggests pseudohypoparathyroidism, but normal somatic features do not preclude this diagnosis. *Monilia* infections of the nails, often with loss of the nails, are characteristic of idiopathic hypoparathyroidism.

Initial laboratory studies should include measurements of the serum magnesium, calcium, phosphorus, creatinine, alkaline phosphatase, and PTH levels. A low or midnormal serum level of PTH in the face of hypocalcemia with a normal serum magnesium level supports a diagnosis of surgical or idiopathic hypoparathyroidism. An elevated serum PTH level in the presence of hypocalcemia strongly suggests the presence of resistance to PTH action (see Table 6).

Ideally, the diagnosis of pseudohypoparathyroidism should be confirmed by assessing the response to exogenous PTH when the patient is normocalcemic. As shown in Figure 1, normal

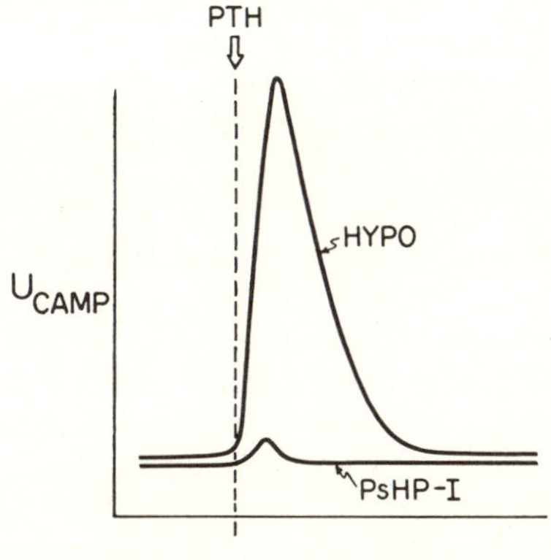

Figure 1. Changes in urinary cAMP (U_{cAMP}) excretion following an acute infusion of PTH in patients with hypoparathyroidism (HYPO) and pseudohypoparathyroidism type I (PsHP-I).

individuals and those with hypoparathyroidism respond to infused PTH with a brisk rise in plasma and urinary cyclic AMP levels and with increased urinary phosphate excretion. Patients with pseudohypoparathyroidism, in contrast, show minimal change in either parameter. (An uncommon subgroup of pseudohypoparathyroidism, designated pseudohypoparathyroidism type II, is characterized by a normal cAMP response to PTH, but no phosphaturia.)

Treatment of Hypocalcemia

Some patients with hypocalcemia can be easily treated merely by withdrawing an offending medication (e.g., colchicine). Patients with magnesium deficiency due to poor nutrition often can correct their hypomagnesmia and hypocalcemia by consuming a hospital diet for a few days; other patients may need magnesium supplements, either orally or parenterally (magnesium sulfate, 1–4 g daily in divided doses).

Patients with chronic hypocalcemia due to either hypoparathyroidism or pseudohypoparathyroidism generally require both calcium and vitamin D supplements, although mild hypocalcemia may sometimes respond to calcium supplements alone. Dietary calcium should total at least 1 g daily (1 qt of milk provides about 1 g of elemental calcium). Additional calcium may be given as calcium carbonate tablets (625 mg each, 40% calcium), calcium lactate tablets (500 mg each, 13% calcium), or calcium gluconate tablets (500 mg each, 9% calcium). Calcium supplement 1–4 g in divided doses may be provided in this fashion. A suitable liquid preparation, NeoCalGlucon (115 mg calcium/5 ml), is also available but is expensive. In patients with marked hyperphosphatemia (>6 mg/dl), it is probably better to give calcium supplements and avoid a high-calcium diet, since dairy products are also rich in phosphorus.

For acute treatment of symptomatic hypocalcemia, intravenous calcium gluconate is the preparation of choice, given as a slow intravenous infusion of 10 ml of a 10% solution over several minutes.

Vitamin D is often given as vitamin D_2 (ergocalciferol), the form of vitamin D produced by plants; it is fully as active in humans as vitamin D_3, cholecalciferol, the form produced in mammalian skin under the influence of sunlight. Vitamin D_2 is usually given in doses of 50,000–100,000 units (1.25–2.5 mg) daily. Vitamin D has a narrow therapeutic index, and toxicity due to hypercalcemia is common.

An alternative preparation, dihydrotachysterol (AT-10, DHT) is more expensive but may be more effective than vitamin D, since it does not require 1-hydroxylation in the kidney for activity. Doses of 0.5–1.0 mg/day are usually sufficient.

Recently, the active metabolite of vitamin D, 1,25-dihydroxyvitamin D_3 (Calcitriol, Rocaltrol: Hoffman-LaRoche, Inc.) has become available commercially. It is active in extremely low doses (0.5–2.5 μg/day). Its main advantages lie in its rapid onset of action and relatively short duration of action; hypercalcemia due to overtreatment is usually corrected by withholding the drug for 24–48 hours. This drug is still regarded as experimental for the treatment of hypoparathyroid states but may be soon approved for this use in the United States.

In treating surgical or idiopathic hypoparathyroidism, the goal should be to maintain the serum calcium level in the low-normal range (8.5–9.0 mg/dl). In the absence of the calcium-retaining effect on the kidney of PTH, renal calcium losses become marked at serum calcium levels of 9.5–10.5 mg/dl; the resulting hypercalciuria may eventually produce nephrolithiasis or nephrocalcinosis. In pseudohypoparathyroidism, normocalcemic hypercalciuria is less of a problem, perhaps because of residual PTH action on the renal tubule. Whatever form of vitamin D is given to treat chronic hypocalcemia, therapy should be monitored carefully to avoid severe or prolonged hypercalcemia. After steady-state control has been achieved, serum calcium, phosphorus, and creatinine levels should be checked every 2–4 months, and the 24-hour urinary calcium level measured every 3–6 months.

Patients who develop moderate hypocalcemia (>7.0 mg/dl) after neck surgery should be treated conservatively with calcium supplements, avoiding vitamin D unless hypocalcemia is protracted. Many such patients eventually recover sufficient parathyroid function to maintain normocalcemia. Postoperative hypomagnesemia may also contribute to hypocalcemia.

Thiazide diuretics decrease urinary calcium excretion and may lead to a reduced need for calcium and/or vitamin D supplements. The diminished urinary calcium losses also decrease the risk of nephrolithiasis.

DISCUSSION CASES

Case 1

A 52-year-old man was admitted to the hospital with complaints of severe back pain and polyuria. Initial laboratory evaluation revealed the following data: serum calcium 11.8 mg/dl, albumin 3.8 g/dl, phosphorus 4.4 mg/dl, creatinine 1.1 mg/dl, chloride 98 mEq/liter, and hematocrit 36%. A chest roentgenogram was normal apart from generalized osteopenia and several vertebral compression fractures; serum PTH determination was sent. A serum protein electrophoresis showed a large paraprotein ''spike'' in the γ-globulin region. A bone marrow aspirate was diagnostic of multiple myeloma.

During his initial hospitalization, he remained in bed most of the time because of back pain. Over the course of 3 days, he became progressively more lethargic and confused and took little food or liquid. His serum calcium level on the third hospital day climbed to 15.1 mg/dl. He was rapidly given 2 liters of physiologic saline intravenously and then furosemide 80 mg every 6 hours. Urine output was closely monitored, and the volume replaced with intravenous saline; potassium supplements were given as needed. Twenty-four hours later, the serum calcium level had fallen to 12 mg/dl. Salmon calcitonin, 8 MRC units/kg, was then given intravenously every 12 hours, along with prednisone 80 mg/day orally. The serum calcium level fell further to 10.1 mg/dl over the next day and remained at this level; furosemide was discontinued and ambulation encouraged. Chemotherapy for myeloma was begun (melphalan); calcitonin and prednisone were discontinued after 1 week. He has remained normocalcemic for 8 months.

Comment

Immobilization and dehydration led to the rapid escalation of hypercalcemia in this patient with myeloma. After acute lowering with fluids and diuresis, the serum calcium level was kept in the normal range with steroids and calcitonin while definitive chemotherapy was begun.

Case 2

A 44-year-old chronically alcoholic man was hospitalized with complaints of muscle weakness, paresthesias, and tetany of 6 weeks duration. He had additionally noted frequent, tan, bulky stools and a 40-lb weight loss over the past 6 months. Neurologic examination was normal except for positive Chvostek's and Trousseau's signs; cataracts were not present. His habitus and intelligence were normal.

Initial laboratory studies revealed the following: serum calcium 5.6 mg/dl, albumin 2.0 g/dl, phosphorus 2.5 mg/dl, magnesium 0.7 mEq/liter, alkaline phosphatase 194 units/liter (normal <110 units/liter), bilirubin 2.8 mg/dl, SGOT 114 units/liter. An abdominal radiograph showed pancreatic calcifications. Stool fat was 19 g/24 hr (normal <5 g/24 hr).

He was initially given intramuscular magnesium sulfate, 1 g b.i.d., and a regular hospital diet (1,000 mg calcium); within 5 days, the serum magnesium level was 1.8 mEq/liter but the serum calcium level was still 6.9 mg/dl with a serum albumin level of 2.75 g/dl. Steatorrhea continued, leading to the institution of therapy with oral pancreatic enzyme supplements. Two weeks later, the serum calcium level was 7.8 mg/dl and the albumin level 4 g/dl. Vitamin D_2 was then given in a dose of 50,000 units/day along with 2 g of calcium (as calcium lactate). The serum calcium level rose to 9.4 mg/dl 2 weeks later. He continued on this therapy for the next 3 months, when he returned complaining of weakness and polyuria. The serum calcium level was now 14 mg/dl. Vitamin D and calcium were discontinued and intravenous fluid given, with normalization of the serum calcium level within 4 days. Therapy was later reinstituted with 10,000 units/day of vitamin D_2. He remained normocalcemic for the next 2 years.

Comment

This patient's initial hypocalcemia was probably due to several factors: dietary deficiency of calcium and vitamin D, intestinal malabsorption of vitamin D and calcium, hypomagnesemia, and decreased hepatic metabolism of vitamin D to 25-hydroxyvitamin D. Correction of the hypomagnesemia improved but did not totally normalize serum calcium. Alleviation of the malabsorption syndrome produced a further increment in the serum calcium level. The initial dose of vitamin D proved to be excessive, with the eventual development of hypercalcemia.

SUGGESTED READING

Hypercalcemia

Aurbach GD, Mallette LE, Patten BM, et al: Hyperparathyroidism: Recent studies. *Ann Intern Med* 79:566–581, 1973.

Avioli LV, Krane SM (eds): *Metabolic Bone Disease*. New York, Academic Press, 1978.

Broadus AE, Rasmussen H: Clinical evaluation of parathyroid function. *Am J Med* 70:475–478, 1981.

Christensson T: Hyperparathyroidism and radiation therapy. *Ann Intern Med* 89:216–217, 1978.

Marx SJ, Attie MF, Levine MA, et al: The hypocalciuric or benign variant of familial hypercalcemia: Clinical and biochemical features in fifteen kindreds. *Medicine* 60:397–412, 1981.

Metz SA, McRae JR, Robertson RP: Prostaglandins as mediators of paraneoplastic syndromes: Review and update. *Metabolism* 30:299–316, 1981.

Scholz DA, Purnell DC: Asymptomatic primary hyperparathyroidism: 10-year prospective study. *Mayo Clin Proc* 56:473–478, 1981.

Skrabanek, P, McPartlin J, Powell D: Tumor hypercalcemia and "ectopic hyperparathyroidism." *Medicine* 59:262–282, 1980.

Stewart AF, Horst R, Deftos LJ, et al: Biochemical evaluation of patients with cancer-associated hypercalcemia: Evidence for humoral and nonhumoral groups. *N Engl J Med* 303:1377–1383, 1980.

Hypocalcemia

Kumar R, Riggs BL: Vitamin D in the therapy of disorders of calcium and phosphorus metabolism. *Mayo Clin Proc* 56:327–333, 1981.

Porter RH, Cox BG, Heaney D, et al: Treatment of hypoparathyroid patients with chlorthalidone. *N Engl J Med* 298:577–581, 1978.

Rude RK, Oldham SB, Singer FR: Functional hypoparathyroidism and parathyroid hormone end-organ resistance in human magnesium deficiency. *Clin Endocrinol* 5:209–224, 1976.

Schneider AB, Sherwood LM: Pathogenesis and management of hypoparathyroidism and other hypocalcemic disorders. *Metabolism* 24:871–898, 1975.

Tommaso CL, Tucci JR: Metabolic studies in a case of hypocalcemia and osteoblastic metastases. *Arch Intern Med* 139:238–240, 1979.

7 ARNOLD S. BRICKMAN

Metabolic Bone Disease

A number of technologic advances in the field of mineral metabolism have greatly improved our knowledge of the diagnosis and treatment of a variety of metabolic bone diseases during the past 5–10 years. Among these advances are the development of sensitive radioimmunoassays for parathyroid hormone (PTH) and calcitonin and competitive binding assays for vitamin D metabolites, particularly 25-hydroxyvitamin D [25(OH)D] and 1,25-dihydroxyvitamin D[1,25(OH)$_2$D]. Perhaps a more immediate development has been the more widespread use of the bone biopsy in diagnosing and following responses to treatment. Evaluation of histomorphometric parameters on undecalcified biopsy specimens and utilization of tetracycline prebiopsy labeling of bone to study dynamic features of bone histology are noteworthy advances. These developments, plus the recent availibility of a number of new therapeutic agents, have resulted in a plethora of new information about a large number of metabolic disorders and offer further hope for cure or management of these conditions.

This chapter will review only a few of the numerous disorders generally considered under the topic of metabolic bone diseases. These will include (1) osteoporoses, (2) osteomalacias, (3) bone disease of primary hyperparathyroidism, and (4) renal osteodystrophy.

THE OSTEOPOROSES

As generally used the term *osteoporosis* is defined as a state in which there is a reduction in the bone mass characteristic of individuals of the same age, sex, and race. Some clinicians also insist on the presence of mechanical failure (fracture of vertebrae, femoral neck or radius) for the full definition and diagnosis of osteoporosis. Moreover, osteoporoses constitute a heterogeneous group of disorders. Radiologically, the condition is perceived as osteopenia with decreased bone density. Since osteopenia results from a large number of disease processes, it is apparent that conventional roentgenology or even densitometric techniques cannot specifically diagnose osteoporosis. The diagnosis must be established by a bone biopsy, although in a number of clinical settings the diagnosis may be presumed with fair certainty (e.g., chronic steroid therapy or a postmenopausal woman who has not received estrogen therapy). Histologically, osteoporosis is characterized by a reduction in the amount of trabecular bone present relative to the total histologic section. The amount of mineralized bone relative to unmineralized bone matrix approximates the normal condition. This contrasts with osteomalacic states in which the amount of unmineralized bone matrix relative to total mineralized bone is increased.

Pathogenesis

The osteoporoses constitute a heterogeneous group of conditions with the development of osteopenia as a common feature. Diverse environmental, nutritional, developmental, and endocrine and metabolic alterations or abnormalities enter into the development of distinctive disorders. A simplified classification of disorders in which osteoporosis may develop is given in Table 1. The pathogenesis of the bone disorder in many if not most of these conditions is poorly understood at the present time. The most common of these conditions in the United States are senile or involutional osteoporosis, osteopenia that develops in the postmenopausal female, and osteoporosis that develops during chronic therapy with glucocorticoids.

The development of involutional osteoporosis occurs in a setting of advancing age. Controversy exists whether this loss of bone represents a normal physiologic aging process or

Table 1 **Classification of Osteoporoses**

Age-related
Senile
Postmenopausal
Nutritional disorders
Calcium deficiency
Vitamin deficiency
Protein malnutrition
Vitamin C deficiency
Endocrine disorders
Hyperparathyroidism
Hyperthyroidism
Cushing's disease or syndrome
Hypogonadism
Diabetes mellitus
Medications or toxins
Heparin
Ethanol
Chemotoxins (e.g., methotrexate)
Miscellaneous
Idiopathic
Immobilization or disuse
Renal osteodystrophy
Chronic acidosis

whether a subset of the aging population experiences bone loss at an accelerated rate. Risk factors such as decreased exercise and poor nutrition, including calcium and vitamin D deficiency, have been identified and undoubtedly are important. However, the not unusual demonstration of advanced osteopenia in otherwise healthy young adults suggests that other factors may be important. One view is that a major factor in the development of involutional osteoporosis is previous failure to acquire a normal skeletal mass during childhood growth and development. Here too, innumerable factors occurring during childhood may be involved, such as poor nutrition, environmental factors, inadequate exercise, childhood illnesses, or hereditary factors.

Two of the more common conditions in which osteoporosis occurs are the postmenopausal state and chronic treatment with glucocorticoids. The pathogenesis of osteoporosis developing during the postmenopausal period is thought to be attributable to estrogen deficiency. The latter appears to alter bone sensitivity to PTH, resulting in a relative increase in resorption (osteoclastic activity) but decreased bone formation (osteoblastic activity). Thus formation and resorption are uncoupled and bone volume is reduced. As a consequence of increased bone resorption and release of calcium, the serum calcium level may rise slightly, resulting in a decrease in PTH secretion. PTH modulates the renal production of $1,25(OH)_2D_3$, the major active hormonal form of vitamin D. Moreover, there is some evidence that estrogens may also directly or indirectly stimulate production of $1,25(OH)_2D_3$. Reduced levels of $1,25(OH)_2D_3$ have been reported to occur with aging and in the postmenopausal state. This presumably explains the decrease in intestinal absorption of calcium frequently demonstrated in this condition.

Glucocorticoids have a complex action on bone and calcium metabolism. A major effect is the direct anti-vitamin D action that results in a decrease in intestinal absorption of calcium. Other information suggests that steroids may also alter the production of $25(OH)D_3$ and possibly $1,25(OH)_2D_3$. Neither action is fully established. The steroid-induced tendency to hypocalcemia may also result in mild hyperparathyroidism which stimulates bone resorption. Augmented resorption (osteolysis) is not coupled to increased bone formation, since glucocorticoids appear to inhibit osteoblastic activity directly. The net effect of these processes is loss of bone volume and the development of osteopenia.

Diagnosis and Laboratory Findings

The diagnosis of osteoporosis is one of exclusion. Although a bone biopsy permits the exclusion of osteomalacia and hyperparathyroid bone disease (osteitis fibrosa), the findings are frequently nonspecific and thus of limited value in the absence of a contributory history of an underlying disease. Similarly, there are no consistent specific abnormalities in serum or urine electrolyte levels. PTH levels are generally reported as normal, but elevated levels have been reported in some subsets of patients. Recently, plasma levels of calcitonin have been reported to be decreased in women with postmenopausal osteoporosis. Levels of this hormone fall in both sexes with advancing age but appear to fall to a greater degree in postmenopausal woman. Treatment with estrogens results in a rise in calcitonin levels in this setting. Plasma levels of $1,25(OH)_2D_3$ also appear to fall with aging and may be even lower in individuals with osteoporosis. None of these findings is specific or of diagnostic value. It is possible however, that following changes in specific parameters, such as urinary hydroxyproline (which provides an index of bone turnover) during treatment may be of value. Thus, both the 24-hour urinary calcium level and the urinary calcium/creatinine ratio in a fasting morning specimen may be elevated in osteoporosis. Levels revert to normal with specific therapies (e.g., estrogens in the postmenopausal woman).

Treatment

Treatment of osteoporosis should be focused on reversing the factors that have been established as contributing to the development of osteopenia. Thus correction of a specific underlying endocrine disorder (Table 1) such as thyrotoxicosis (excess thyroid hormone) or Cushing's disease will stabilize and reduce bone loss and even result in regaining some of the lost bone mineral. However, in the more common conditions, such as postmenopausal osteoporosis and involutional osteopenia, responses to therapy are much less certain. General approaches to therapy include rehabilitative physical therapy, mobilization and exercise programs, and attention to diet and pharmacologic agents.

Estrogen Therapy

It is clearly established that estrogen replacement therapy reduces the rate of bone loss in the postmenopausal woman. This occurs in either the setting of the natural menopause or following surgical castration at an earlier age. Parameters of increased bone loss such as increased urinary calcium excretion and hydroxyproline excretion are quickly normalized with ethinyl estradiol (0.2 mg) or conjugated equine estrogens (0.625 mg) given cyclically for 21 days of each month. It is probable that even lower doses of these estrogens will be effective in reducing bone loss. This is an important concern in view of the association between treatment with estrogens and the development of uterine carcinoma.

Calcium and Vitamin D

The use of oral calcium supplements that raise total daily intake to 1,500 mg of calcium or greater has also been shown to reduce the accelerated rate of bone loss in postmenopausal osteoporosis. Administration of pharmacologic doses of vitamin D have been used to augment calcium absorption but appear to have little other value. Information concerning the experimental use of more potent vitamin D sterols such as $25(OH)D_3$ and $1,25(OH)_2D_3$ is limited. However, preliminary observations suggest that both compounds may be effective in halting or possibly in some cases reversing bone loss in steroid-induced osteopenia.

Fluoride

Fluoride (sodium fluoride, 25–50 mg/day) stimulates osteoblastic activity and bone formation. Thus use of this salt, often in combination with vitamin D and calcium supplements, has been advocated by a number of investigators. However, the newly formed bone may be structurally inferior to normal bone because of the presence of fluoroapatite in bone matrix. In toxic quantities, fluoride therapy may result in osteomalacia. Such complications with fluoride therapy may be significantly reduced by its administration in a cyclic manner. Stimulation of new bone formation is heralded by a rise in the plasma levels of bone alkaline phosphatase. This generally occurs within 3–6 weeks of initiation of therapy. At this point administration of fluoride may be discontinued and use of calcium and vitamin D supplements continued to facilitate new bone mineralization. When alkaline phosphatase levels fall toward baseline levels, the course of treatment with fluoride can be resumed. This approach may prevent the development of features of fluorosis.

Other approaches to therapy, including the use of calcitonin, androgens, and diphosphonates, remain experimental at this time, since there is insufficient information concerning clinical efficacy to warrant their widespread use at this time.

OSTEOMALACIAS

Osteomalacia is a general term referring to defective mineralization of bone resulting in the accumulation of undecalcified bone matrix (osteoid). When this disorder occurs in childhood (before fusion of the epiphyseal plates), the condition is called *rickets*. The latter is characterized in its severest form by epiphyseal dysplasia, impaired growth of long bones, and a variety of bony deformities.

The most common causes of osteomalacia are conditions of altered vitamin D metabolism or depletion and phosphate-wasting states with hypophosphatemia and phosphate depletion. Other less common causes include treatment with mineralization inhibitors (diphosphonates), fluorosis, trace metal toxicity (cadmium), and rare conditions in which there are abnormalities in bone cell metabolism and collagen formation.

Disordered Vitamin D Homeostasis

Table 2 lists a number of conditions in which altered vitamin D homeostasis results in the development of osteomalacia. In general these can be separated into two classes: (1) disorders in which circulating levels of specific vitamin D are reduced and, (2) conditions in which there appears to be a resistance to vitamin D metabolites in one or more target organs.

Vitamin D-Resistant States

Newer knowledge concerning the metabolism of vitamin D has altered our concept of vitamin D resistance. It is now clear that impaired metabolism of vitamin D at one or more

Table 2 **Causes of Rickets/Osteomalacia: Altered Vitamin D Metabolism**

Hereditary disorders
Type I vitamin D-dependent rickets (1α-hydroxylase deficiency)
Type II vitamin D-dependent rickets
Vitamin D-resistant rickets or osteomalacia (X-linked, familial, sporadic)?
Acquired abnormal metabolism
Chronic liver disease (cirrhosis, primary biliary cirrhosis)
Chronic renal disease
Nephrotic syndrome
Chronic acidosis?
Oncogenic osteomalacia (tumor-associated)
Medications
Anticonvulsants
Glutethimide
Malabsorption of vitamin D
Small-bowel disorders (sprue, short-bowel syndrome)
Pancreatic insufficiency
Disruption of bile salt metabolism

sites explains wholly or at least in part the so-called resistance to vitamin D in disorders such as hypoparathyroidism and chronic renal failure. In the former condition, the absence of PTH as well as the tendency to hyperphosphatemia result in impaired renal conversion of 25(OH)D_3 to 1,25$(OH)_2D_3$. Pharmacologic doses of vitamin D_3 or D_2 are generally administered in the treatment of hypoparathyroidism; however, doses of 1–5 mg/day (40,000–200,000 units) of these relatively inactive sterols produce little change in circulating levels of the major metabolite, 1,25$(OH)_2$D. The physiologic responses during long-term treatment with vitamin D are a consequence of its metabolism to 25(OH)D in the liver. The latter appears to act at the intestine and perhaps bone on a mass action basis. Thus the requirement for pharmacologic doses of vitamin D is a reflection of the low biologic activity of this prohormone, the slow rate of conversion to 25(OH)D, and the tightness of enzymatic regulation of 1,25$(OH)_2$D formation. In contrast, in chronic renal failure loss of functional renal mass underlies the reduced capacity to form 1,25$(OH)_2$D. In both hypoparathyroid states and in end-stage renal failure, seemingly physiologic doses of 1,25$(OH)_2D_3$ (Rocaltrol, Hoffman-La Roche, Inc.) are highly active in stimulating intestinal absorption of calcium and correcting hypocalcemia.

However, it is now clear that true peripheral resistance to vitamin D metabolites such as 1,25$(OH)_2D_3$ doses occurs in several clinical settings. Type II vitamin D-dependent rickets is such a disorder. In this condition osteomalacia develops in a setting of high circulating levels of 1,25$(OH)_2D_3$. In the few cases reported treatment with pharmacologic doses of this metabolite (10–25 μg/day) may be required to correct hypocalcemia; in some patients even these doses are ineffective. Recent studies with cultured fibroblasts from skin biopsy specimens of patients with this disorder indicate the presence of decreased receptor binding for 1,25$(OH)_2D_3$. Another probable example of peripheral vitamin D resistance occurs in association with the osteomalacia developing during long-term anticonvulsant therapy. In this disorder circulating levels of 25(OH)D_3 are low, but 1,25$(OH)_2D_3$ levels are normal or high. The low levels of 25(OH)D_3 may be explained by altered hepatic microsomal metabolism of D_3, but the high levels of 1,25$(OH)_2D_3$ suggest the possibility that peripheral resistance to this and perhaps other vitamin D sterols plays a role in the pathogenesis of anticonvulsant osteomalacia.

Osteomalacia as a Consequence of Vitamin D Deficiency

Osteomalacia associated with low circulating levels of vitamin D metabolites occurs in three general settings: (1) inadequate dietary intake including both malnutrition and lack of sufficient solar (ultraviolet light) exposure; (2) gastrointestinal malabsorption states; (3) altered vitamin D metabolism, primarily in the liver or kidney. In these settings low circulating levels of both 25(OH)D_3 and 1,25$(OH)_2D_3$ are the usual finding. However, as mentioned above, in some disorders such as anticonvulsant osteomalacia plasma 25(OH)D_3 levels are low but 1,25$(OH)_2D_3$ levels are high or normal. Similarly, normal or high levels of 1,25$(OH)_2D_3$ have been reported in some cases of apparent nutritional osteomalacia. Such observations have several possible implications. First, it seems possible that metabolites other than 1,25$(OH)_2D_3$ may be important in the development of vitamin D deficiency bone disease. Second, peripheral resistance to 1,25$(OH)_2D_3$ may occur in some of these conditions. Finally, the normal or even elevated levels of 1,25$(OH)_2D_3$ may be a transient event in the natural history and pathogenesis of the disorder and low levels will develop subsequently. Much more information concerning vitamin D homeostasis in these conditions is required to clarify our knowledge of the development of these disorders.

Each of the types of disorders listed in Table 2 is discussed in greater detail in more extensive reviews (see Suggested Reading). Brief comments here will be restricted to three conditions.

Primary Biliary Cirrhosis

Malabsorption of vitamin D occurs in several clinical settings (Table 2). Among these is disruption of the normal bile salt metabolic pathway. Several vitamin D metabolites—including $25(OH)D_3$ and $24,25(OH)_2D_3$—have been shown to undergo enterohepatic circulation. Disruption of this pathway can result in excessive loss of these metabolites and development of osteomalacia. This has been demonstrated to occur in primary biliary cirrhosis. Here, however, the condition is further complicated by the development of hepatocellular disease with impaired metabolism of vitamin D_3 to $25(OH)D_3$. Treatment with large parenteral doses of vitamin D_3 may be ineffective in preventing the development of bone disease or be ineffective in completely healing disease once it has developed. The latter suggests the possibility of peripheral resistance to vitamin D sterols in some forms of hepatic disease.

Vitamin D-dependent Rickets Type I

This rare metabolic disorder is inherited as an autosomal recessive disease. Osteomalacia develops in the presence of normal circulating levels of $25(OH)D_3$ but low levels of $1,25(OH)_2D_3$. Patients usually require pharmacologic doses of vitamin D for treatment, but small doses of $1,25(OH)_2D_3$ usually correct the hypocalcemia and malabsorption of calcium. This condition is now thought to occur as a consequence of the deficiency of the enzyme responsive for $1,25(OH)_2D_3$ formation (25-hydroxyvitamin D-1α-hydroxylase deficiency). The fact that in some cases greater than physiologic doses of $1,25(OH)_2D_3$ are needed to correct the disorder has raised the speculation that other defects in vitamin D homeostasis may be present in some patients with this condition.

Tumor-associated Osteomalacia (Oncogenic Osteomalacia)

Osteomalacia has been recognized in an increasing number of patients with underlying malignancies. The usual presentation is bone pain associated with hypophosphatemia and varying degrees of hypocalcemia, both of which are resistant to correction with conventional vitamin D therapy. Frequently, osteopenia and occasionally pseudofractures are seen on roentgenograms, but metastatic lesions are absent. The majority of cases reported have been associated with large mesenchymal tumors both benign and malignant. However, recently, tumor-associated osteomalacia has been recognized in patients with prostatic cancer and other malignancies. Two views concerning the pathogenesis of this disorder are that the tumors produce a phosphaturic substance that promotes phosphate wasting and depletion and that the tumors produce an inhibitor of $1,25(OH)_2D_3$ synthesis. Circulating levels of the latter are low and with removal or ablation of the tumor return to normal with healing of the osteomalacia and reversal of biochemical abnormalities. In cases where surgical removal of the tumor is not feasible, administration of $1,25(OH)_2D_3$ has resulted in varying degrees of clinical improvement.

Osteomalacia Associated with Hypophosphatemic States

Osteomalacia or rickets occurs in a number of settings in which apparent phosphate depletion occurs in association with hypophosphatemia. The most common causes include renal phosphate-wasting states, intestinal malabsorption of phosphorus, and dietary phosphorus restriction. These are summarized in Table 3.

Table 3 **Causes of Rickets/Osteomalacia: Hypophosphatemic Disorders**

Hereditary (renal phosphate wasting)
Vitamin D-resistant rickets or osteomalacia (X-linked familial, sporadic)
Fanconi syndrome
Acquired
Primary hyperparathyroidism?
Oncogenic osteomalacia
Malabsorption (chronic use of phosphate-binding antacids, gastrointestinal disorders)
Malnutrition
Chronic hemodialysis (low phosphate dialysate)

Familial X-Linked Hypophosphatemia

This disorder, also referred to as primary hypophosphatemia or vitamin D resistant rickets (VDRR), remains the most common cause of rickets and osteomalacia in the United States today. The salient biochemical features of this condition include hypophosphatemia, renal phosphate wasting as a consequence of a low threshold for phosphorus reabsorption (TmP_i/GFR) and normal serum calcium and PTH levels. In contrast to the Fanconi syndrome, which may occur in several clinical settings and varieties, neither aminoaciduria nor renal tubular acidosis is present in classical VDRR. The pathogenesis of hypophosphatemia is attributable to defective epithelial cell transport of phosphorus manifested in both the kidney and intestine. Plasma levels of $1,25(OH)_2D_3$ are either low or normal, suggesting a concomitant defect in regulation of synthesis of this metabolite since hypophosphatemia of the degree present in this condition would be expected to stimulate renal 25-hydroxyvitamin D-1α-hydroxylase activity. In addition to X-linked and autosomal recessive forms of VDRR, sporadic forms also occur commonly. It is uncertain whether or not the pathogenesis of all these disorders is the same. However, the treatment of these conditions is similar—administration of oral phosphate supplements (up to 3 g/24 hr in divided doses) and pharmacologic doses of vitamin D. In this setting the vitamin D both augments intestinal absorption of phosphorus and promotes skeletal mineralization.

Diagnostic Features

Clinical Features

The clinical manifestations of osteomalacia depend on the duration of disease, the age of onset, and the severity of the disorder. Skeletal pain is common particularly in the spine, ribs, and lower extremities. Bone tenderness is also frequently present. Proximal muscle weakness and tenderness may be present in some individuals. In children with rickets, bony deformities (craniotabes, frontal bowing, thickening of the ribs, bowing of the long bones) and short stature are frequently observed because the disease process involves rapidly growing and remodeling bone. Such deformities are unusual in adult-onset disease.

Radiologic Features

Roentgenograms of bone often resemble those of osteoporosis, with diffuse osteopenia. The classic finding, pathognomonic of osteomalacia, is the pseudofracture (Looser zones, milkman fractures). These tend to occur symmetrically and bilaterally at sites such as the pubic and ischial rami, the long bones such as the femoral shaft and head, ribs, and scapulae. In children, radiologic features include the finding of the deformities mentioned above as well as typical abnormalities at growing epiphyses, widening of the growth plates, and fraying of the metaphyses.

Bone Biopsy

On iliac crest bone biopsy, the major histologic finding is an accumulation of unmineralized osteoid. Both the amount of surface area and the width of osteoid lamellae covering mineralized bone are increased. When tetracycline labeling procedures are carried out, both the amount of tetracycline uptake by osteoid and the rate of mineralization are decreased (e.g., mineralization lag time is increased). This distinguishes osteomalacia from other disorders such as thyrotoxicosis and primary hyperparathyroidism in which osteoid volume may also be increased as a result of increased bone turnover, but the rates of formation and mineralization are increased. In addition to features of a mineralization defect, evidence of secondary hyperparathyroidism, including osteoclastosis and marrow space fibrosis, is usually present. However, the latter findings are generally not observed in osteomalacia associated with hypophosphatemia and phosphate-wasting states.

Biochemical Features

The laboratory findings in osteomalacia differ according to duration of disease and etiology. In patients with disorders attributable to deficient or disordered vitamin D metabolism, hypocalcemia and the features of secondary hypoparathyroidism are likely as the disease increases in severity. Low plasma levels of $25(OH)D_3$ are considered the best index of vitamin D depletion. Levels of $1,25(OH)_2D_3$ vary from low to normal.

In contrast, osteomalacia in chronic hypophosphatemic disorders is rarely associated with hypocalcemia, and features of secondary hyperparathyroidism are generally not present. Varying degrees of aminoaciduria and increased hydroxyproline excretion may be found in both forms of the disease.

Treatment

Therapy for osteomalacia varies with etiology. In nutritional disorders small amounts of vitamin D_2 or D_3 (100–400 units, 2.5–10 μg) given orally daily will produce rapid therapeutic responses. To facilitate more rapid clinical responses, larger doses are often utilized along with oral calcium and phosphorus supplements. Biochemical responses to treatment may include an acute lowering of serum calcium and phosphorus; the latter, however, usually rises rapidly along with alkaline phosphatase levels.

When irreversible malabsorptive states are present, parenteral vitamin D therapy may be required. Doses vary according to clinical response. In some cases pharmacologic oral doses of 100,000–200,000 units daily may be effective if malabsorption is less severe.

As previously mentioned, treatment with $1,25(OH)_2D_3$ has been applied in specific disease states where levels of this metabolite are low, such as vitamin D-dependent rickets type I. Patients frequently respond to physiologic or near-physiologic doses (0.5–1 μg/day) of this drug. Similar observations have been made in nutritional osteomalacia. However, the use of $1,25(OH)_2D_3$ in these disorders is still regarded as experimental by the Food and Drug Administration.

In chronic hypophosphatemic diseases, the mainstay of therapy is the use of oral phosphate supplements. The goal is to achieve normal levels of serum phosphorus. Studies have shown that round-the-clock therapy with oral supplements can restore normophosphatemia, dramatically improving linear growth velocity in children with this condition. Vitamin D therapy can be used as an adjunct to improve both phosphorus and calcium absorption and to further promote mineralization. Vitamin D may also reduce the likelihood of the development of hypocalcemia and secondary hyperparathyroidism during oral phosphate therapy.

Duration of treatment of osteomalacia will vary with clinical response and etiology. Lifelong therapy may be required in certain metabolic disorders, while short-term therapy may suffice in nutritional disease states.

PRIMARY HYPERPARATHYROIDISM

The clinical presentation of metabolic bone disease in primary hyperparathyroidism appears to have undergone considerable change. Hyperparathyroidism in cases diagnosed before 1950 was associated with features of severe bone disease (osteitis fibrosa cystica generalisata) in as many as 50% of patients. In cases studied between 1965 and 1975, fewer than 10% of patients could be stated to have this severe form of bone disease. Presently, the most common presenting form of bone disease, detected on roentgenograms, is diffuse osteopenia, present in approximately 20% of patients.

Detection of bone disease in patients with primary hyperparathyroidism is generally a function of the rigorousness of the techniques used. In recent series, biochemical screening with measurement of alkaline phosphatase levels in patients with this disease showed elevation in perhaps only 10–20% of patients, similar to the incidence of positive findings on routine skeletal roentgenograms. More sensitive radiologic techniques (radiographic morphometery or magnification studies of fine-grain X-ray films) and bone densitometric studies show abnormalities consistent with hyperparathyroidism in 40–50% of cases. It has been reported that bone-scanning techniques may detect abnormalities in perhaps 50–60% of patients.

However, the bone biopsy remains the most sensitive assessment of both the presence of changes consistent with hyperparathyroidism and, in the opinion of some specialists, the actual diagnosis of the disorder. Recent studies have indicated that the diagnosis of this disorder can be made in 90–97% of cases based on histomorphometric analysis. The predominant histologic findings include coupled increases in osteoclastic and osteoblastic activity (increased active resorption and formation surfaces) and increased osteoid width and/or surface distribution (reflecting an increased appositional rate). In more severe disease, marrow space fibrosis and woven bone are present. The number and size of bone trabeculae may be decreased, particularly in individuals with significant osteopenic disease. The presence of so-called osteocytic osteolysis (resorption of bone by osteocytes) in hyperparathyroidism seems to remain conjectural at the present time. Finally, rare cases of primary hyperparathyroidism may involve osteomalacia. Here, the bone appositional rate and mineralization are markedly decreased. Such patients may have either low or normal serum levels of calcium, which revert to hypercalcemia during treatment with vitamin D.

The factors responsible for the different patterns of bone disease in primary hyperparathyroidism remain to be elucidated. Clearly, patients with more severe and long-standing hyperparathyroidism seem more likely to have more severe bone disease. However, this has not always proven to be the case. Moreover, at present, it remains unclear why patients with primary hyperparathyroidism seem to segregate into those with renal stone disease and those with more severe metabolic bone disease. Those with the former tend to have disease of longer duration, and if bone disease is present, it tends to be of the osteopenic variety. Alterations in vitamin D metabolism may explain at least in part the different clinical presentations of hyperparathyroidism. Patients with nephrolithiasis have been shown to have elevated levels of $1,25(OH)_2D_3$, augmented intestinal calcium absorption, and marked hypercalciuria. It is possible that other alterations in vitamin D homeostasis, as yet poorly understood, may contribute to the development of different patterns of bone disease. Additional possible contributory factors include underlying renal function, sex hormone status (menopausal and estrogen therapy status), concomitant diseases, or treatment with agents such as thiazide diuretics, nonsteroidal antiinflammatory agents, propranolol, and cimetidine. The latter agents are known to alter directly or indirectly bone responsiveness to PTH or to perhaps influence PTH secretion.

Treatment

In general, treatment of hyperparathyroid bone disease is treatment of the primary disorder. However, although surgical removal of an adenoma, or subtotal parathyroidectomy in the case of hyperplasia, may result in a cure, there is currently increased interest in medical management. At present insufficient information is available to judge what effects such therapy may have on the natural history of the underlying bone disease. Oral phosphorus supplements generally in doses of 1–2 g of elemental phosphorus have been given to patients with hyperparathyroidism and recurrent nephrolithiasis, with good control of stone disease. Effects on skeletal homeostasis have not yet been reported. Estrogen therapy may improve the degree of hypercalcemia and even mask the diagnosis of hyperparathyroidism. The mechanism at least in part may reflect the anti-PTH-like effects of estrogen on bone. Since estrogen therapy is invariably used in the peri- or postmenopausal setting, the possible effects of such therapy on the natural history of underlying parathyroid bone disease is entirely unknown. Finally, dichloromethylene diphosphonate has recently been used experimentally in the treatment of primary hyperparathyroidism. The effect of this agent is lowering serum calcium is thought to be due to its inhibitory effects on osteoclastic resorption. The consequence of such therapy would be to decrease bone calcium loss. Again, the long-term consequences of such therapy on bone disease in primary hyperparathyroidism are entirely unknown at the present time.

RENAL OSTEODYSTROPHY

The term *renal osteodystrophy* encompasses a heterogeneous group of metabolic bone diseases found in individuals with end-stage or progressive renal failure. The pathogenesis of these disorders is multifactorial. However, two disturbances in mineral homeostasis appear to play a central role in development of the most commonly encountered types of bone disease, the development of secondary hyperparathyroidism and one or more alterations in vitamin D homeostasis.

According to one major school of thought, secondary hyperparathyroidism develops as a consequence of the tendency to phosphorus retention that occurs with progressive loss of renal function (Bricker hypothesis). Incremental rises in serum phosphorus levels result in small (perhaps virtually undetectable) decreases in serum calcium levels, which stimulate PTH secretion. Initially, these perturbations are small. The elevated levels of PTH facilitate urinary excretion of the retained phosphorus and readjustment of serum calcium and phosphorus levels. With progressive loss of nephron function, there is greater phosphorus retention and a progressive rise in the levels of PTH representing a higher state of production and secretion. Eventually, hyperphosphatemia and hypocalcemia ensue.

A second group of investigators has emphasized the primary role of impaired vitamin D metabolism in the development of secondary hyperparathyroidism. With progressive renal functional deterioration there is reduced renal production of $1,25(OH)_2D_3$. This contributes to the development of relative malabsorption of calcium (and phosphorus). Formation or metabolism of other vitamin D analogs such as $25(OH)D_3$ and $24,25(OH)_2D_3$ may also be impaired. These abnormalities constitute a state of relative or absolute vitamin D deficiency and result in the development of renal osteomalacia. Both the malabsorption of calcium and the skeletal resistance to PTH present in osteomalacia contribute to the appearance of hypocalcemia.

Clearly features of both phosphate retention and altered vitamin D metabolism contribute to the development of uremic bone disease. Neither hypothesis alone explains all the features of renal osteodystrophy.

Types of Bone Disease in Chronic Renal Failure

Several types of metabolic bone disease are typically seen in patients with end-stage renal failure. These are summarized as follows: (1) mild lesions (mild hyperparathyroidism), (2) osteitis fibrosa (severe hyperparathyroidism), (3) osteomalacia, (4) mixed histologic lesions (variable features of both hyperparathyroidism and osteomalacia). In addition to these groups there may be additional categories of disease perhaps representing further complications of the disorders listed above, such as osteosclerosis and conventional disorders such as postmenopausal osteoporosis developing in a patient with uremia.

The only reliable technique for establishing diagnosis of the type of bone disease is a bone biopsy. This procedure, performed with quantitative assessment of histomorphometric parameters in the biopsy specimen, allows a reasonable classification of the type of bone disease present. This has proven to have both therapeutic as well as prognostic value. The additional determination of dynamic features of bone activity through the use of tetracycline labeling of bone before the biopsy procedure is of particular value. Table 4 gives an abbreviated classification of types of bone disease based on these measurements and also indicates the usual levels of calcium and PTH found in such settings.

Table 4 **Histologic and Biochemical Features of Various Types of Uremic Bone Disease**

	Mild	*Osteitis Fibrosa*	*Mixed*	*Osteomalacia*	*Vitamin D-Resistant Osteomalacia*
Serum calcium level	N[a]	N/↑	N/↓	↑[b]	↑
PTH level	↑	↑↑	↑↑	↑	N/↓
Mineralization rate	N	N	↓[c]	↓↓	↓↓
Bone appositional rate	N	N/↑	↓	↓	↓

[a]N, normal
[b]↑, increased
[c]↓, decreased.

Mild Lesion

The earliest type of bone disease seen in progressive renal failure appears histologically as a so-called mild lesion. Clinically, individuals with this type of bone biopsy are generally assymptomatic, skeletal roentgenograms are usually normal or only slightly abnormal (e.g., mild osteopenia), and biochemical parameters are generally indicative of mild secondary hyperparathyroidism. Likewise, histologically the features are those of mild PTH excess, with minimal marrow space fibrosis.

Osteitis Fibrosa

It is probable that the mild histologic lesion progresses with time (as a function of the duration of uremia or hemodialysis) to the lesions of osteitis fibrosa, osteomalacia, or a mixed histologic picture. Osteitis fibrosa represents a more severe form of hyperparathyroid bone disease. Bone resorption (osteoclastosis) and formation are both markedly increased, generally in a coupled fashion thus reflected in an increase in bone appositional rate and a shortened mineralization lag time. PTH levels are usually markedly elevated. Clinically, patients with this disease are more likely to have skeletal pain and tenderness. Roentgenograms may show severe subperiosteal (cortical) resorption, "brown tumors," cysts, osteopenia, and focal osteosclerosis. Overt hypercalcemia and hyperphosphatemia are likely, although not invariably present. Serum PTH levels are usually markedly elevated. Elevated levels of bone alkaline phosphatase are a fair index of the severity of underlying skeletal disease.

Osteomalacia and Mixed Histologic Lesions

These two types of bone disease differ from each other in the degree of histologic manifestation of features of hyperparathyroidism. Patients with a relatively pure form of osteomalacia tend to have lower circulating levels of PTH and correspondingly little evidence of marrow space fibrosis. The mixed histologic lesion closely resembles the histologic picture of nutritional osteomalacia; PTH levels may be markedly elevated, and significant marrow fibrosis is present. In both types of disease the bone appositional rate and mineralization rate are low. Clinically, patients with these disorders may manifest skeletal pain and tenderness. Some patients have severe, incapacitating muscle pain, tenderness, and weakness. The latter appears to be a form of metabolic myopathy attributable either to the secondary hyperparathyroidism or vitamin D deficiency. Serum levels of both calcium and phosphorus generally range from low to normal. Indeed, hypophosphatemia and phosphorus depletion as a consequence of overzealous management with phosphate-binding antacids have been implicated in the pathogenesis of osteomalacia in some individuals.

Vitamin D-Resistant Osteomalacia

A less common but clinically very challenging uremic bone disease is a form of osteomalacia resistant to conventional treatments with vitamin D analogs. Patients with this disorder in general have undergone long-term treatment with hemodialysis. Many have had previous extensive treatment with vitamin D, and some have undergone parathyroid surgery. Low levels of PTH attributable to previous surgery or possibly parathyroid gland failure are invariably found. Clinically, patients are severely incapacitated with skeletal pain, tenderness, and frequently pathologic fractures. Hypercalcemia even in the presence of low or undetectable levels of PTH is usually present. The pathogenesis of this disorder is poorly understood, but both low levels of PTH and high levels of bone aluminum have been implicated. Prognosis is frequently poor, although some treatment successes have occurred.

Treatment of Renal Osteodystrophy

The major therapeutic modalities in the treatment of renal osteodystrophy are control of hyperphosphatemia, adequate intake of calcium through diet and dialysate, use of vitamin D compounds, and parathyroid surgery.

Dietary restriction of phosphorus and the use of phosphate-binding antacids are the mainstays of control of serum phosphorus levels. Overzealous use of these modalities can lower serum phosphorus levels to the point of phosphate depletion. Treatment doses must be individualized.

Available forms of vitamin D compounds in the United States include vitamin D_2 or D_3, dihydrotachysterol, $25(OH)D_3$ (Calcitriol), and $1,25(OH)_2D_3$. The latter two compounds have the advantages of relatively rapid onset and offset of action, as well as greater potency than vitamin D_2 or D_3. Doses must be individualized, but for $25(OH)D_3$ starting doses may range from 50–200 μg/day, while lower doses are generally used during maintenance therapy; starting doses of $1,25(OH)_2D_3$ usually range from 0.5 to 1.0 μg/day, but larger doses are occasionally used. Maintenance doses vary with response to treatment. Conventional pharmacologic doses of vitamin D_2, D_3, and DHT are usually required.

Indications for treatment with vitamin D in renal failure include correction of hypocalcemia, management of secondary hyperparathyroidism, treatment of osteomalacia when hyperparathyroidism is present, and treatment of proximal muscle myopathies. Vitamin D therapy is invariably required in children.

Parathyroid surgery (subtotal parathyroidectomy) should be reserved for individuals who have clinically overt secondary hyperparathyroidism. Features include hypercalcemia, uncontrollable hyperphosphatemia, progressive soft tissue calcification, itching, and associated symptoms of bone pain.

DISCUSSION CASES

Case 1

Description

A 51-year-old man complains of generalized weakness, muscle aches and bone pain. Physical examination reveals demonstrable weakness bilaterally in the upper arms and legs, as well as tenderness over both humeri and tibiae. His personal medical history and physical examination are otherwise noncontributory. There is no family history of a similar disorder. Routine blood tests reveal the following pertinent abnormalities: creatinine 0.9 mg/dl, alkaline phosphatase 156 IU/ml (normal $<$105 IU/ml), calcium 8.9 mg/dl, phosphate 1.8 mg/dl.

Question

1. Discuss the differential diagnosis of metabolic bone disease in this patient.

Answer

This patient appears to have some form of osteomalacia. The diagnosis is suggested by the clinical features of diffuse bone pain and tenderness. The muscle symptoms of pain, tenderness, and weakness are classically found in patients with rickets or osteomalacia and appear to be attributable to a vitamin D sensitive myopathy. Hypocalcemia is not invariably present even in moderate bone disease, whereas a low serum phosphorus level is invariably present. Alkaline phosphatase levels are variable. Among entities that might be considered are the following: (1) sporadic hypophosphatemic osteomalacia, (2) tumor-associated osteomalacia, (3) primary hyperparathyroidism with osteomalacia, (4) toxicity due to various trace elements, such as fluorosis or cadmium toxicity, is also a possible disorder but is usually indicated by an exposure or environmental toxicity history. Of the first three diagnoses the first diagnosis is probably most likely. This disorder is similar to X-linked hypophosphatemia but lacks the positive family history. Hypocalcemia is usually absent, and the disorder may appear during adulthood as an osteomalacic syndrome. In tumor-associated osteomalacia hypocalcemia (vitamin D-resistant) is usually present, and tumors, either malignant or benign, are usually demonstrable. This condition is associated with prostatic carcinoma, a less likely diagnosis in a 51-year-old man. Primary hyperparathyroidism may rarely occur with concomitant osteomalacia. In this setting serum calcium levels are usually normal but rise to the hypercalcemic range during effective therapy with vitamin D.

Question

2. What additional diagnostic studies would be helpful in clarifying the diagnosis in this patient?

Answer

Roentgenogram findings of pseudofractures would confirm the diagnostic impression of osteomalacia but would not specify the cause. Measurement of the PTH level would determine whether or not secondary hyperparathyroidism is present. PTH levels are usually normal in primary phosphate-wasting forms of osteomalacia (as are serum calcium levels). In the presence of a normal PTH level the calculation of percent tubular reabsorption of phosphate $(1 - C_{PO_4}/C_{Cr}) \times 100$ or the threshold of phosphate resorption may be of diagnostic value. Both these parameters are low in phosphate-wasting states (as well as hyperparathyroid states). A low level of 25(OH)D suggests the presence of either malabsorption of vitamin D or ingestion of a drug that alters hepatic metabolism of vitamin D or 25(OH)D. Plasma levels of $1,25(OH)_2D_3$ would likely be normal or even possibly slightly elevated in sporadic hypophosphatemia or primary hyperparathyroidism, respectively. However, $1,25(OH)_2D$ levels are invariably low in tumor-associated osteomalacia. Finally, a bone biopsy processed as an undecalcified specimen will provide the ultimate diagnostic confirmation of osteomalacia and provide information of the presence or absence of hyperparathyroidism (primary or secondary).

Question

3. Discuss treatment of osteomalacia in this patient.

Answer

In osteomalacia developing as a consequence of hypophosphatemia and phosphate depletion, treatment with oral phorphorus supplements is the first line of therapy. Doses vary as a function of the control of hypophosphatemia but usually involve administration of 2–4 g/day of elemental phosphorus in divided doses. Vitamin D in the form of vitamin D_2 or D_3, as well as modest oral calcium supplements, may also be administered to facilitate skeletal remineralization. In tumor-associated osteomalacia extreme vitamin D resistance may be encountered, in which case the use of dihydrotachysterol may be useful (1–2.5 mg/day). Treatment with calcitriol in doses of 1–5 μg/day has been used with success on an experimental basis.

Case 2

A 63-year-old man has been treated with hemodialysis for 3 years. At the dialysis unit he complains of rib pain over the right chest wall. A roentgenogram reveals fractures of the fifth and sixth ribs. He states that the pain developed following a severe coughing spell. He is an extremely compliant individual, sticks to his protein restriction diet, and faithfully takes aluminum hydroxide antacids as recommended by his internist. The following serum biochemical tests are reported: creatinine 14.3 mg/dl, BUN 64 mg/dl, calcium 8.9 mg/dl, phosphate 1.7 mg/dl, alkaline phosphatase 286 IU/ml, PTH 643 μEq/ml (normal <100 μEq/ml, N-terminal assay) 25(OH)D 10 ng/ml.

Question

1. Discuss the diagnostic considerations concerning metabolic bone disease in this patient.

Answer

Diagnosis of the type of metabolic bone disease cannot be established definitively without a bone biopsy in this patient. However, the presence of the extremely low serum phosphate level in a dialysis patient suggests the possibility of iatrogenic phosphorus depletion. The serum level of 25(OH)D is also lower than would be expected in the average dialysis patient in the western United States. A low level of 25(OH)D also points toward a possible diagnosis of underlying osteomalacia. Withdrawal or reduction of aluminum hydroxide treatment will permit the phosphate levels to return to normal. If the serum calcium level falls, this will also support the presence of either osteomalacia or a mixed histologic picture. The levels of PTH and alkaline phosphatase would be of no help in differential diagnosis of the type of renal osteodystrophy in this case.

Question

2. Discuss management of this patient.

Answer

Parathyroid surgery would be contraindicated. The bone biopsy is likely to indicate either osteomalacia or a mixed histologic picture in this patient. Aluminum hydroxide treatment should be temporized, allowing serum phosphorus levels to seek a normal level. In the presence of osteomalacia (suspected or confirmed), particularly if, as is highly likely the serum calcium level falls, should be managed with some form of vitamin D therapy. Available agents of particular usefulness include $25(OH)D_3$ (Calcifediol, UpJohn Company) and $1,25(OH)_2D_3$ (Calcitriol/Rocaltrol, Hoffman-La Roche, Inc.).

SUGGESTED READING

Avioli LV, Krane SM (eds): *Metabolic Bone Disease,* vol 1 and 2. New York, Academic Press, 1978.

Marx SJ, Spiegel AM, Brown EM, et al: A familial syndrome of decrease in sensitivity to 1,25-dihydroxy-vitamin D. *J Clin Endocrinol Metab* 47:1303–1310, 1978.

Purnell DC, Scholz DA, Smith LH, et al: Treatment of primary hyperparathyroidism. *Am J Med* 56:800–809, 1974.

Sherrard DJ, Baylink DJ, Wergedahl JE, Maloney N: Quantitative histological studies on the pathogenesis of uremic bone disease. *J Clin Endocrnol Metab* 39:119–128, 1974.

Sitrin M, Meredith S, Rosenberg IH: Vitamin D deficiency and bone disease in gastrointestinal disorders. *Arch Intern Med* 135:886–888, 1978.

Thompson DL, Frame B: Involutional osteopenia: Current concepts. *Ann Intern Med* 85:789–803, 1976.

8 STEWART A. MIDDLER

Addison's Disease and Cushing's Syndrome

Adrenocortical physiology and the syndromes of glucocorticoid hyposecretion and hypersecretion are the subjects of this chapter. The hyposecretory states to be considered include primary adrenocortical insufficiency (Addison's disease), secondary adrenocortical failure due to hypothalamic-pituitary disease, and hypothalamic-pituitary suppression. Adrenocortical hypersecretion includes the many causes of Cushing's syndrome.

ADRENOCORTICAL PHYSIOLOGY

The human adrenal cortex is anatomically and functionally segregated into three zones. The outermost zona glomerulosa secretes the potent salt-retaining mineralocorticoid aldosterone. It is controlled mainly by the renin–angiotensin system, with only minor influences by adrenocorticotropin (ACTH). Destructive diseases of the cortex impair both aldosterone and glucocorticoid secretion. This combined defect is responsible for the manifestations of Addison's disease.

The zona fasciculata is the site of production of cortisol, the major glucocorticoid of humans. This steroid has diverse metabolic effects, including the stimulation of gluconeogenesis and acceleration of protein catabolism. It also may have a "permissive" effect on other hormone systems, such as the catecholamine pressor response. The zona fasciculata is dependent on ACTH stimulation for continued cortisol secretion.

The innermost zona reticularis produces mainly the androgenic adrenal steroids such as dehydroepiandrosterone (DHEA) and its sulfate, and androstenedione. These are weak androgens compared to testosterone, but in prepubertal males and adult females they provide the major source of androgen activity. Axillary and pubic hair growth in the normal woman is felt to be dependent on these steroids.

Adrenocorticotropin

In the absence of ACTH secretion, the zona fasciculata rapidly atrophies, and cortisol secretion falls to zero. ACTH is formed by basophilic pituitary corticotrophs as part of a much larger polypeptide hormone, pro-opiomelanocortin. This molecule contains the amino acid sequences of ACTH and β-lipotropin (β-LPH), as well as endorphins and several melanotropic substances. After numerous enzymatic cleavages, ACTH and β-LPH appear in the circulation. The former may provide most of the melanocyte-stimulating hormone activity in humans.

The measurement of ACTH by radioimmunoassay requires that blood be drawn into a plastic heparinized syringe and centrifuged rapidly in a cold plastic or siliconized glass tube, and the plasma immediately frozen.

The 39-amino-acid ACTH molecule is secreted in a pulsatile manner into the circulation under hypothalamic control. It is regulated by a biologic clock that is responsible for a diurnal variation, with an apex occurring about 1 hour after awakening in the morning, followed by a gradual decline with a nadir between 3 and 8 hours after the onset of sleep. These pulsatile increments in serum ACTH levels are followed almost immediately by a parallel increase in serum cortisol levels. From 12 to 30 mg of cortisol are produced daily, and this may increase to 200–300 mg in response to severe stress.

The circadian secretion of ACTH may be altered by a stress-related increase in a hypothalamic corticotropin-releasing factor (CRF). Glucocorticoids suppress ACTH by both a direct feedback on the corticotrophs and by inhibiting CRF release.

Most circulating cortisol is bound to a specific hepatic protein called cortisol-binding globulin or transcortin. Because estrogens rapidly stimulate transcortin production, cortisol levels rise in pregnancy and after the administration of exogenous estrogens.

Cortisol is metabolized in the liver, conjugated with glucouronide, and excreted in the urine as various end products. These are quantitated clinically as 17-hydroxycorticosteroids (17-OHCS) with a normal range of 3–7 mg/day per gram of creatinine excreted. The 17-ketogenic steroid (17-KGS) excretion is somewhat higher, since it includes several other steroid metabolites including pregnanetriol. 17-Ketosteroid excretion (17-KS) reflects mainly adrenal androgen secretion and has little place in the evaluation of hypercortisolism except in attempting to differentiate adrenal carcinoma from adenoma (vide infra). It has no value in work-ups for patients for adrenocortical insufficiency.

ADRENOCORTICAL INSUFFICIENCY

Thomas Addison first described primary adrenocortical failure in 1855. Its dramatic clinical presentation with progressive hyperpigmentation, profound asthenia, anorexia, gastrointestinal disturbances, weight loss, orthostatic hypotension, hyperkalemia, hypokaliuria, hyponatremia and, in the extreme, cardiovascular collapse, is a striking demonstration of the physiologic importance of adrenocortical function. Appropriate therapy with salt and water repletion, and treatment with glucocorticoids and mineralocorticoids, will lead to rapid recovery in those who have what was considered a fatal disease 40 years ago.

The clinical presentation as just described represents only the most flagrant cases of Addison's disease. Lesser degrees of adrenal hypofunction, secondary adrenal atrophy, and a larger number of conditions that simulate this disease may present challenges in differential diagnosis to even the most expert physicians.

The causes of Addison's disease include bilateral adrenalectomy, tuberculosis, nontuberculous granulomatous diseases, and autoimmune adrenalitis. Until 1950, tuberculosis was the major cause of Addison's disease, although in recent series, it accounts for less than 15% of cases.

Nontuberculous granulomatous diseases have been reported in small numbers to have caused adrenal failure, including histoplasmosis, blastomycosis, coccidioidmycosis, and sarcoidosis. Histoplasmosis frequently involves the adrenals when it disseminates; however, destruction of enough of the gland (90–100%) needed to produce the Addisonian syndrome is unusual.

Metastatic carcinoma, particularly from lung and breast, involves the adrenals not uncommonly; however, hormonal insufficiency rarely occurs.

At the present time, the most common cause of Addison's disease is primary adrenal atrophy or autoimmune adrenalitis. Pathologically, the adrenals are atrophic and are infiltrated with lymphocytes, plasma cells, epithelial cells, and fibrosis. Autoimmune endocrine disease is discussed in Chapter 18, but several comments are pertinent here. Over 50% of patients with primary adrenal atrophy have demonstrable circulating antibodies to adrenal tissue. These antibodies may be present months to years before the development of adrenal insufficiency. On the other hand, antiadrenal antibodies are found infrequently in tuberculous adrenalitis or in normal controls (less than 5%).

The association of autoimmune adrenalitis with lymphocytic thyroiditis (Schmidt's syndrome), as well as other autoimmune endocrine and nonendocrine diseases, is well documented. These include insulin-dependent diabetes mellitus, hypoparathyroidism, premature ovarian failure, Graves' disease, pernicious anemia, myasthenia gravis, alopecia totalis, and vitiligo. The diathesis of autoimmune endocrinopathy may be familial in many instances (Chapter 18).

Other much rarer causes of adrenal failure include amyloid infiltration, adrenal hemorrhage in endotoxic shock or with use of anticoagulants, familial insensitivity to ACTH, and adrenoleukodystrophy. The latter is a rare X-linked disorder affecting the cerebral white matter with adrenocortical degeneration appearing in childhood.

Clinical Manifestations

Over 80% of Addisonian patients have hyperpigmentation due to the hypersecretion of ACTH and perhaps other pigmentary hormones derived from pro-opiomelanocortin. This may be manifested by generalized increased darkening of the skin, areolae, nevi, and recent surgical scars, or by localized areas of hyperpigmentation over flexor surfaces, in body creases, and on the buccal mucous membrane.

Weakness and fatiguability occur in the vast majority of Addisonian patients. Rest and a good night's sleep may restore strength, but stamina rapidly wanes as the day progresses. This has been said to contrast with psychogenic asthenia, which is often unrelieved by rest. Anorexia and weight loss are almost universal. Other gastrointestinal complaints include nausea, vomiting, chronic diarrhea, and acute abdominal pain which may be associated with an adrenal crisis.

Postural hypotension and tachycardia, sometimes with lightheadedness or syncope, is due to mineralocorticoid insufficiency and salt depletion. Excessive perspiration or gastrointestinal fluid losses aggravate this condition.

Other clinical manifestations of interest are microcardia on chest roentgenograms and hardening of the ear cartilage and its occasional calcification.

Adrenal Crisis

Acute adrenocortical failure can occur after abrupt steroid withdrawal or during an intercurrent infection in a patient with chronic adrenal failure. Severe hypotension, tachycardia, hyperpyrexia, dehydration, azotemia, abdominal pain, and coma progressing to death may rapidly ensue in the absence of definitive treatment.

Table 1 **Laboratory Abnormalities Associated with Addison's Disease**

Hyponatremia
Hyperkalemia
Elevated BUN and creatinine levels
Normocytic anemia
Eosinophilia
Lymphocytosis
Hypercalcemia
Hypoglycemia

Laboratory Abnormalities

The *sine qua non* in the diagnosis of Addison's disease is the demonstration of abnormally low cortisol secretion and an inadequate response to exogenous ACTH. Baseline plasma ACTH levels are usually high-normal to distinctly elevated. Multiple other laboratory studies may be abnormal as the pathophysiologic consequence of glucocorticoid and mineralocorticoid deficiency (Table 1).

Although common, electrolyte abnormalities are by no means universal in patients with Addison's disease. Hyponatremia results from sodium loss due to aldosterone deficiency and gastrointestinal losses as well as a dilutional effect because of impaired free water clearance. Hyponatremic Addisonian patients usually have inappropriately elevated urine sodium levels which help distinguish them from patients with primary sodium depletion or congestive heart failure, where urinary sodium is quite low. The syndrome of inappropriate antidiuretic hormone secretion (SIADH) (Chapter 3) may also cause hyponatremia with high urine sodium concentrations; however, the BUN and uric acid levels are usually quite low in SIADH, the opposite of what is seen in Addison's disease. Hyperkalemia is generally not seen with SIADH.

The hyperkalemia and metabolic acidosis of Addison's disease are a consequence of aldosterone deficiency and the resultant impairment of distal nephron exchange of sodium for potassium and hydrogen ions. The differential diagnosis of hyperkalemia is limited to only a few disorders, including end-stage renal failure, potassium-retaining diuretics, very rare disorders of renal tubular potassium transport, and hypoaldosteronism. Hypoaldosteronism may be due to panadrenocortical failure or may be an isolated defect (Chapter 9).

Diagnostic Studies

Earlier tests, such as impaired excretion of a water load or the eosinopenic response to an ACTH infusion, are now of only historical interest.

In general, a measurement of the baseline serum cortisol level or its diurnal variation is not sufficiently specific or sensitive and may be normal in Addison's disease; however, measurements of cortisol levels in an acutely ill hypotensive patient where the diagnosis is suspect can often be diagnostic. Blood for cortisol and ACTH measurements may be drawn, and the patient then treated presumptively with saline and parenteral glucocorticoids. A good therapeutic response and a subsequent laboratory report of an inappropriately low cortisol level (and an elevated ACTH level, when available) can be considered diagnostic proof of Addison's disease.

Most diagnostic tests are performed on patients not acutely ill. In general, they involve measuring the response of serum cortisol or urinary cortisol or 17-OHCS to ACTH injection. Synthetic $^{1-24}$ corticotropin polypeptide, or cosyntropin (Cortrosyn, Synacthen), has replaced the use of animal pituitary extracts.

Cosyntropin, 0.25 mg, is given intravenously or intramuscularly, and blood for cortisol testing is drawn at 0, 30, and 60 minutes. A normal response is a doubling of the serum cortisol level, with an increment of at least 7.0 μg/dl or a maximal level of at least 19–20 μg/dl.

Patients who have secondary adrenocortical deficiency due to hypothalamic-pituitary diseases or prolonged pituitary suppression may also be unresponsive to acute ACTH stimulation. Under these circumstances, plasma ACTH levels are low or in the midnormal range and are never elevated. Prolonged ACTH stimulation will, however, demonstrate adrenocortical responsiveness. Cosyntropin, 0.25 mg, is given as an intravenous infusion in normal saline over 8 hours daily for 3 days. On the last day, urinary free cortisol, 17-OHCS, or 17-KGS levels should be 2 to $2\frac{1}{2}$ times greater than baseline values and above the upper range of normal values. Some investigators also rely on the response of serum cortisol after prolonged ACTH infusion. A continuous 48-hour infusion of ACTH has also been used to document secondary adrenocortical insufficiency.

The hypothalamic-pituitary-adrenal axis may also be tested by the response to insulin-induced hypoglycemia, pyrogen, or vasopressin injection. For most clinical purposes, these tests have little to recommend them, although cortisol secretion may be efficiently evaluated if the tests are performed for other purposes (e.g., testing growth hormone secretion; see Chapter 2).

Metyrapone testing may be of some usefulness in differentiating primary from secondary adrenal failure. This drug inhibits cortisol production by blocking the enzyme that converts 11-deoxycortisol (compound S) to cortisol, resulting in increased secretion of the former and decreased secretion of the latter. This reduction in the circulating cortisol level lessens the feedback inhibition of ACTH secretion. The increase in the ACTH level stimulates steroidogenesis, which is measured by the serum level of compound S. In order to have a normal response to metyrapone, the subject must have an intact hypothalamic-pituitary-adrenal axis.

A short metyrapone test involves administering 2.5–3.0 g orally at 11:00 PM and measuring the serum compound S level at 8:00 AM. A value of 8.0 μg/dl or greater is considered a normal response. If the test is abnormal, a simultaneous serum cortisol level must be checked to ensure that adequate enzymatic blockage of its production has occurred.

The prolonged metyrapone test requires that 750 mg be given every 4 hours for six doses. Serum compound S may be measured as above, or the total urinary 17-OHCS concentration, which includes the metabolites of 11-deoxycortisol, can be quantitated. On the day of the test or the following day, this value should be at least twice the baseline value. Acute adrenocortical insufficiency may be precipitated by this test; caution must be taken.

Supraphysiologic doses of glucocorticoids may cause hypothalamic-pituitary-adrenal suppression of variable duration and intensity. The maximum safe dose and duration are not known. A week of moderate dose prednisone can be given without major concern. Beyond about 2 weeks, adrenal insufficiency may occur and persist for weeks or months. Single daily doses of prednisone are less likely to cause suppression than multiple daily doses. Patients treated with alternate-day therapy with up to 40 mg of prednisone are the least likely to have hypothalamic-pituitary-adrenal suppression.

One approach to avoiding adrenal insufficiency after prolonged suppression, either endogenously or exogenously, is to taper the pharmacologic doses as permitted by the underlying disease state and the patient's clinical response. When the equivalent of 20 mg of cortisol per day is reached (approximately 5 mg of prednisone), cortisol is given daily in the morning. Since it has a much shorter half-life than the synthetic glucocorticoids, it will not suppress the early morning rise in ACTH secretion. The cortisol dose is tapered over 4 weeks to 10 mg each morning. After several more weeks, a morning serum cortisol level is measured. This value represents endogenous secretion. When it is greater than 10 μg/dl, the cortisol supplementation can be discontinued except during times of physiologic stress. After several weeks off all supplementation, a short cosyntropin test can be used to demonstrate resumption of adrenocortical responsiveness. A normal result predicts a normal cortisol response to acute surgical stress.

It is good practice to admonish all patients withdrawn from moderate dose glucocorticoid therapy about the need for steroid coverage during physiologic stress for periods up to 1 year later.

Treatment

Maintenance therapy for adrenocortical failure requires the administration of glucocorticoids equivalent to 20–30 mg/day of cortisol. This is frequently given in a dose of 20 mg in the morning (or 25 mg as cortisone acetate) with one-half as much being given at noon or in the evening. An occasional patient will find that using a t.i.d. regimen of the same total daily dose is better. Many patients do quite well taking 5.0 mg of prednisone each morning. The adequacy of cortisone or cortisol treatment may be documented by measuring serum cortisol levels 30–60 minutes after the morning dose and just before the evening dose. Appropriate levels are 25–30 μg/dl, and 6.0 μg/dl, respectively.

The glucocorticoid dose should be doubled for moderate medical illnesses, such as influenza or gastroenteritis. More severe stresses, such as serious pneumonia, myocardial infarction, or general surgery, may require 100–300 mg/day.

Patients and their families should have access to an injectable glucocorticoid such as methylprednisolone (Solu-Medrol) or hydrocortisone hemisuccinate (Solu-Cortef) for emergency use if they cannot take oral medication. Patients should carry or wear medical identification specifying their need for glucocorticoids.

Secondary adrenal insufficiency does not require mineralocorticoid treatment. Addisonian patients need 0.05–0.2 mg/day of fluorohydrocortisone (fludrocortisone; Florinef) and a liberal salt intake to prevent hyperkalemia and salt depletion. Dose adjustment is made by determination of orthostatic changes in blood pressure and pulse and in the serum sodium and potassium levels. There is sufficient mineralocorticoid activity in 150 mg of cortisol so that patients receiving such doses do not need additional therapy.

Adrenal crisis with hyperpyrexia, shock, vomiting, and severe dehydration should be treated with large volumes of normal saline (usually 3–4 liters in the first 24 hours). A rapid infusion of 100 mg of hydrocortisone hemisuccinate is given followed by an additional 200 mg over the next 24 hours. Rapid improvement in blood pressure and clinical symptoms are expected over the next several hours.

Summary

Addison's disease is a constellation of signs and symptoms due to failure of secretion of cortisol and aldosterone. In its florid expression it is easily diagnosed by anyone familiar with its manifestations. It is a rare disease and in its milder forms the symptoms may be quite nonspecific. Most patients with fatigue, asthenia, relative hypotension, or nausea who are evaluated for Addison's disease will be found not to have it. A screening approach with a short cosyntropin test or an overnight metyrapone test will separate most patients who require further evaluation. X-ray examination of the sella turcica, determination of plasma ACTH levels by radioimmunoassay, and perhaps prolonged (48-hour or 3-day) ACTH infusions can then be used for a more definitive diagnosis.

Once primary adrenal failure is diagnosed, antiadrenal antibody tests, x-ray examination looking for adrenal calcification, a tuberculin skin test, and possibly a search for other autoimmune diseases can be undertaken.

If secondary adrenocortical failure is diagnosed (by an abnormal metyrapone response with a normal adrenocortical response to a 3-day ACTH infusion), then studies must be performed to determine its cause (Chapter 2). Appropriate replacement therapy, thorough patient education, and attention to increased steroid requirements during periods of stress should all lead to the return of the patient to vigorous good health and, ultimately, an excellent prognosis.

CUSHING'S SYNDROME

The pathophysiologic consequences of sustained hyperglucocorticoidism is Cushing's syndrome (CS). When it is due to eutopic pituitary ACTH hypersecretion, it is known as *Cushing's disease* (CD), although some endocrinologists reserve this term for cases involving pituitary macroadenomas. In addition, this syndrome may be caused by exogenous steroid administration, ectopic ACTH secretion, or autonomously functioning lesions of the adrenal cortex, including adenomas, carcinomas, and bilateral nodular hyperplasia. The clinical manifestations vary depending on the degree of concomitant secretion of androgens and mineralocorticoids. Table 2 lists the major features of CS.

Etiology

The frequency of causes of CS is listed in Table 3.

Table 2 **Signs and Symptoms of Cushing's Syndrome**

Protein wasting	Muscle atrophy and myopathy; fatigue; thin skin; abdominal pink striae, as well as striae over the breasts, buttocks, and thighs; easy bruisability; growth retardation in children
Abnormal fat distribution	Centripetal obesity, moon facies, dorsal ("buffalo") hump, supraclavicular fat pads, widening of the superior mediastinum
Hematologic changes	Leukocytosis, lymphopenia, eosinopenia, erythrocytosis, capillary fragility with ecchymosis
Carbohydrate intolerance	Diabetes mellitus
Skeletal disorders	Osteoporosis, aseptic necrosis of the hip, hypercalciuria, nephrolithiasis
Dermatologic changes	Acne, facial plethora, downy hair growth, striae, ecchymosis
Immunologic dysfunction	Opportunistic infections such as tuberculosis, systemic fungi, and pneumocystis carinii
Psychoneurotic disorders	Psychosis, depression
Mineralocorticoid excess	Hypertension, hypokalemia, alkalosis, edema
Androgen excess	Hirsutism, virilization, acne, erythrocytosis

Table 3 **Causes of Cushing's Syndrome**

Cushing's disease (bilateral adrenal hyperplasia)	65%
Adrenal adenoma	10%
Adrenal carcinoma	10%
Bilateral nodular hyperplasia	Rare
Ectopic ACTH	15%

Cushing's Disease

This disorder is clearly caused by abnormalities of hypothalamic-pituitary control of ACTH secretion. Some investigators have postulated a primary hypothalamic dysfunction; however, apparent cure after selective removal of an ACTH-secreting pituitary adenoma argues against this. About 10–15% of CS patients have pituitary macroadenomas at the time of examination, and another 10–20% develop obvious pituitary tumors with hyperpigmentation and marked ACTH hypersecretion after bilateral adrenalectomy (Nelson's syndrome). The true incidence of microadenomas is unknown; however, recent studies utilizing transsphenoidal microsurgery have suggested that it might be as high as 100%.

Adrenal Tumors

Adrenal adenomas are unilateral 98% of the time. They rarely occur ectopically in the spleen, ovary, or testes. When they secrete enough cortisol to produce CS, they rarely produce excessive androgens or mineralocorticoids. This is in contrast to adrenocortical carcinomas which often cause a very high secretion of these other adrenal steroids; hence elevated urinary 17-KS, serum DHEA-sulfate, or 11-deoxycortisol levels in a patient with an adrenal tumor suggest that the tumor is malignant. Adrenal adenomas are well described, but infrequent findings in the syndrome of multiple endocrine neoplasia type I (Chapter 17).

Adrenocortical carcinomas are usually large (greater than 6.0 cm in diameter and greater than 100 g) at presentation and frequently palpable. Although they may occur at any age, they are the most common cause of CS in children (65%). Metastases occur in the liver, vena cava, lung, and, rarely, bone and brain. Spontaneous infarction or hemorrhage into large primary tumors or hepatic metastases may occur. At diagnosis, about 25% are curable, 25% recur after surgery, and 50% are nonresectable.

Bilateral Nodular Hyperplasia

This rare disorder usually behaves endocrinologically like an adrenal tumor. ACTH levels may be undetectable, and cortisol secretion may not be suppressed in response to the usual doses of exogenous glucocorticoids; however, this is highly variable, and easily detectable ACTH levels with suppressible adrenal function, as in CD, have been reported. It has been suggested that the disorder begins as a pituitary-dependent CS that later develops into autonomous bilateral adenomata.

A striking finding in a few young patients with this disorder has been the apparent lack of the usual stigmata of CS but marked osteoporosis.

Ectopic ACTH Syndrome

Many nonpituitary tumors have been described that secrete ACTH and result in bilateral adrenal hyperplasia. These are summarized in Table 4.

Unfortunately, only about 10% of patients have curable tumors at presentation.

Table 4 **ACTH-Secreting Nonpituitary Tumors**

Lung carcinoma (mostly oat cell or undifferentiated)	55%
Thymoma	15%
Pancreatic carcinoma (usually islet cell)	10%
Pheochromocytoma	3%
Bronchial adenoma	2%
Others (medullary thyroid carcinoma, parotid, liver, ovary, breast, esophagus, kidney, testes, stomach, and other carcinomas)	15%

Serum ACTH levels in the ectopic syndrome are usually markedly elevated. This, perhaps along with other melanotropic fragments of pro-opiomelanocortin, accounts for the frequently observed hyperpigmentation in this disorder. It should be noted that elevated ACTH levels without CS due to biologically inactive "big" ACTH occur in many patients with cancer.

The clinical presentation of these patients may not be accompanied by many of the usual stigmata of CS. Weakness and hypokalemic alkalosis may be the sole endocrine manifestations, perhaps because of the rapid downhill course and lack of sufficient time for the other sequelae to occur. The progression of the underlying tumor often dominates the clinical course. Chapter 2 presents further details of the ectopic ACTH syndrome.

Diagnosis

Diagnostic evaluation involves three major steps: the documentation of inappropriate or autonomous hypercortisolism, differentiating tests to determine the etiology of the syndrome, and localization procedures to determine the site of abnormal hormone production.

The most reliable and definitive test for documenting CS is the low-dose dexamethasone suppression test. After giving 0.5 mg of dexamethasone every 6 hours for eight doses, the 17-OHCS level on the second day (while the patient is still receiving dexamethasone) should normally be 2.5 mg/g of creatinine or less, and the urine free cortisol level less than 19–25 μg. False positive results (i.e., lack of suppression) occur about 3% of the time, particularly in severely depressed patients.

Screening tests with somewhat less diagnostic accuracy include measurement of the elevated urine free cortisol level and the overnight dexamethasone suppression test. The urine free cortisol level is abnormal in virtually all patients with CS but the test has a significant incidence (3%) of false positive results, particularly in hospitalized or stressed individuals. The overnight dexamethasone suppression test is performed by giving 1.0 mg of the drug at 11:00 PM to 12:00 AM, and measuring the plasma cortisol level 8 hours later. A normal response is a fall in serum cortisol levels to 5.0 μg/dl or less. This study is abnormal in 98% of patients with CS. False positive results occur in 1% of nonstressed outpatients, in 13% of obese patients, in as many as 25% of hospitalized patients, and in most patients with endogenous depression. Estrogen and diphenylhydantoin will interfere with this last test. Estrogen causes a false positive test result by elevating transcortin levels (vide supra), and diphenylhydantoin by increasing dexamethasone clearance.

Differential Tests

ACTH Levels. Patients with adrenal tumors and most with bilateral nodular hyperplasia have ACTH levels that are undetectable. Since ACTH assays may have significant "noise" in the low-normal range, it is necessary that the physician be familiar with the laboratory being utilized and interpret these studies with caution. This single test separates patients with adrenal tumors or those with autonomous bilateral nodular hyperplasia from patients with eutopic or ectopic ACTH hypersecretion. In CD, the ACTH levels range from midnormal to 3 to 10 times the normal range. Most, however, are below 200 pg/ml. With an ectopic ACTH-secreting tumor levels range from high-normal to 30 times normal and are frequently above 200 pg/ml; however, there is a significant overlap in these two groups. A single plasma ACTH determination costs about $90.00.

High-Dose Dexamethasone Suppression. When dexamethasone is given at 2.0 mg every 6 hours for eight doses, almost all CD patients will suppress ACTH secretion. A 40–50% reduction in 17-OHCS excretion or urine free cortisol levels on the second day occurs in about 93% of CD patients. In contrast, only 3% of adrenal tumors have reportedly produced false positive responses. False positive suppression may also occur with ectopic ACTH secretion, particularly from bronchial adenomas. Cyclic hypersecretion of cortisol by adrenal tumors (periodic hormonogenesis) may explain some of the apparent positive responses to dexamethasone suppression and the rare patient who seems to have a paradoxical increase in steroid excretion in response to exogenous glucocorticoid.

Although some patients with bilateral nodular hyperplasia will not suppress with 8.0 mg of dexamethasone, they may respond to 16–24 mg/day. This may also be true of rare patients with CD who have a higher feedback suppression "set point."

Other Tests. The diagnostic value of a metyrapone test (750 mg every 4 hours for six doses) is flawed by a false positive response in 15–20% of adrenal tumors. An increment of 10 mg/day or doubling of the 17-OHCS excretion is considered consistent with CD.

Likewise, the infusion of ACTH in CD produces a dramatic increase in cortisol secretion, but many adrenal tumors may have ACTH receptors and thus will respond in this test.

Insulin-induced hypoglycemia is not a commonly used test in patients with CS. In normal individuals, it causes an elevation of serum cortisol levels, but about 80% of patients with CS do not respond. The test is useful in diagnosing patients who have an elevated serum cortisol level because of depression or the alcohol pseudo-Cushing's syndrome (vide infra). These patients show normal increases in serum cortisol levels in response to insulin-induced hypoglycemia.

As noted above, 17-KS excretion and serum DHEA-sulfate and 11-deoxycortisol levels are more likely to be elevated in adrenocortical carcinoma than in benign adenomas; however, several large carcinomas have shown normal 17-KS excretion.

Localization

Once CD is diagnosed, polytomograms of the sella turcica and high-resolution computed tomography (CT) scans utilizing coronal sections may demonstrate pituitary microadenomas. The macroadenomas are frequently seen on plain views of the sella.

Abdominal ultrasound and CT scanning provide a high degree of accuracy in localizing adrenal tumors. Many centers can now identify normal-sized adrenal glands with CT scanners and thus can demonstrate unilateral or bilateral enlargement. Arteriography or venography may occasionally be of preoperative value for the surgeon. Bilateral adrenal vein sampling for cortisol to localize unilateral tumors is not as widely needed as before the newer imaging techniques became available.

Scans of the adrenals using radioiodinated cholesterol uptake are utilized at some centers with the appropriate facilities.

When the ectopic ACTH syndrome is suspected, chest roentgenograms, chest tomography, or chest CT scans will disclose 65–70% of the responsible tumors.

Differential Diagnosis

Innumerable patients with obesity, hypertension, and diabetes mellitus are evaluated for suspected CS. Special mention needs to be made of those with severe depression who may have abnormal diurnal variation of serum cortisol levels and a blunted response to dexamethasone suppression. The usefulness of insulin-induced hypoglycemia in this situation is noted above.

Alcoholic pseudo-Cushing's syndrome is a newly described entity in active alcoholics who may have physical stigmata of CS, abnormal diurnal variation in cortisol levels, and abnormal low-dose dexamethasone suppression, but a normal response to insulin hypoglycemia. The abnormal pituitary-adrenal function disappears after alcohol withdrawal.

Treatment

Adrenal Tumors

Removal of an adrenal adenoma cures the disease. Prolonged suppression of the pituitary and the contralateral adrenal requires prolonged administration and slow withdrawal of exogenous glucocorticoids (vide supra).

Adrenal carcinomas that are unresectable or recur may show biochemical and occasionally anatomic evidence of regression with *o,p′*-DDD (Mitotane) therapy. Metyrapone and aminoglutethimide can also be used to treat hypercortisolism by blocking cortisol biosynthesis.

Bilateral nodular hyperplasia requires bilateral adrenalectomy for cure. The later occurrence of Nelson's syndrome has been described.

Ectopic ACTH Syndrome

Patients with curable disease usually have thymomas or bronchial adenomas. *o,p′*-DDD, metyrapone, and aminoglutethimide have all been used to reduce steroid hypersecretion.

Cushing's Disease

Bilateral adrenalectomy has been the preferred treatment for many years. There have been conflicting reports as to whether prophylactic pituitary irradiation lowers the incidence of Nelson's syndrome. Conventional pituitary irradiation cures only about 20% of adults; however, it seems to be highly effective for children and adolescents (80%). The true incidence of postirradiation hypopituitarism is controversial.

o,p′-DDD has been used alone in low doses (3–6 g/day) and in higher doses (8–12 g/day) with and without pituitary irradiation. Glucocorticoid replacement and mineralocorticoids are required when higher doses are used. If the drug is tolerated (nausea, vertigo, ataxia), it can control the disease in most patients and cure some. Long-term follow-up is still inadequate.

Several centers have returned to transsphenoidal microsurgery for CD even in the absence of radiographically demonstrable tumors. In expert hands, it has led to cure after selective adenectomy or hypothesectomy in almost all patients. Morbidity and mortality seem better than with bilateral adrenalectomy. ACTH levels may be suppressed for many months, and thus glucocorticoid replacement is required. The long-term follow-up in terms of possible recurrence or Nelson's syndrome is still in question.

Cyproheptadine, presumably through its antiserotoninergic effect at the hypothalamic-pituitary level, is successful in reducing cortisol levels in about 40% of patients; however, it may cause drowsiness and weight gain, and hypercortisolism recurs on drug withdrawal. Rarely, patients have been described who respond to bromocriptine suppression of ACTH.

Summary

Figure 1 summarizes a diagnostic approach for patients with suspected CS. Definitive diagnosis usually requires the demonstration of abnormal cortisol suppression with the low-dose dexamethasone suppression test. It must be kept in mind that mild or early cases may have normal test results and may have to be restudied several times over various intervals. Urinary 17-OHCS excretion persistently above 2.5 mg/g of creatinine after 0.5 mg every 6 hours on the second day of dexamethasone administration is highly suggestive of CS. Patients with pituitary-dependent disease (CD) may show clear-cut suppression of baseline steroid excretion, even over 50%, but these levels will almost always remain above 2.5 mg/g of creatinine.

After hypercortisolism is documented, measurement of the plasma ACTH level will divide patients into two groups: low plasma ACTH levels in those with primary adrenocortical disease including adenomas and carcinomas, and elevated plasma ACTH levels in those with ACTH hypersecretion, including CD and the ectopic syndrome. The plasma ACTH level and the response to the high-dose dexamethasone suppression should allow the correct diagnosis in the vast majority of patients. The differentiation of benign from malignant adrenal tumors is frequently made at surgery. Bilateral nodular hyperplasia may escape definitive diagnosis by this

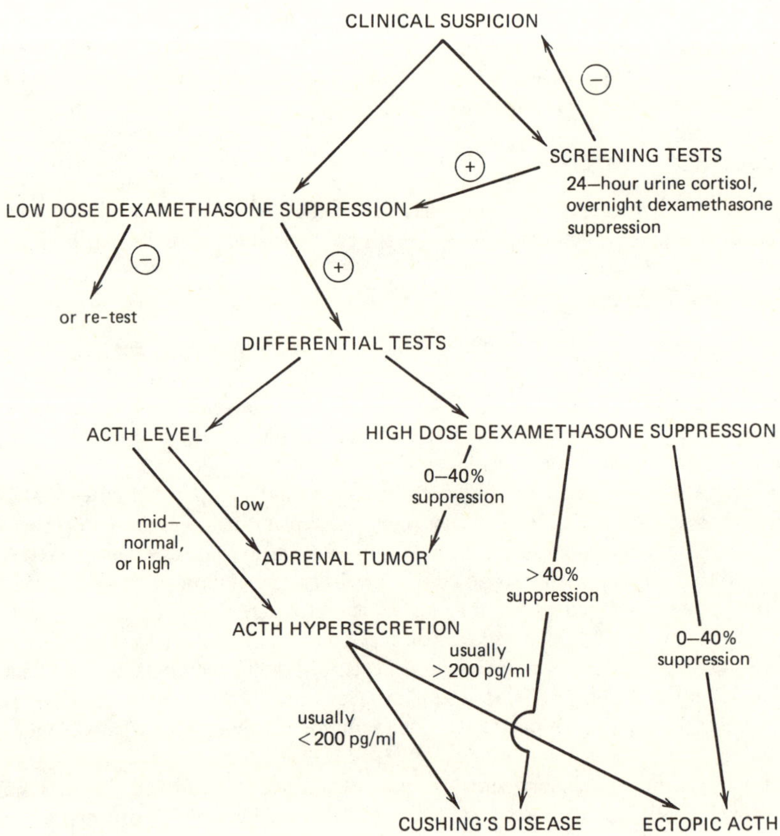

Figure 1. Workup of suspected Cushing's syndrome.

schema; however, bilateral adrenal enlargement on CT scanning for a suspected adrenal tumor or the discovery of multiple adenomas at the time of surgery may help identify this very unusual lesion.

DISCUSSION CASES

Case 1

A 21-year-old woman developed exophthalmos, painless goiter, hyperthyroidism, and an elevated level of antithyroid antibodies. Radioiodine uptake was low. Hypothyroidism spontaneously occurred 2 months later. She was treated with L-thyroxine.

A cosyntropin test was done at age 24 because of hyperpigmentation, but she otherwise felt well. Her serum cortisol level was 8–9 μg/dl, both before and after cosyntropin administration. The basal plasma ACTH level was 350 pg/ml (normal 20–100 pg/ml). Hydrocortisone, 20 mg every morning and 10 mg every evening, was prescribed. The following summer, she developed syncope and hyperkalemia after excessive perspiration.

Comment

This patient developed three autoimmune diseases: exophthalmos, Hashimoto's thyroiditis (Hashitoxicosis), and Addison's disease. Although the basal cortisol level was in the normal range, hyperpigmentation had developed and the ACTH level was distinctly elevated. As expected, exogenous ACTH did not elevate the serum cortisol level further. The need for mineralocorticoid was not appreciated until the patient experienced excessive salt loss through perspiration.

Case 2

After recent hospitalization for depression and anxiety a 30-year-old woman had normal values for serum cortisol levels over a 2-year period. She was later evaluated for weakness, weight gain, easy bruising, moon facies, and severe anxiety with paranoid features. Urine 17-OHCS levels were 24, 33, and 43 mg/24 hr. On 0.5 mg of dexamethasone every 6 hours, for 2 days, 17-OHCS levels were 36 and 29 mg/day. On 2.0 mg every 6 hours, 17-OHCS values were 8.8 and 4.0 mg/day. The basal plasma ACTH level was 210 pg/ml (normal 20–100 pg/ml).

The urine free cortisol level was 921 μg/24 hr (normal 20–90 μg/24 hr). On cyproheptadine, this value fell to normal (48, 72, and 43 μg/24 hr). One year after pituitary irradiation, the cyproheptadine was discontinued, and the urine cortisol level again became elevated. Despite normal sella polytomograms, a transsphenoidal adenectomy was performed and a small adenoma was removed. Postoperatively, replacement cortisol was required for 6 months until normal pituitary-adrenal responsiveness returned.

Comment

This case of CD went undiagnosed, although suspected, for 2 years, because of confusion brought about by the psychiatric component and the fact that basal serum cortisol levels were persistently normal. Crapo points out that there are no highly reliable criteria for ruling out CD based on basal serum values. Once the urine cortisol and 17-OHCS levels were measured, the diagnosis was easily confirmed. There was no suppression of 17-OHCS on low-dose dexamethasone, and a clear-cut fall on high-dose suppression.

The effectiveness of cyproheptadine and the subsequent cure after a selective transsphenoidal adenectomy suggest that the cyproheptadine either directly suppressed the microadenoma or inhibited hypothalamic stimulation of this tumor. There is in vitro data suggesting a direct effect on pituitary adenomas of this drug. CD has not recurred in $2\frac{1}{2}$ years since adenectomy.

Case 3

As a 14-year-old boy, the patient had been treated with a subtotal thyroidectomy for Graves' disease. In 1966, at age 35, he developed profound fatigue. Two months later, there was an "influenzal illness" with chills, fever, and headache followed by abdominal pain, vomiting, constipation, and a blood pressure of 90/60. Addison's disease was diagnosed on the basis of urinary 17-KS measurements of 1.8 and 3.2 mg/24 hr (normal 10–20 mg/24 hr). The serum sodium concentration was 125 mEq/liter and hyperkalemia was noted. He was given intramuscular deoxycorticosterone acetate (DOCA) which normalized the serum potassium level and actually produced hypokalemia and hypertension. The patient did fairly well until 1972 when he became dehydrated following an upper respiratory infection. He was admitted to another hospital where he was treated with cortisone acetate, 25 mg in the morning, and fluorohydrocortisone, 0.1 mg daily. The DOCA, however, was continued. The hypertension and headaches worsened, and antihypertensives were eventually prescribed.

The mineralocorticoids were later discontinued, and only cortisone was given. Because of periodically elevated serum potassium levels, the cortisone dose was increased to 40 mg daily. When seen in July of 1979 the patient had been off mineralocorticoids for 2 years. He had severe fatigue and paresthesias of the extremities. His blood pressure was 112/85, seated and standing. There was mild bilateral proptosis and periorbital edema. Laboratory studies revealed the following: serum creatinine 2.0 mg/dl, BUN 42 mg/dl, sodium 130 mEq/l, potassium 6.0 mEq/1, adjusted serum thyroxine (T_4) 1.9 μg/dl (normal 5–13 dl), serum TSH greater than 100 μU/ml (normal, less than 4 μU). Hydrocortisone was prescribed at 15 mg every morning and 10 mg every evening and fluorohydrocortisone, 0.1 mg every other day. After adequate treatment of adrenal insufficiency, L-thyroxine was started and gradually increased to 0.15 mg/day. On this regimen, the blood pressure has remained at about 125/90, the sodium and potassium levels are normal, the serum creatinine is 1.5 mg/dl, and the BUN level is 16 mg/dl. The serum T_4 level is normal. The patient feels better than he has in 14 years.

Comment

The salient features of this amazing story include a history of Graves' disease associated with Addison's disease presumably due to autoimmune adrenalitis. Antiadrenal antibodies measured in 1979 were negative. Multiple errors in the patient's original management are obvious.

17-KS is generally a poor test for Addison's disease, since it does not reflect glucocorticoid secretion, and adrenal unresponsiveness to ACTH was never documented; however, the hyperkalemia and its subsequent correction with mineralocorticoid substantiate the diagnosis of primary adrenal failure.

This man's treatment was obviously inappropriate, since a mineralocorticoid (DOCA) was initially prescribed even to the point of toxicity manifested by hypertension, headache, and hypokalemia. He was then given a glucocorticoid which was inappropriately increased in an attempt to control the hyperkalemia that recurred after the mineralocorticoid was discontinued. In the midst of this confusion, his physicians neglected the fact that the patient was more than

20 years post-subtotal thyroidectomy for Graves' disease and had developed rather profound hypothyroidism. The institution of rather straightforward hormonal replacement therapy in this patient has made a remarkable difference in his state of health and well-being.

SUGGESTED READING

Anderson PB, Fein SH, Frey WG III: Familial Schmidt's syndrome. *J Am Med Assoc* 224:2068–2070 1980.

Bigos ST, Somma M, Rassio E, et al: Cushing's disease: Management by transsphenoidal pituitary microsurgery. *J Clin Endocrinol Metab* 50:348–354, 1980.

Brown RD, et al: Cushing's disease with periodic hormonogenesis: One explanation for paradoxical response to dexamethasone. *J Clin Endocrinol Metab* 36:445–451, 1973.

Byyng, RL: Withdrawal from glucocorticoid therapy. *N Engl J Med* 295:30–32, 1976.

Carroll BJ, et al: Plasma dexamethasone concentration and cortisol suppression response in patients with endogenous depression. *J Clin Endocrinol Metab* 51:433–437, 1980.

Crapo L: Cushing's syndrome: A review of diagnostic tests. *Metabolism* 28:955–977, 1979.

Gold EM: The Cushing syndromes: Changing views of diagnosis and treatment. *Ann Intern Med* 90:829–844, 1979.

Graber AL, Ney RL, Nicholson WE, et al: Natural history of pituitary-adrenal recovery following long-term suppression with glucocorticoids. *J Clin Endocrinol Metab* 25:11–16, 1965.

Imura H: Ectopic hormone syndromes. *Clin Endocrinol Metab* 9:235–260, 1980.

Jennings AS, Liddle GW, Orth DN: Results of treating childhood Cushing's disease with pituitary irradiation. *N Engl J Med* 297:957–962, 1977.

Kahlet H, Binder C: The value of an ACTH test in assessing hypothalamic-pituitary-adrenocortical function in glucocorticoid treated patients. *Br Med J* 2:147–149, 1973.

Lamberts SW, Klijn FG, de Jong FH, et al: Hormone secretion in alcohol induced pseudo-Cushing's syndrome. *J Am Med Assoc* 242:1640–1643, 1979.

Linfoot, JA: *Recent Advances in the Diagnosis and Treatment of Pituitary Tumors*. New York, Raven Press, 1979.

Lufton JP, Mahoudeau JA, Bouchard P, et al. Treatment of Cushing's disease by *o,p'*-DDD. *N Engl J Med* 300:459–464, 1979.

Moore TJ, Dluhy RG, Williams GH, et al. Nelson's syndrome: Frequency, prognosis, and effect of prior pituitary irradiation. *Ann Intern Med* 85:731–734, 1976.

Oki S, Nakao K, Issey T, et al: Concomitant secretion of adrenocorticotropin, beta-endorphin and gamma melanotropin from perfused pituitary tumor cells of Cushing's disease. *J Clin Endocrinol Metab* 52:42–49, 1981.

Suda T, Demura H, et al: Anterior pituitary hormones in plasma and pituitaries from patients with Cushing's disease. *J Clin Endocrinol Metab* 51:1048–1053, 1980.

9 MICHAEL L. TUCK

Disorders of Aldosterone Secretion

PRIMARY ALDOSTERONISM

Introduction

Adrenal causes of hypertension are quite rare, yet are extremely important in that they represent in most cases curable forms of hypertension. Also, they serve as models for gaining further understanding of other types of hypertensive processes. The human adrenal cortex secretes several steroids with predominately mineralocorticoid properties, the most important being aldosterone. These steroids by definition bind to specific receptor sites in the kidney and other tissues that regulate electrolyte transport. Several precursor steroids including 11-deoxycorticosterone, corticosterone, 18-hydroxycorticosterone, and 18-hydrodeoxycorticosterone manifest variable degrees of mineralocorticoid potency. Deoxycorticosterone is the most potent of the nonaldosterone steroids, demonstrating about one-thirtieth the potency of aldosterone. The major adrenal glucocorticoid, cortisol, has minimal mineralocorticoid potency under normal conditions, but in excessive amounts can take on enhanced mineralocorticoid activity. Aldosterone and other mineralocorticoids act to augment sodium reabsorption in exchange for potassium or hydrogen ion excretion in the distal nephron. Primary aldosteronism serves as the major example of a mineralocorticoid excess syndrome and implies autonomous hypersecretion by the adrenal gland of this steroid. The term *primary* signifies that the hypersecretion of aldosterone has its origin within the adrenal gland, whereas in various forms of *secondary* aldosteronism the stimulus is extraadrenal in origin. There are two major pathologic forms of primary aldosteronism. Until recently it was thought that most cases of primary aldosteronism were due to a single or, infrequently, multiple aldosterone-producing adrenal adenomas. However, it is currently recognized that between 15 and 30% of all cases involve bilateral adrenal cortical hyperplasia as the source of excessive aldosterone production. In rare cases primary aldosteronism is caused by an adrenal carcinoma or multiple adenomata, and it has been reported in the absence of demonstrable adrenal histological changes.

Incidence

No accurate figure for the incidence of primary aldosteronism in the hypertensive population has been established. At one extreme, a recent retrospective survey of the frequency of surgical treatment of aldosterone-producing adenomas at a large clinic revealed a 0.01% incidence or one case in 10,000 patients with hypertension. In contrast, a recent prospective report on 1,036 hypertensive subjects carefully screened for primary aldosteronism revealed an unexpectedly high 2.2% prevalence rate. This study also reported that 6 of 76 black hypertensive patients (8%) had primary aldosteronism. Given the problems with prevalence rates, the knowledge that the disease is difficult and expensive to diagnose, requiring special testing procedures, makes it difficult to establish how carefully hypertensive subjects should be evaluated for primary aldosteronism.

Clinical Features

Most pathophysiologic findings in primary aldosteronism can be accounted for by the effects of this mineralocorticoid on sodium and potassium transport. The physiologic actions of aldosterone include increased renal tubular reabsorption of sodium with concomitant secretion of potassium or hydrogen ions. Although the site of action of aldosterone is the renal distal convoluted tubule, it also acts on similar electrolyte transport mechanisms in salivary and sweat glands and the gastrointestinal tract mucosa. The subcellular mechanism of action of aldosterone is similar to that of most steroid hormones, with specific binding to cytoplasmic receptors in target tissue and subsequent nuclear interaction of a hormone–receptor complex to activate transcription and subsequent induction of specific proteins. It is uncertain whether aldosterone-induced protein controls sodium entry into the apical cell membrane or acts on the Na,K-ATPase membrane pump in the basal membrane. Excessive aldosterone production in primary aldosteronism causes arterial hypertension in all patients. Factors other than volume expansion, such as arteriolar sodium content and vascular and sympathetic reactivity, may also contribute to the genesis of hypertension in primary aldosteronism. Blood pressure elevation, contrary to previous beliefs, is not mild; severe and sustained hypertension is the rule. Malignant hypertension, however, is rare in this disease. Many patients have only hypertension and lack other symptoms, confusing the clinical differentiation of this disease from the larger essential hypertensive population. Aldosterone excess increases renal tubular secretion of potassium, producing intra- and extracellular depletion of this electrolyte. Many symptoms in primary aldosteronism can be accounted for by potassium depletion. Potassium maintains excitability of nerve and muscle tissue by affecting the electrical potential difference across the cell membrane. A prominent complaint in primary aldosteronism is muscle weakness and fatigue, more pronounced in the lower extremities and occasionally progressing to complete paralysis. Weakness and fatigue are the most common symptoms in this disease. Potassium depletion, particularly if severe, produces a renal concentrating defect. Patients frequently have nocturnal polyuria sometimes associated with polydipsia. Polyuria and polydipsia are frequently resistant to vasopressin administration, but potassium repletion completely reverses the symptoms. Chronic hypokalemia also alters the electrical potential of myocardial cells, leading to the electrocardiographic findings of the widened Q-T interval and U waves in this disease. Hypokalemia may cause the diminished glucose tolerance seen in about 50% of patients with primary aldosteronism. Potassium exerts a direct effect on insulin release from pancreatic beta cells and may also influence insulin action. Aldosterone excess results in a mild metabolic alkalosis which is not due to a direct aldosterone effect but seems best correlated with the degree of hypokalemia in these patients. Physical examination of patients with primary aldosteronism is characterized by a paucity of findings. There are few typical physical stigmata of this disease. Arterial hypertension is the most constant finding, and accompanying prolonged blood pressure elevation there may be mild to moderate hypertensive retinopathy and left ventricular hypertrophy. Evidence of edema is almost always absent. Prolonged hypokalemia can blunt certain circulatory reflex responses, so that postural hypotension with bradycardia can occur. In general, it is almost impossible to differentiate these patients from those with essential hypertension based on clinical findings.

Laboratory Tests

The major biochemical criteria for the diagnosis of primary aldosteronism include:

1. Hypokalemia with inappropriate kaliuresis.
2. Suppressed plasma renin activity.
3. Elevated aldosterone levels that fail to be suppressed by volume expansion.

No single test of the above-listed biochemical abnormalities has enough reliability for potential screening of hypertensive patients. Thus one must rely on fulfillment of two or, better, all three criteria to avoid diagonistic errors.

Potassium

Serum potassium levels are below 3.5 mEq/liter in most patients with primary aldosteronism. Many experts recommend serum potassium determinations as the screening procedure for detecting this disorder. Spontaneous or unprovoked hypokalemia of 2.7 mEq/liter or less in hypertensive patients is in most instances due to primary aldosteronism. Normokalemic primary aldosteronism has been reported in most large study groups. A recent report described serum potassium levels above 3.5 mEq/liter in 11 of 51 patients (22%) with an established diagnosis of primary aldosteronism. Several reports have suggested that salt loading in such patients will reduce the serum potassium level below 3.5 mEq/liter. Others advise examining urinary potassium excretion, with a serum potassium level less than 3.5 mEq/liter and urinary excretion greater than 30 mEq/24 hr being inappropriately high and indicative of aldosterone excess. A number of hypertensive subjects receive or have taken diuretics, resulting in diuretic-induced hypokalemia. After cessation of diuretic therapy urinary potassium excretion promptly falls below 30 mEq/24 hr in diuretic-induced potassium depletion. Conversely, in mineralocorticoid-induced hypokalemia potassium excretion persists at greater than 30 mEq/24 hr. Thus serum and 24-hour urine potassium determinations offer a reasonable and practical screening procedure for primary aldosteronism. The potassium ion is itself a determinent of aldosterone production, with low potassium levels turning off aldosterone secretion. Thus chronic hypokalemia in this disorder may itself reduce tumor production of aldosterone, which in turn would reduce potassium excretion and partially correct the hypokalemia.

Plasma Renin Activity

Aldosterone secretion is regulated by three control mechanisms: the renin–angiotensin system, operating through volume-mediated changes; potassium ion; and ACTH. Under most conditions the renin–angiotensin system predominates and operates via changes in extracellular fluid volume. Renin is a proteolytic enzyme released from the juxtaglomerular cells of the renal afferent arterioles in response sodium restriction, upright posture, and diuretic administration. Released renin acts on a circulating α_2-globulin to cleave the decapeptide, angiotensin I, which is rapidly metabolized by specific converting enzymes (located mainly in the lung) to the octapeptide, angiotensin II. Angiotensin II then directly stimulates the production of aldosterone in the zona glomerulosa region of the adrenal cortex. Angiotensin II is rapidly degraded by several angiotensinases, and a seven-amino-acid heptapeptide metabolite (angiotensin III) is also capable of releasing aldosterone. Released aldosterone acts on the distal tubule to increase sodium retention and restore effective blood volume.

Normally plasma renin activity increases with volume depletion induced by sodium restriction, hemorrhage, upright posture, or diuretic administration. Likewise, volume expansion suppresses plasma renin activity, and the chronic hypervolemia of primary aldosteronism accounts for the markedly suppressed renin levels seen in this disease. Several methods of volume depletion have been used to evaluate renin responsiveness, the most physiologic being 5 days of marked dietary sodium restriction (10 mEq sodium daily) combined with 4 hours of upright posture. A more practical method of testing renin response is administration of a potent diuretic such as furosemide, 60–80 mg orally at 8:00 AM, with measurement of plasma renin activity after 3–4 hours of ambulation. This outpatient procedure can delineate low or suppressed renin levels from normal renin levels. In a recent modification of this protocol, using 1 day of sodium restriction and 40 mg furosemide, a suppressed plasma renin activity (<2.0 ng angiotensin I/ml/hr) after diuretic was found in 46 of 51 (94%) patients with primary aldosteronism. Thus, as a single test, demonstration of suppressed plasma renin activity offers high sensitivity for the diagnosis of primary aldosteronism. This advantage is attenuated by its low specificity since 20–30% of the essential hypertensive population have low or suppressed levels of renin.

Aldosterone Measurements

Aldosterone is secreted from the zona glomerulosa cells of the adrenal cortex, and with normal sodium and potassium intake about 50–250 μg is secreted daily. Aldosterone is secreted in only microgram amounts, is weakly bound to plasma proteins, and is very rapidly inactivated by the liver and kidney. As a result the circulating levels of this hormone are exceedingly low and in the past have been difficult to measure. Thus the more common index of aldosterone has been the measurement of urinary excretion rates. Aldosterone excretory rates measure the acid-labile metabolite of aldosterone in a 24-hour urine specimen; this represents approximately 10% of total daily aldosterone production. Plasma aldosterone levels can now be measured by radioimmunoassay techniques available at most medical centers. The normal range for plasma aldosterone with a regular sodium intake is approximately 5–10 ng/100 ml, and for urinary excretion 10–25 μg/24 hr. However, a word of caution is necessary in interpreting these values. Aldosterone levels vary with time of day, dietary sodium and potassium intake, postural status, and stress conditions of the patient. It is now also recognized that plasma and urinary aldosterone concentrations decrease with advancing age, as does plasma renin activity. In patients over the age of 50 years, aldosterone levels are 30–50% lower than in subjects aged 19–29 years. Thus, in a 60-year-old hypertensive subject, a urinary aldosterone level in the range 10–15 μg/24 hr could signify primary aldosteronism.

Based on the above considerations, it is not surprising that aldosterone levels in primary aldosteronism have been reported as being in the normal range. A recent study reported that 31% of patients with primary aldosteronism had aldosterone excretion rates of less than 20 μg/day. Other investigators have felt that a basal supine plasma aldosterone 8:00 AM value above a certain level (12 ng/dl in one series) is diagnostic of primary aldosteronism. In general, if aldosterone levels in urine and plasma are high, especially if either suppressed renin activity or hypokalemia accompanies these values, the patient has primary aldosteronism. Values overlapping into the normal range will frequently occur, requiring more extensive testing in certain cases. There is some evidence that, at a certain point in this disorder, chronic hypokalemia may itself reduce aldosterone production by the adrenal tumor. Potassium repletion in some patients will return aldosterone levels to their previous elevated state. Therefore, in most patients and especially in those with a serum potassium level below 3.0 mEq/liter, potassium repletion (200 mEq potassium diet for 5 days and/or 60–120 mEq KCl elixir p.o. daily) should be carried out before measurements of aldosterone are made.

An alternative approach has been to examine the effect of volume expansion on aldosterone levels in primary aldosteronism to test for suppressibility of aldosterone. This is based on the knowledge that aldosterone production is relatively autonomous in primary aldosteronism and, since renin is suppressed, there is loss of volume-mediated changes. However, it should be noted that aldosterone-producing tumors do not show complete autonomy, since response to other trophic factors such as potassium and ACTH are retained in this disease. Acute or chronic volume expansion by most methods will not suppress aldosterone levels in primary aldosteronism. In contrast, in normal subjects and in other forms of hypertension adequate volume expansion will result in a 50–80% fall in aldosterone levels from the baseline level. Volume expansion of a magnitude adequate to cause suppression may be performed by oral salt loading (200–300 mEq sodium intake for 5 days), infusion of normal saline (2 liters over 4 hours), or administration of a potent mineralocorticoid (deoxycorticosterone acetate, i.m. 10 mg b.i.d., or fludrocortisone, p.o. 200 μg t.i.d) for 3 days.

Of these procedures the saline infusion study appears to be the most practical (4 hours) and has good diagnostic accuracy, making it the volume-expanding procedure of choice at our institution. One recent large series reported that the saline suppression test yielded the highest sensitivity (0.77) as a single diagnostic test for primary aldosteronism when a postsaline value of plasma aldosterone of greater than 8.5 ng/dl was used as an indicator for primary aldosteronism. Another recent series of 51 patients reported that plasma aldosterone concentration in all subjects who received saline remained above 10 ng/dl. It should be noted that patients should be potassium-repleted if the baseline serum potassium value is less than 3.0 nEq/liter, as saline loading induces a marked kaliuresis in this disorder. Certain patients with evidence of a milder form of primary aldosteronism exhibit a normal aldosterone suppression by volume expansion. This condition has been termed indeterminate hyperaldosteronism. A rare and sometimes familial form of primary aldosteronism with adrenocortical hyperplasia exhibits complete suppression of clinical and biochemical abnormalities by glucocorticoid administration.

Adenoma Versus Hyperplasia

In cases of established primary aldosteronism a preoperative distinction between an aldosterone-producing adenoma (APA) and bilateral adrenal hyperplasia (BAH) should be made. Patients with a single adenoma usually respond favorably to surgery, whereas those with BAH are rarely cured following subtotal or even total adrenalectomy. The explanation for the persistence of hypertension following surgery in BAH is as obscure as the etiology, especially considering that the biochemical abnormalities remit. There are few clinical and routine biochemical differences between these two distinct pathologic and perhaps pathophysiologic entities. It is agreed, however, that the BAH group have a biochemically less severe disease with less renin suppression and hypokalemia and milder elevations of aldosterone levels. Such group statistical differences offer little insight into individual patient considerations where overlap is the rule.

Important differences in the control of tumor aldosterone production in APA and BAH provide biochemical tests to help differentiate these disorders. APA appears quite responsive to ACTH, whereas angiotensin II has little effect on aldosterone production. ACTH thus appears to be the major regulator of aldosterone production in these tumor cells. The opposite pertains to BAH, where angiotensin II is the major regulator. Patients with APA have a circadian rhythm of aldosterone levels that correlates with fluctuations in plasma ACTH and cortisol levels and is abolished by dexamethasone administration.

These differences in aldosterone tumor regulation form the basis of the postural response test. Patients remain supine, and initial samples for plasma aldosterone are taken at 8 AM, and then are ambulatory for 4 hours with repeated sampling. Since plasma renin activity is markedly suppressed in APA, the normal renin increment with orthostasis is abolished and plasma aldosterone levels show a paradoxical decline along with reductions in ACTH and cortisol levels in response to ambulation and the passage of time. Patients with BAH show a normal increase (greater than 25% of the baseline value) in aldosterone levels with upright posture, accounted for by a partially intact renin response and enhanced adrenal gland sensitivity to angiotensin II. Infusion of angiotensin II into patients with BAH shows a prompt aldosterone response, whereas in APA there is no aldosterone response to this agent. The level of a biosynthetic precursor of aldosterone, 18-hydroxycorticosterone, has been reported to be elevated in patients with APA, and its level is six times higher in APA than in BAH. Levels of plasma 18-hydroxycorticosterone greater than 100 ng/dl obtained at 8 AM while patients are recumbent are indicative of an APA; levels in BAH are less than 100 ng/dl. A lower aldosterone/deoxycorticosterone ratio was also noted in patients with APA, but the potential usefulness of this test must await further studies.

The accuracy of these biochemical tests in identifying adrenal pathology in primary aldosteronism is good but not acceptable as the single preoperative determinant. Recent series report that 23 of 32 (72%) patients with APA had an anomalous postural decline in plasma aldosterone levels. Thus a higher diagnostic yield is seen by combining the postural response test with one or more of the several adrenal localizing procedures.

Major advances in the technology for localizing adrenal gland pathology in the past 10 years have enhanced preoperative precision in differentiating APA and BAH. The three procedures that emerge as the best choices are retrograde adrenal venography and adrenal venous sampling for aldosterone measurements, adrenal scanning with special radionuclide agents and computerized axial tomography (CAT). It is not clear which of these procedures is the best choice, as all have certain limitations. Adrenal venography is an invasive procedure, requires technical skill, and is accompanied by some morbidity. Radionuclide adrenal scanning requires special isotopes given in relatively high doses, and is time-consuming and variable in accuracy. Abdominal CAT scanning offers simplicity and safety but only recently with advanced instrumentation and improved resolution has the efficacy of this procedure been evaluated. All these procedures suffer from the standpoint of poor resolution in detecting aldosterone-producing adrenal tumors, since a significant proportion of tumors are less than 0.8 cm in diameter.

In limited situations when technical expertise is available retrograde catheterization of the adrenal veins with venography and venous sampling for aldosterone has a diagnostic accuracy of 50–75% in localizing APA. Some feel that the reliability of this procedure is increased by the administration of ACTH intravenously to lessen artifactual errors due to episodic secretion of aldosterone. Cortisol levels are also monitored to ensure proper placement of catheters; this is especially important in the right adrenal vein which is difficult to localize. In APA aldosterone concentrations in adrenal venous plasma from the uninvolved side range from 100 to 400 ng/dl, whereas in the involved gland levels range from 500 to 4,000 ng/dl, giving a clearly distinct 26:1 mean ratio between the two sides. Significant morbidity has been related to intraadrenal hemorrhage during venography and more generally to the invasive nature of this procedure.

Adrenal scintigraphy or imaging with ^{131}I-19-iodo-cholesterol is a noninvasive localizing procedure and can detect adrenal tumors as small as 9 mm in diameter. Its overall detection rate for APA is about 75–94%. Recently one group reported that, although the procedure was useful in detecting APA, it was not helpful in always differentiating an adrenal adenoma from hyperplasia. Others have reported that adrenal scanning was unsuccessful in 47% of patients in correctly identifying the adrenal lesion. In this series the scan showed bilateral uptake in 12 patients in whom unilateral adenomas were found at surgery. The reliability of adrenal scanning is enhanced by preadministration of dexamethasone to suppress isotopic uptake by normal ACTH-dependent adrenal tissue. Large doses of radioisotope must be administered, so that iodine therapy must be given to block ^{131}I uptake by the thyroid gland. The iodocholesterol scan requires 6 days to complete. A newer scanning agent ^{131}I-6β-iodomethyl-19-norcholesterol(NP-59) has a faster rate of adrenal accumulation, so that imaging can be done in 48 hours. Limitations on the availability of these isotopes hamper their general applicability.

The most promising radiologic advance for visualizing adrenal gland pathology is CAT. The procedure has the advantages of being noninvasive, not requiring isotope administration, and rapidity of results. The major limitation has been the resolving power of CAT scans in detecting small aldosterone-producing tumors. Currently this procedure can quite accurately visualize tumors greater than 1.0 cm in diameter. One recent series reported that 12 of 16 patients with unilateral adenoma suspected by biochemical testing had CAT scan demonstrations of the lesion. The remaining 4 patients had suspicious lesions or abnormalities that could not be classified. The advent of the next generation of CAT scanners with a thinner slice thickness should further improve adrenal localization and make this the procedure of choice.

Treatment

Based on current knowledge it seems prudent to recommend surgery in patients with APAs and medical therapy in the bilateral hyperplasia group. The surgical procedure at most centers is a transabdominal rather than a lumbar approach with careful exposure and inspection of both adrenal glands. Most adenomas are small, often less than 1 cm in diameter, and twice as many occur on the left as on the right side. Usually the gland containing the tumor is excised, but some surgeons prefer simple resection of the adenoma. Sometimes no tumor tissue is located and a subtotal or total adrenalectomy is necessary. One recent series reports surgical results for 40 patients with a unilateral solitary adenoma of approximately 68% correction of hypertension and significant improvement in blood pressure in the remainder. Since ACTH and cortisol remain intact in primary aldosteronism, pre- and postoperative steroid replacement is usually not needed. However, a very important preoperative consideration is potassium repletion which can in most cases be accomplished with oral potassium supplementation. As an alternative method, preoperative treatment with the mineralocorticoid antagonist spironolactone has been advocated. Since this compound is a competitive antagonist of aldosterone, high doses (400–600 mg daily) are needed to normalize potassium and blood pressure preoperatively. It has been proposed that normalization of blood pressure with spironolactone predicts the success of surgery. Likewise, it has been stated that pretreatment with spironolactone restores renin responsiveness and hastens recovery of aldosterone production by the remaining normal suppressed adrenal tissue.

The approach in patients with bilateral hyperplasia consists of medical therapy. This is supported by a current report of a surgical cure rate (normalization of blood pressure) of only 18% in BAH. Spiropolactone seems to be the obvious choice, but in BAH the results have been variable and long-term evaluation of this therapy is not available. In addition, long-term spironolactone treatment is frequently accompanied by impotence and gynecomastia in males and menstrual disorders in females. Spironolactone behaves not only as an aldosterone antagonist but also blocks aldosterone biosynthesis in normals and in patients with primary aldosteronism. This effect correlates with the appearance of "spironolactone bodies" in the tumor cells. The reduction in aldosterone levels with biosynthetic blockage could eventuate in reducing doses of spironolactone and minimizing the antiandrogenic side effects. Unfortunately aldosterone levels may return toward pretreatment levels after several months' therapy as the blockage is overridden by rising renin levels.

Recently amiloride has been shown to be a successful therapeutic agent in the treatment of primary aldosteronism. Amiloride is a potassium-sparing diuretic that acts on renal tubular cells independently of aldosterone activity. In 19 patients given amiloride (40 mg/day) blood pressure was well controlled in the majority and normokalemia restored in all subjects. Side effects were negligible, including the absence of any antiandrogenic effects.

Miscellaneous Aldosterone Disorders

Several clinical disorders with hypertension can biochemically mimic primary aldosteronism (Table 1). These include some forms of Cushing's syndrome, excessive licorice ingestion, two types of congenital adrenal hyperplasia, Liddle's syndrome, and low-renin essential hypertension. In some of these cases patients have secondary aldosteronism, the elevation of aldosterone being secondary to activation of the renin–angiotensin system. Thus the most direct test for differentiating primary from secondary aldosteronism is measurement of plasma renin activity. The most common form of secondary aldosteronism associated with hypertension is malignant or accelerated hypertension associated with very high levels of renin and aldosterone, frequently accompanied by marked hypokalemia. Hyperreninism in malignant hypertension is due to renal damage leading to release of renin from the ischemic kidneys. Renal vascular hypertension should theoretically produce secondary aldosteronism, since most recent evidence implicates

Table 1 **Biochemical Characteristics of Aldosterone Disorders**

Disorder	*Renin Level*	*Aldosterone Level*	*Serum Potassium Level*
Primary aldosteronism	Low	High	Low
Edematous disorders	High	High	Low
Malignant hypertension	High	High	Low
Renovascular hypertension	Normal or high	Normal or high	Normal or occasionally low
Congenital adrenal hyperplasia (11- and 17-hydroxylase deficiency)	Low	Low	Low
Cushing's syndrome	Normal or low	Normal or low	Normal or low
Liddle's syndrome	Low	Low	Low
Bartter's syndrome	High	High	Low
Licorice ingestion	Low	Low	Low
Low-renin essential hypertension	Low	Normal or low	Normal

this as a renin-dependent form of hypertension. Yet hyperaldosteronism and hypokalemia are uncommon in this disorder, as the majority of cases have a normal peripheral renin level. Cushing's syndrome and, in particular the ectopic ACTH syndrome, can produce hypertension and hypokalemia suggesting primary aldosteronism. In most cases the physical stigmata of hypercortisolism or the presence of a tumor producing ACTH directs attention toward the proper diagnosis. Certain forms of congenital adrenal hyperplasia, including the 11β- and 17α-hydroxylase deficiency syndromes result in hypertension and hypokalemia. The hypertension and hypokalemia respond to glucocorticoid therapy. There is also a rare form of hyperaldosteronism occurring mostly in children where glucocorticoid therapy can correct the hypertension and hypokalemia. Another remote consideration in Liddle's syndrome, which is a familial disorder of increased sodium retention resulting in hypertension and hypokalemia. This abnormality is attributed to increased activity of the nonaldosterone-dependent site of distal tubular sodium and potassium exchange. Equally rare causes of hypertension and hypokalemia are certain tumors producing either renin or a mineralocorticoid. Excessive ingestion of licorice can mimic primary aldosteronism by producing hypertension, hypokalemia, and a suppressed renin level. Licorice contains a flavoring agent, glycyrrhizic acid, which in excess acts as a mineralocorticoid by competitively binding to the aldosterone receptor site in the kidney. Finally, approximately one-fourth of patients with essential hypertension may demonstrate low levels of plasma renin activity. However, the differential diagnosis rests on the fact that the vast majority of this group are normokalemic and have aldosterone levels in the normal to low range. One provocative study has proposed that low-renin essential hypertensive patients may represent individuals in a very early phase of primary aldosteronism. Several patients with suspected or indeterminant primary aldosteronism and BAH at certain times in their clinical course demonstrated features common to those of the low-renin essential hypertension group.

MINERALOCORTICOID DEFICIENCY SYNDROMES

Previously, the most common cause of hypoaldosteronism was that associated with primary adrenal insufficiency with hypocortisolism due to destruction of the adrenal cortex. There also exists a very rare form of congenital adrenal hyperplasia with specific enzymatic blockage of the conversion of 18-hydroxycorticosterone to aldosterone (methyl oxidase II defect). The features of this syndrome have been variable, appearing as volume and sodium depletion, hyperkalemia, and shock in some and as asymptomatic hyperkalemia in others. The syndrome has been best described in isolated, nomadic tribes with a high rate of consanguinity. Levels of plasma renin activity are high in response to volume deficiency. Specific diagnosis is made by measurements of the ratio of the urinary metabolites of 18-hydroxycorticosterone to aldosterone, a procedure limited to special centers.

Perhaps the leading causes of hypoaldosteronism today are certain forms of renal disease leading to impaired renin formation or secretion. This syndrome has been termed *hyporeninemic hypoaldosteronism* and is most often associated with mild to moderate renal insufficiency, especially in older individuals with variable degrees of hyperkalemia. The most consistent underlying renal disorder has been diabetic nephropathy, although it has also been found in certain interstitial nephropathies. Various disorders of renin release have been proposed, including destruction of the juxtaglomerular apparatus, sympathetic nervous system defects, and chronic volume expansion. None of the tests that stimulate aldosterone and renin release are effective in this disorder. Treatment includes careful replacement of mineralocorticoids using the synthetic agent fluorohydrocortisone (Florinef), 0.05–0.15 mg daily, potassium restriction, and diuretic therapy.

DISCUSSION CASES

Case 1

Description

A 38-year-old woman had a history of hypertension of 4 years' duration. Initial treatment was with hydrochlorothiazide, 50 mg b.i.d., but blood pressure control was inadequate and she discontinued the medication because of extreme fatigue and weakness. Her symptoms improved, but 2 years later a blood pressure of 180/116 necessitated hospitalization. Evaluation included a normal physical examination, an intravenous pyelogram, and routine laboratory tests. The serum K^+ was 3.6 and Na^+ 143 mEq/liter. The patient was discharged and treated with hydrochlorothiazide, 50 mg b.i.d., and alpha-methyldopa, 250 mg t.i.d. Over the next year blood pressure control was marginal, and she stopped treatment because of recurrent weakness and muscle cramps in her extremities. She was hospitalized after her physician noted a serum K^+ measurement of 2.3 mEq/liter. There was no family history of hypertension, diabetes, or renal disease. She denied intake of other medications or licorice ingestion. Other symptoms included occasional frontal headaches, light-headedness, and nocturnal frequency two to three times per night.

Physical examination revealed the following: Blood pressure 180/112, supine, 162/102 upright. Pulse 88. Funduscopic: arteriolar narrowing, no hemorrhages. Cardiovascular: PMI minimally sustained, forceful in midclavicular line; S_4 noted; no murmurs; peripheral pulses 3+ and equal. Pulmonary: clear on ausculatation. Abdomen: no organomegaly or masses; no bruits. Extremities: moderate weakness in proximal muscles of the lower extremities.

Laboratory results were as follows: Hemoglobin 14.2 g/dl; WBC 6,400/mm^3 with normal differential; BUN 16 mg/dl; creatinine 1.2 mg/dl; FBS 115 mg/dl, 2-hour p.c. 162 mg/dl; urine specific gravity 1.020; urine protein trace; Serum: sodium 142 mEq/liter; potassium 2.2 mEq/liter; chloride 96 mEq/liter; CO_2 33 mEq/liter.

The patient was placed on a 120 mEq Na^+/100 mEq K^+ diet for 5 days for the following studies:

1. Supine position: plasma renin activity (PRA) 0.1 ng/ml per hour (8:00 AM, overnight recumbency), plasma aldosterone, 24 ng/dl, plasma cortisol 9.8 μg/dl.
2. Upright position (4 hours): PRA 0.28 ng/ml per hour, aldosterone 11 ng/dl, cortisol 7.2 μg/dl.
3. 24-hour urine collection: Na^+ 103 mEq/24 hr, K^+ 68 mEq/24 hr (serum K^+ 2.6 mEq/liter), aldosterone excretion 62 μg/24 hr (normal 8–20 μg/24 hr).

CAT revealed a left adrenal gland mass and a normal right adrenal gland. Because of hypokalemia and severe muscle weakness, the patient was given spironolactone, 300 mg/day, and discharged to await surgery. After 5 weeks the patient demonstrated normal muscle strength, her serum potassium level was 4.1, and her blood pressure was 136/90. Spironolactone was discontinued, and 4 days later she underwent a left adrenalectomy by transabdominal surgery, demonstrating a 2.1-cm adenoma. One week following surgery, her blood pressure was 126/88 and her serum potassium level was 4.1 mEq/liter.

Question

1. What additional testing could have been considered to confirm the diagnosis?

Answer

A saline suppression test would have been the procedure of choice if the baseline results had been equivocal. The patient would most likely have demonstrated less than a 50% decline in plasma aldosterone levels from baseline values after the 4-hour infusion. This patient, however, demonstrated unequivocal elevations of aldosterone, suppression of renin, and hypokalemia with disproportionate kaliuresis, negating the need for further biochemical testing.

Question

2. Did the patient's response to spironolactone aid in the diagnosis and predict the response to surgery?

Answer

Normalization of *both* blood pressure and serum potassium levels after 4–6 weeks' therapy with spironolactone in 200–400 mg/day dosages is believed by most to be unique to primary aldosteronism. Since some patients with primary aldosteronism due to bilateral hyperplasia respond to spironolactone but not adrenal surgery, this therapeutic trial is not always predictive of operative results.

Question

3. The plasma aldosterone response to upright posture in this patient indicates which form of adrenal pathology?

Answer

The decline in plasma aldosterone with upright posture indicates an aldosterone-producing adenoma. Patients with BAH have an increase in plasma aldosterone levels. This test is about 80% predictive but should not be used as the sole criterion to judge surgical versus medical therapy.

Case 2

Description

A 44-year-old man has diabetes mellitus of 20 years' duration and has been taking NPH insulin 40 units every morning. Recent problems include proximal muscle weakness in the lower extremities and frequent palpitations. He has had moderate renal insufficiency and background diabetic retinopathy for 3 years. Control of blood glucose has been considered adequate for the past 2 years, with fasting levels ranging from 142 to 166 mg/dl. The patient is hospitalized because of EKG abnormalities and hyperkalemia.

Physical examination revealed the following: Blood pressure 160/98 supine, 144/80 upright. Pulse 92 supine, 96 upright. Funduscopic: multiple microaneurysms, scattered waxy exudates; no proliferative changes. Cardiac: irregular rhythm with multiple ectopic beats; no murmurs but S_4 noted. Lungs: clear on ausculatation. Abdomen: no organomegaly or masses. Pulses: bilateral reduction of posterior tibial and dorsalis pedis. Extremities: no edema, mild muscle weakness lower extremities. Neurologic: normal.

Laboratory results were as follows: Hemoglobin 13.6 g/dl; WBC 6,200/mm^3; BUN 23 mg/dl: creatinine 1.6 mg/dl; chest X-ray, normal; FBS 158 mg/dl, urine specific gravity 1.010 protein 4+; RBC 0; Serum: sodium 139 mEq/liter; potassium 6.4 mEq/liter; chloride 104 mEq/liter; CO_2 18 mEq/liter; ECG: peaked T waves with decreased amplitude of R waves; frequent atrial premature contractions.

With constant ECG monitoring, the patient received 20 g kayexalate every 4 hours for 2 days until his serum K was 4.7 mEq/L. He was then placed on 120 mEq Na/40 mEq K diet for the following studies:

1. Supine position 8:00 AM: Plasma aldosterone 2.6 ng/dl, plasma renin activity 0.3 ng/ml per hour, plasma cortisol 14 μg/dl.
2. Upright posture for 4 hours: plasma aldosterone 2.8 ng/dl, plasma renin activity 0.2 ng/ml per hour.
3. A 24-hour urine collection: aldosterone excretion rate 2 μg. Cosyntropin, 0.25 mg i.m., showed no aldosterone response but normal cortisol increments.

Question

1. What is the cause of hyperkalemia in this patient?

Answer

The patient has hyporeninemic hypoaldosteronism; the low aldosterone levels prevent adequate potassium excretion. This syndrome is common in diabetes mellitus, especially in patients with diabetic renal disease. The cause of low renin levels in these patients is unknown but could be due to diabetic exudative infiltration of renin-releasing juxtaglomerular cells, sympathetic nervous system dysfunction, or chronic volume expansion.

Question

2. With aldosterone deficiency in this syndrome why are sodium levels normal?

Answer

Because of the multiple other mechanisms for sodium conservation besides aldosterone, a near-normal serum sodium is found. Conversely, potassium depends mainly on the aldosterone-sensitive Na^+/K^+ exchange mechanism for external disposition.

Question

3. What would be appropriate long-term therapy to maintain normal potassium levels in this patient?

Answer

As there is no current mechanism for restoring normal renin and aldosterone secretion in this subject, other methods are utilized. Replacement with the synthetic mineralocorticoid fluorohydrocortisone (Florinef) 0.05–0.15 mg daily is appropriate therapy. This may aggravate hypertension in a previously hypertensive patient such as this individual. The second choice is a loop diuretic (e.g., furosemide) in doses to promote adequate sodium excretion combined with a low potassium intake and/or small doses of Florinef. Diuretic therapy often corrects hypertension which should be vigorously controlled in all diabetic subjects.

SUGGESTED READING

Conn JW: Primary aldosteronism, in Genest J, Koiw E, Kuchel O. (eds): *Hypertension—Physiopathology and Treatment,* New York, McGraw-Hill Book Co, 1977, p 768.

Biglieri EG, Schambelan M: The significance of elevated levels of plasma 18-hydroxycorticosterone in patients with primary aldosteronism. *J. Clin Endocrinol Metab* 49:87–91, 1979.

Ganguly A, Dowdy AJ, Luetscher JA, Melada GA: Anomalous postural response of plasma aldosterone concentration in patients with aldosterone-producing adrenal adenoma. *J Clin Endocrinol Metab* 36:401–418, 1973.

Ganguly A, Pratt JH, Yune HY, Grim CE, Weinberger MH: Detection of adrenal tumors by computerized tomographic scan in endocrine hypertension. *Arch Intern Med* 139:589–594, 1979.

Hert SM, Teates DC, Tegtmeyer CJ, Vaughan ED, Ayers CR, Carey RM: Identification and differentiation of surgically correctable hypertension due to primary aldosteronism. *Am J Med* 67:397–402, 1979.

Hogan MJ, McRae J, Schambelan M, Biglieri EG: Location of aldosterone-producing adenomas with ^{131}I-19-iodocholesterol. *N Engl J Med* 294:410–414, 1976.

Miles JM, Wahner HW, Carpenter PC, Salassa RM, Northcutt RC: Adrenal scintiscanning with NP-59, a new radioiodinated cholesterol agent. *Mayo Clin Proc* 54:321–330, 1979.

Schambelan M, Brust NL, Chang BCF, Slater KL, Biglieri EG: Circadian rhythm and effect of posture on plasma aldosterone concentration in primary aldosteronism. *J Clin Endocrinol Metab* 43:115–131, 1976.

Streeten DHP, Tomycz N, Anderson GH: Reliability of screening methods for the diagnosis of primary aldosteronism. *Am J Med* 67:403–414, 1979.

Vetter H, Siebenschein R, Studer A, Witassek F, Furrer J, Glanzer K, Siegenthaler W, Vetter W: Primary aldosteronism: Inability to differentiate unilateral from bilateral adrenal lesions by various routine clinical and laboratory data and by peripheral plasma aldosterone. *Acta Endocrinol* 89:710–725, 1978.

Weinberger MH, Grim CE, Hollifield JW, Kem DC, Ganguly A, Kramer NJ, Yune HY, Wellamn H, Donohue JP: Primary aldosteronism: Diagnosis, localization, and treatment. Ann Intern Med 90:386–395, 1979.

Wisgerhof M, Carpenter PC, Brown RD: Increased adrenal sensitivity to angiotensin II in idiopathic hyperaldosteronism. *J Clin Endocrinol Metab* 47:938–946, 1978.

10 JAMES R. SOWERS

Pheochromocytoma

Pheochromocytoma is a relatively rare, most often histologically benign tumor of the sympathetic nervous system that secretes excessive amounts of norepinephrine and epinephrine into the bloodstream. Ninety percent of these tumors occur in the adrenals (more often the right than the left). Eight percent are found in other chromaffin tissue within the abdomen, and only 2% are located extraabdominally in the thorax or neck. About 10% are bilateral or multiple in adults, 35% are multiple in children, and between 6 and 10% are malignant. Familial pheochromocytomas almost always occur in the adrenal medulla and are bilateral in at least 70% of cases. Pheochromocytomas may appear at any age, but the highest frequency occurs in the fourth and fifth decades; approximately 10% occur in children. In adults there appears to be a slight predilection for females, as in several large series 53–60% of tumors occurred in women; in children, however, almost two-thirds of pheochromocytomas occur in males. Although the precise incidence of pheochromocytoma is unknown, at least 0.1% of the population with persistent diastolic hypertension probably has this tumor. This figure was determined by Manger and Gifford in an encyclopedic coverage of pheochromocytoma. A relatively high incidence of pheochromocytoma (0.09%) found in two large series of consecutive autopsies of patients dying of any cause suggest that many of these tumors may cause only minimal clinical manifestations.

CLINICAL PRESENTATION

The symptoms in adults with pheochromocytoma are listed in Table 1.

The clinical signs of pheochromocytoma encountered in 76 patients are listed in Table 2.

The three most commonly experienced symptoms in pheochromocytoma patients with either paroxysmal or persistent hypertension are headache, excessive generalized sweating, and palpitations. Often symptoms appear in a dramatic, explosive manner when the tumor suddenly discharges catecholamines into the circulation. In general, patients with paroxysmal hypertension have more severe symptoms than those with sustained hypertension. However, about 50% of patients with sustained hypertension experience a sudden onset of symptoms, usually associated with episodic increases in hypertension. Clinical features may suggest the predominant hormone

Table 1 **Symptoms of Pheochromocytoma**

Symptom	*Occurrence* (%)
Common	
Headache	72–92
Sweating	60–70
Palpitations with or without tachycardia	51–73
Nervousness	35–40
Weight loss	40–70
Chest or abdominal pain	22–48
Nausea with or without vomiting	26–43
Weakness or fatigue	15–38
Less common	
Visual disturbance	3–21
Constipation	0–13
Paresthesias, pains in arms	0–11
Polydypsia, polyuria	0–2
Flushing	~18
Dyspnea	11–19
Dizziness	3–11
Convulsions (grand mal)	3–5
Bradycardia (noted by patients)	3–8
Warmth without or without heat intolerance	13–15
Tightness in throat	~8
Tinnitus, dysarthria, gagging	3

secreted by the tumor. Patients whose tumors secrete mainly epinephrine (almost always an adrenal tumor) have disproportionate systolic hypertension (due to increased cardiac output), tachycardia, sweating, and flushing. Several reports have appeared of hypotensive crises in patients in whom a pheochromocytoma secreted predominantly, if not entirely, epinephrine. Predominantly dopamine-secreting pheochromocytomas should be suspected as the cause of normotensive crises in which dopamine counteracts the vasoconstrictor effects of norepinephrine. Symptomatic episodes have been noted to occur as infrequently as once every few months to as often as 25 times daily and to persist for from less than a minute to as long as 1 week. About 75% of patients with pheochromocytoma experience one or more attacks weekly, and the remainder have one or more attacks daily. Attacks lasting less than 15 minutes occur in half of patients, and attacks less than 1 hour in 80%. Typically, attacks become more frequent, but not necessarily more severe, with the passage of time. They may be elicited by pressure in the area of the tumor; postural changes; exercise; anxiety; ingestion of foods or alcoholic beverages containing tyramine, such as cheese, beer, and wine; hyperventilation; sneezing; smoking; the Valsalva maneuvers; sexual intercourse; straining at stool; bladder distension; micturition; certain odors; administration of drugs such as histamine, glucagon, epinephrine, tyramine, methacholine, nicotine, succinylcholine, ACTH, phenothiazines, and saralasin and other angiotensin II analogs; and angiography, intubation, anesthesia, parturition, or operative procedures.

Table 2 **Clinical Signs of Pheochromocytoma**

Blood pressure changes—seen in 98% of patients

- Sustained hypertension in 50–60%, with superimposed paroxysms in 50%. Hypertension is intermittent only in 2–50%. rarely, there is paroxysmal hypotension or hypertension alternating with hypotension
- Hypertension induced by a physical maneuver such as exercise, postural change, or palpation and massage of flank or mass elsewhere
- Orthostatic hypotension with or without postural tachycardia
- Paradoxical blood pressure response to some antihypertensive drugs and marked pressor response with induction of anesthesia

Other signs of catecholamine excess

- Hyperhydrosis
- Tachycardia or reflex bradycardia, forceful heartbeat, arrhythmia
- Pallor of face and upper part of body (seen in 28–60%)
- Anxious, frightened, troubled appearance
- Hypertensive retinopathy (seen in 50–70%)
- Dilated pupils; very rarely exophthalmos, lacrimation, scleral pallor or injection; pupil may not react to light
- Leanness or underweight
- Tremor
- Raynaud's phenomenon or livedo reticularis; occasionally, puffy, red cyanotic hands in children; skin of extremities wet, cold, clammy, and pale; gooseflesh; occasionally cyanotic nail beds
- Fever

Mass lesion—palpable tumor in abdomen (rare), neck pheochromocytoma or chemodectoma, thyroid carcinoma (in MEN-II), or thyroid swelling (very rare and seen only during hypertensive paroxysms)

Signs caused by encroachment on adjacent structures or by invasion and pressure effects of metastases

Manifestations related to complications or coexisting diseases or syndromes:

- Sudden death after minor trauma
- Arrhythmias, tachycardia, unexplained hypotension, or cardiac arrest following induction of general anesthesia
- Congestive heart failure with or without cardiomyopathy
- Fever, leukocytosis, and sustained hypotension simulating gram-negative shock
- Myocardial infarction
- Cerebrovascular accident
- Azotemia
- Ischemic enterocolitis with or without megacolon
- Dissecting aneurysm
- Hypertensive encephalopathy
- Severe preeclampsia during pregnancy; fever, shock, or sudden death pre- or postpartum
- Cholelithiasis

The most common symptom is headache which occurs in 92% of patients with paroxysmal and 72% of patients with sustained hypertension. The headaches are characteristically throbbing in nature, are bilateral, and are usually very severe during a paroxysm of hypertension. Most often they are occipital or frontal, but at times they are generalized. They may awaken the patient, and frequently they are accompanied by nausea and vomiting. Sweating occurs in 60–70% of patients and is usually greater in the upper part of the body. The most profuse sweating occurs during paroxysmal attacks of hypertension. Palpitations with or without tachycardia are the third most common symptoms occurring in 73 and 51% of patients with paroxysmal or sustained hypertension, respectively. Gastrointestinal complaints are common and include nausea, vomiting, and epigastric pain. The incidence of cholelithiasis is increased markedly in pheochromocytoma. Chronic elevation of catecholamines impairs intestinal motility, leading to constipation in many patients. Megacolon and ischemic enterocolitis, as well as intestinal obstruction, have been reported. Vasoconstrictive effects of catecholamines may be manifested as paresthesias, arm pain, and even Raynaud's phenomenon. These symptoms are seen most commonly in patients with paroxysmal hypertension. Intermittent claudication, ischemia, and leg ulcerations have also been reported.

When pheochromocytomas occur in childhood or in pregnancy, or when the tumor arises in the urinary bladder, certain unusual manifestations are often evident. Over 90% of children with pheochromocytoma have sustained hypertension. Visual complaints, vasomotor disturbances, generalized sweating, nausea, vomiting, and weight loss occur more frequently in children than in adults. Impaired growth is often a striking feature. Polydipsia, polyuria, and convulsions occur in about 25% of children with pheochromocytoma but are rarely observed in adults. The puffy, red cyanotic appearance of the hands seen in 11% of these children is not observed in adults. Pregnancy complicated by pheochromocytoma may be misdiagnosed as toxemia of pregnancy, preeclampsia, or a ruptured uterus when the patient goes into shock during or immediately after labor.

Of extra-adrenal pheochromocytomas, about 10% occur in the bladder wall. A bladder pheochromocytoma should be suspected if the patient has typical micturitional attacks, namely, headaches, palpitations, or nausea during or right after voiding. Painless hematuria has been noted in 65% of the cases, hypertension in 60%, and micturitional attacks in 47%.

At least 50% of adult patients with pheochromocytoma have sustained hypertension, whereas the remaining 40–50% experience paroxysms of hypertension alternating with relatively normotensive intervals. Investigators have reported a few patients with a functioning pheochromocytoma, but no hypertension. It has been observed that some of these patients become hypertensive or die suddenly after an invasive procedure or during mild trauma. Some have made the observation that orthostatic hypotension occurring in a hypertensive patient taking no medications should make one think of pheochromocytoma. The drop is usually to normal or slightly below normal, but occasionally to shock range. Postural tachycardia is usually present.

In Manger and Gifford's series, 53% of patients with sustained hypertension had grade III or IV and 40% had grade I or II hypertensive retinopathy, and only 5% had normal fundi. These retinal changes almost always improve after blood pressure is controlled and the pheochromocytoma removed. Pallor of the face and upper part of the body was noted in 60 and 28% of patients with paroxysmal and sustained hypertension, respectively. Some investigators found elevated body temperature (1–2°C) in two-thirds of patients with pheochromocytoma. Temperature elevation may be present even when the patient is free of a paroxysmal attack. The elevation in temperature is due to the heat production of the hypermetabolic state and impaired heat loss due to peripheral vasoconstriction. A palpable mass in the abdomen may be seen in 10–14% of patients with pheochromocytoma.

FAMILIAL SYNDROMES ASSOCIATED WITH PHEOCHROMOCYTOMA

Familial pheochromocytoma in association with medullary carcinoma of the thyroid, parathyroid hyperplasia or adenoma and, rarely, bilateral adrenocortical hyperplasia has been designated multiple endocrine neoplasia (MEN) type IIa. The coexistence of pheochromocytoma, medullary thyroid carcinoma, mucosal neuromas, thickened corneal nerves, alimentary tract ganglioneuromatosis, and frequently a Marfanoid habitus constitutes still another familial entity, MEN type IIb, also designated type III. Neurofibromatosis, or von Recklinghausen's disease, with or without café au lait spots, occurs in about 5% of patients with pheochromocytoma; the incidence of pheochromocytoma in neurofibromatosis may be less than 1%. Rarely, pheochromocytoma occurs in association with von Hippel-Lindau disease (cerebellar hemangioblastoma and retinal angioma) or acromegaly.

DIFFERENTIAL DIAGNOSIS

Important differential diagnostic possibilities are described in Table 3.

LABORATORY DIAGNOSIS

In general, the following groups of patients should be screened for pheochromocytoma: all patients with severe sustained or paroxysmal hypertension (grades 3 and 4 retinopathy) of unknown etiology or resistant to treatment; all hypertensive children; all patients with MEN-IIa or IIb and their first-degree relatives, even if asymptomatic and normotensive; patients with hypertension and diabetes mellitus or hypermetabolism; patients experiencing hypertensive episodes during induction of anesthesia, radiologic procedures, parturition, and in association with antihypertensive therapy, especially with β-adrenergic blocking agents, ganglionic blockers or guanethidine; patients with unexplained circulatory shock during anesthesia, during pregnancy, during delivery, or during the puerperium, after surgery or after administration of phenothiazine drugs; patients with apparent toxemia of pregnancy; patients with unexplained pyrexia; and patients with radiographic evidence of a suprarenal mass.

BIOCHEMICAL TESTS

At present, the most useful tests for pheochromocytoma are:*

a. A 24-hour urine test for total metanephrines (normal <0.9 mg/24 hr).
b. A 24-hour urine test for vanillylmandelic acid (VMA) (normal <6.5–10 mg/24 hr).
c. A 24-hour urine test for free catecholamines (normal <100–200 μg/24 hr).
d. A determination of plasma catecholamine levels after 30 minutes supine resting (normal: norepinephrine <1,000 pg/ml and epinephrine <100 pg/ml.

*The normal ranges may vary somewhat from laboratory to laboratory.

Table 3 **Differential Diagnosis of Suspected Pheochromocytoma**

All hypertension (sustained and paroxysmal)
Anxiety, tension states, psychoneurosis, psychosis
Diabetes mellitus
Paroxysmal tachycardia
Hyperdynamic circulatory state
Menopause (flushing, sweating)
Vasodilating headache (migraine and cluster headaches)
Coronary insufficiency syndrome
Acute hypertensive encephalopathy
Hyperthyroidism
Renal parenchymal or renal arterial disease with hypertension
Focal cerebral arterial insufficiency
Intracranial lesions, with or without increased intracranial pressure
Autonomic hyperreflexia
Diencephalic seizure and syndrome
Toxemia of pregnancy
Hypertensive crises associated with monoamine oxidase inhibitors
Carcinoid syndrome
Hypoglycemia
Mastocytosis
Familial dysautonomia
Acrodynia
Neuroblastoma, ganglioneuroblastoma, ganglioneuroma
Acute infectious disease
Rare causes of paroxysmal hypertension (acute porphyria, lead poisoning, tabetic crisis, encephalitis, clonidine withdrawal, hypovolemia with inappropriate vasoconstriction, pulmonary artery fibrosarcoma, pork hypersensitivity, dysregulation of hypothalamus, tetanus, Guillain-Barré syndrome, factitious)
Fortuitous circumstances simulating pheochromocytoma

Measurement of total metanephrines (metanephrine plus normetanephrine) in a 24-hour urine specimen is the most reliable screening method for detecting pheochromocytoma; more than 95% of patients have elevated excretion of total metanephrines.

The determination of plasma catecholamines (with single- and double-isotope derivative methods) yields sensitive data. The advantages of plasma catecholamine determinations are that (1) blood can be conveniently collected before and immediately after an attack, spontaneous or provoked, and values correlate well with blood pressure changes; (2) specific determinations of norepinephrine, dopamine, or epinephrine help in localizing the site of the tumor. Bravo et al. have presented data indicating that measurement of resting supine plasma catecholamine levels using a relatively sensitive radioenzymatic assay was more useful than a 24-hour test for urinary VMA or for urinary metanephrine or both. In a study on 24 patients with surgically documented pheochromocytomas, they reported only one patient who did not have increased plasma catecholamine levels. In contrast, urinary VMA values were normal in 11 patients, urinary metanephrine in 5, and both urinary metabolites in 3 of 22 patients in whom they were measured. However, many conditions may elevate plasma catecholamines to the range seen in patients with pheochromocytoma: volume depletion, exercise, acidosis, smoking, hypotension, hypoglycemia, increased intracranial pressure, anoxia, marked obesity, renal failure, hemolysis, hyperbilirubinemia, methyldopa, L-dopa, large doses of histamine or glucagon. Since so many factors may elevate plasma catecholamines, measurement of urine metanephrine levels is the preferred screening test. Plasma catecholamines are particularly valuable in (1) selective blood sampling at different anatomic levels to localize extraadrenal tumors that cannot be located by abdominal exploration; and (2) the diagnosis of a pheochromocytoma that secretes episodically. Recently a study was conducted to determine the best screening test for early diagnosis of pheochromocytoma in patients with MEN-II. In a large family with MEN-II measurement of 24-hour urinary catecholamine levels revealed an increased urinary epinephrine fraction as the dominant or sole abnormality. Indeed, it was found that a urinary epinephrine level greater than 20 μg/24 hr was diagnostic of pheochromocytoma in this syndrome.

Occasionally, a provocative test with glucagon or histamine is necessary in the diagnosis of a paroxysmally secreting pheochromocytoma. Since side effects are more pronounced with histamine than with glucagon, the glucagon test should be performed initially. Both provocative tests suffer from disadvantages of false positive and false negative responses and occasional pressor crises.

RADIOLOGIC PREOPERATIVE LOCALIZATION

Nephrotomography, adrenal arteriography, adrenal venography, ultrasound, and 19-[^{131}I]-iodocholesterol scintigraphy have all been used to visualize pheochromocytomas that are adrenal in origin. Recently, computerized axial tomography (CAT) has proved to be the radiologic method of choice in the preoperative localization of pheochromocytomas. Some have found that this noninvasive procedure has the same degree of detectability and false positivity as selective angiography, 91 and 9% respectively. Intrathoracic pheochromocytomas (2% occur above the diaphragm) may be detected as a paravertebral posterior mediastinal mass on oblique chest roentgenograms. Fluoroscopy plus oblique views of the chest to look at the paravertebral sulcus are useful in detecting small tumors. CAT techniques are also useful in demonstrating intrathoracic and intracranial tumors. Central venous sampling for catecholamines followed by adrenal venography is helpful in the following circumstances: (1) when all other means fail to localize the tumor, including abdominal exploration; (2) for patients with extraadrenal pheochromocytomas; (3) for malignant metastasis; (4) for multiple pheochromocytomas; (5) for recurrent tumors. A group of investigators have recently reported the use of an ^{131}I-labeled adrenergic agent in imaging small adrenal and extraadrenal tumors not detected by CAT. This method offers considerable promise as a replacement for invasive techniques in localizing small, occult tumors.

EMERGENCY MANAGEMENT OF PHEOCHROMOCYTOMA

Acute therapy in patients with known or highly suspected pheochromocytoma includes the following: (1) bed rest; (2) elevation of the head of the bed to take advantage of the orthostatic drop in blood pressure occurring in these patients; (3) phentolamine, an α-adrenergic blocker, 2–5 mg i.v. every 5 minutes until blood pressure has been stabilized. Phentolamine, 2–5 mg i.v., can be given every 2–4 hours to maintain control until longer-acting preparations are given.

Continuous infusion with sodium nitroprusside, 100 mg in 500 ml 5% dextrose in water, can also be used to control blood pressure acutely. For arrhythmias the treatment is propranolol, 1–2 mg i.v. over a 5- to 10-minute period. Later this drug may be given orally 20–40 mg every 6 hours. Propranolol should not be given until α-adrenergic blockage is achieved.

PREOPERATIVE MANAGEMENT

Phenoxybenzamine hydrochloride, a long-acting α-adrenergic blocker, should be initiated at a dose of 20–30 mg/day and increased by 10–20 mg/day. A dose of 40–100 mg/day is usually required for blood pressure stabilization. Recently approved for use is metyrosine (α-methyl-L-tyrosine), an inhibitor of tyrosine hydroxylase. It is used in the preoperative preparation of these patients and for the management of such patients when surgery is contraindicated or all functioning tumor cannot be removed. This drug is administered initially in a dose of 250 mg q.i.d. with daily increments of 250–500 mg. The maximum recommended dosage is 4 g/day. An oral fluid intake of at least 2 liters is recommended to prevent urine crystal formation. Again, if cardiac arrhythmias occur, propranolol, 20–40 mg every 6 hours, is indicated.

Since patients with MEN-II are likely to harbor bilateral pheochromocytomas, the likelihood of total adrenalectomy necessitates the administration of steroids (e.g., cortisone acetate, 200 mg i.m. 2 days before, 1 day before, and on the day of the procedure). In MEN-II with associated hyperparathyroidism with hypercalcemia, one should avoid dehydration during the perioperative period, as this may aggravate hypercalcemia. It should be noted that some oppose complete alpha blockage prior to surgery, as this eliminates the ability of the surgeon to use elevations in blood pressure as a guide in locating the tumor.

OPERATIVE MANAGEMENT

Close monitoring during surgery is an absolute necessity and includes ECG, central venous pressure, continuous arterial pressure readings, and a Swan-Ganz catheter to assess intravascular volume replacement. Morphine and phenothiazines should be avoided, and sodium thiopenthal is the best induction agent. Halothane, methoxyflurane, and enflurane all depress the spontaneous release of catecholamines from the adrenal medulla and the secretion evoked by splanchnic nerve stimulation. Enflurane does not sensitize the heart to catecholamine-induced dysrhythmias, and halothane raises the dysrhythmic threshold for catecholamines. Therefore, enflurane and halothane are the logical anesthetic agents. Hypertensive crises may be heralded by ventricular arrhythmias. Phentolamine in 5-mg boluses may be used in treating the hypertension. Propranolol may be used to treat dysrhythmias but may slow recovery by suppressing cardiovascular homeostatic mechanisms. Increasing the depth of halothane anesthesia or administration of intravenous lidocaine as a 75- to 100-mg bolus are equally effective in suppressing the ventricular dysrhythmias.

The anterior transperitoneal approach is mandatory when operating for an intraabdominal pheochromocytoma, since these tumors may be multiple and extraadrenal. Because of the high incidence of coexisting cholelithiasis (20%), the gallbladder should be carefully examined during exploration. Postoperative hypotension, tachycardia, and decreased urinary output may indicate inadequate correction of the large blood volume deficit, an acute medical problem such as myocardial infarction, cardiac failure, sepsis, or retroperitoneal bleeding. Postoperative hypertension may result from fluid overload, pain, residual pheochromocytoma tissue, or inadvertent ligation of a renal artery. Severe hypoglycemia has been reported in patients within 2 hours postoperatively; it is transient, perhaps because of increased insulin release, and should be treated with infusion of dextrose in water. The 5-year survival rates for patients with benign tumors is 96%, whereas it drops to 44% for patients with malignant pheochromocytomas. Approximately 75% of patients are normotensive following surgical removal, while the remainder show sustained hypertension without evidence of residual tumor. The cause of this sustained hypertension remains uncertain.

DISCUSSION CASES

Case 1

Description

A 39-year-old man is admitted with a history of palpitations, tremors, and a 10-pound weight loss over several months. The patient works as an auto mechanic and has been in prior good health. There is no history of diabetes, hypertension, or hyperthyroidism. The patient denies drug abuse and takes no medication. The patient's family history includes a father who has hypertension which is controlled with medication, and a brother who has been treated for hyperparathyroidism. Recently an uncle has had an operation for "thyroid cancer." In the emergency room the patient's blood pressure was 170/104, and it increased to 200/120 after he was advised that he should be hospitalized.

His initial examination revealed a pulse of 106. There were no postural changes in blood pressure. The funduscopic exam revealed grade I hypertensive retinopathy. The remainder of the exam was normal.

Laboratory studies revealed the following: WBC 7,800 mm^3 with normal differential; hemoglobin 16.2 g/dl; sedimentation rate 10 mm; BUN 14 mg/dl; creatinine 1.0 mg/dl; FBS 145 mg/dl; urinalysis: specific gravity 1.016; protein, trace; glucose, negative; WBC 0; RBC 0. Sodium 140 mEq/liter; chloride 103 mEq/liter; CO_2 27 mEq/liter; potassium 4.5 mEq/liter; calcium 11.3 mg/dl; phosphate 2.7 mg/dl. Chest roentgenogram, normal; EKG, sinus tachycardia; IVP, normal; Urinary metanephrines 6.5 mg/24 hr (normal <0.9 mg/24 hr).

Question

1. What further diagnostic studies for pheochromocytoma should be performed?

Answer

Clinical and biochemical studies suggest pheochromocytoma. Measurement of the urinary metanephrine levels in a 24-hour specimen is probably the screening test of choice, as there are fewer false positive and false negative values than with the tests for urinary catecholamines or VMA. Confirmatory evidence should then be provided by obtaining basal plasma catecholamine values, as this test is a highly sensitive predictor of the presence of pheochromocytoma. It is important to remember that the patient should be prepared properly before plasma catecholamines are drawn. They are collected on ice through an indwelling venous line in a patient who has been supine for at least 30 minutes. In addition, in patients with paroxysmal hypertension, efforts should be made to obtain the blood samples during a hypertensive episode.

In addition to biochemical studies, preoperative localization is usually attempted. At present CAT appears to be the method of choice for localization of both adrenal and extraadrenal tumors.

Ultrasound has proven useful at some centers, particularly in detecting larger tumors. Angiography is also helpful in localizing but is an invasive procedure associated with an increased risk of hypertensive crisis. Scintigraphic localization with meta-[^{131}I] iodobenzylguanidine, an analog of guanethidine, has been recently proposed as offering a safe and reliable method of detecting tumors not detected by a CAT scan. Occasionally, when other methods of localization have failed, selective venous sampling for determination of catecholamines has proven helpful.

Question

2. Does this patient have sporadic or familial phenochromocytoma?

Answer

The patient has hypercalcemia and a family history suggestive for MEN-IIa. MEN-IIa is a syndrome of medullary carcinoma of the thyroid, pheochromocytoma, and chief cell parathyroid hyperplasia. It is inherited as an autosomal dominant, and affected family members may manifest one or more of the endocrine neoplasms. It is important for the surgeon to know whether the pheochromocytoma is thought to be familial or sporadic, as familial pheochromocytoma is frequently multicentric and often bilateral. If bilateral adrenalectomy is anticipated, preparations for steroid coverage should be made. If the patient is found to have MEN-II, all first-degree family members should be screened and followed for the possibility of their involvement.

Question

3. What are the sites of extraadrenal pheochromocytomas?

Answer

The incidence of extraadrenal pheochromocytoma is approximately 10%. The majority of these occur in the abdomen and involve the paraganglia of the sympathetic nervous system and the organ of Zuckerkandl. Tumors may also involve the ovaries, testes, or bladder. Occasionally pheochromocytoma originates in the chest or, rarely, the neck. It appears that extraadrenal pheochromocytomas have a greater tendency to become malignant and for this reason have a worse prognosis than malignant adrenal pheochromocytomas.

Case II

Description

A 45-year old woman is found to have a pheochromocytoma of the right adrenal. Her preoperative course is uneventful. During surgery her operative course is stormy and complicated by cardiac arrhythmias, a period of sustained high blood pressure, and hypotension that occurs after the tumor is removed. Postoperatively the patient remains hypotensive.

Question

1. What are the possible causes for this patient's hypotension?

Answer

Following removal of a pheochromocytoma postoperative hypotension may ensue as a result of the sudden fall in the level of circulating catecholamines. This can be prevented or reversed by adequate infusion of fluids and/or blood combined with careful cardiovascular monitoring. The continued effects of preoperative catecholamine blockage with various agents may also adversely affect postoperative blood pressure. To avoid this problem these agents are often discontinued the night prior to the operation. In addition, acute medical problems, such as myocardial infarction, sepsis, congestive heart failure, or continued bleeding are other possible sources of hypotension that should be considered.

Question

2. What factors might be responsible if the patient remained hypertensive postoperatively?

Answer

Several factors could be involved. The patient may have been fluid-overloaded during the surgery. A renal artery may have been inadvertently ligated or residual pheochromocytoma left. In addition, up to one-quarter of cured patients may continue to have hypertension postoperatively, probably because of the coexistence of essential hypertension. This is usually seen in patients with pheochromocytoma who have had sustained hypertension preoperatively and is uncommon in those with paroxysmal hypertension.

SUGGESTED READING

Bergman SM, Sewars HF, Javadpour N: Postoperative management of patients with pheochromocytoma. *J Urol* 120:109, 1978.

Bravo EL, Tarazi RC, Gifford RW, Stewart BH: Circulating and urinary catecholamines in pheochromocytoma. *N Engl J Med* 301:28, 1979.

Feldman JM, Blalock JA, Zern RT, Wells SA: The relationship between enzyme activity and the catecholamine content and secretion of pheochromocytomas. *J Clin Endocrinol Metab* 49:445, 1979.

Harrison TS, Freier DT: Pitfalls in the technique and interpretation of regional venous sampling for localizing pheochromocytoma. *Surg Clin North Am* 54:339, 1974.

Hume DM: Pheochromocytoma in the adult and in the child. *Am J Surg* 99:458–490, 1960.

Huebner AD, Reed PA: Secreting tumor chromaffin tissue. *Ann Surg* 158:216–221, 1963.

Juan D: Pheochromocytoma: Clinical manifestations and diagnostic tests. *Urology* 17:1, 1981.

Kaufman JF: Pheochromocytoma and tricyclic antidepressants. *J Am Med Assoc* 229:1282, 1974.

Kirkendahl WM, Liechty RD, Culp DA: Diagnosis and treatment of patients with pheochromocytoma. *Arch Intern Med* 115:529, 1965.

Laursen K, Damgaard-Peterson K: CT for pheochromocytoma diagnosis. *Am J Radiol* 134:277, 1980.

Louis WJ, Doyle AE, Heath WC, Robinson MJ: Secretion of dopa in phaeochromocytoma. *Br Med J* 4:325, 1972.

Manger W, Gifford RW Jr: *Pheochromocytoma.* New York, Springer-Verlag, 1977.

Minno AM, Bennett WA, Kvale WF: Pheochromocytoma: A study of 15 cases diagnosed at autopsy. *N Engl J Med* 251:959, 1954.

Munson ES, Tucker WK: Doses of epinephrine causing arrhythmia during enflurane, methoxyflurane and halothane anesthesia in dogs. *Can Anaesth Soc J* 22:469, 1975.

Ochi K, Yoshioka S, Morita M, Takeuchi M: Pheochromocytoma of bladder. *Urology* 17:228, 1981.

Rosati LA, Augur HA Jr: Ischemic enterocolitis in pheochromocytoma. *Gastroenterology* 60:581, 1971.

Schegel GG: Recklinghausen's neurofibromatosis and pheochromocytoma. *Schweiz Med Wochenschr* 90:31, 1960.

Smithwich RH, Greer WER, Robertson CW, Wilkins RW: Pheochromocytoma: A discussion of symptoms, signs and procedures of diagnostic value. *N Engl J Med* 242:252, 1950.

Sutton D: The radiological diagnosis of adrenal tumors. *Br J Radiol* 48:237, 1975.

Stewart BH, Bravo EL, Haaga J, Meaney TF, Tarzai R: Localization of pheochromocytoma by computed tomography. *N Engl J Med* 299:490, 1978.

Teply JF, Lawrence GH: Pheochromocytoma. *Am J Surg* 140:107, 1980.

Thomas JE, Rooke ED, Kvale WF: The neurologists experience with pheochromocytoma: A review of 100 cases. *J Am Med Assoc* 197:754, 1966.

11

GLENN D. BRAUNSTEIN

Ectopic Hormone Secretion

The paraneoplastic syndromes comprise the signs, symptoms, and biochemical abnormalities occurring in cancer patients that are not due to the mass effects of the primary neoplasm or metastases. There are a variety of such remote effects of cancer, and the major categories are listed in Table 1. It has been estimated that at any one time 20% of patients with cancer will have a paraneoplastic syndrome and that 75% of all cancer patients will develop such a syndrome during the course of their disease. Among the most frequent of the paraneoplastic syndromes are the endocrine manifestations due to ectopic hormone production.

Ectopic hormone production was originally defined as the secretion of a hormone by a neoplasm derived from a tissue or organ that does not normally produce the hormone. Conversely, eutopic hormone production referred to the secretion of a hormone by a neoplasm derived from a tissue or organ that normally produces the hormone. However, in recent years a number of investigators have provided *in vivo* and *in vitro* evidence that many different nonendocrine human tissues are capable of producing small quantities of hormones. These minute amounts of hormones detected in nonendocrine tissues may have a biologic function or may merely represent vestigial protein production. Nevertheless, the isolation of hormones from nonendocrine tissues has altered our concept of ectopic hormone production. Thus *ectopic hormone production* describes a quantitative abnormality rather than a qualitative one and may be redefined as the excessive secretion of a hormone by a neoplasm derived from a tissue or organ that is not the known physiologic source of the circulating hormone.

Clinical Importance

There are many reasons why ectopic hormone production is of clinical importance. The recognition of a syndrome may lead to the diagnosis of an occult tumor weeks, months, and, occasionally, years before the tumor otherwise becomes clinically apparent. This is especially true in patients with the ectopic ACTH syndrome associated with bronchial carcinoid tumors or thymic tumors. Similarly, the syndrome of tumor-induced osteomalacia characteristically occurs with the metabolic disturbance antedating the discovery of the tumor. Ectopic hormone syndromes are also of importance, because the patient may succumb to the metabolic effects

Table 1 **Paraneoplastic Syndromes**

Ectopic hormone syndromes
Skin and connective tissue syndromes
Dermatomyositis
Acanthosis nigricans
Ichthyosis
Hypertrophic osteoarthropathy
Amyloidosis
Secondary gout
Polyarthritis
Neuromyopathies
Central nervous system
Amyotrophic lateral sclerosis-like syndrome
Progressive multifocal leukoencephalopathy
Peripheral nerve disorders
Myasthenia (Eaton-Lambert)
Polymyositis
Dementia
Hematologic and vascular syndromes
Anemia
Erythrocytosis
Hypercoagulable state
Leukemoid reactions
Hyperviscosity
Platelet abnormalities
Gastrointestinal tract syndromes
Malabsorption
Exudative enteropathy
Miscellaneous
Fever
Anorexia—cachexia
Acid-base and electrolyte disorders
Nephrotic syndrome

of the hormone excess rather than to the neoplasm. This is best exemplified by patients who develop a hypercalcemic crisis as a result of the production of humoral factors by a tumor. Finally, the measurements of the hormones produced by the tumor may serve as a tumor marker in following the effects of therapy and detecting disease recurrence.

Criteria of Ectopic Hormone Production

Several criteria for the diagnosis of ectopic hormone production have been defined. First, by definition, excessive quantities of the circulating hormone must be present in a patient with a neoplasm derived from a tissue that is not the normal physiologic source of the hormone. Second, there should be a persistence of the excessive serum hormone concentration or endocrine syndrome following removal or suppression of the normal endocrine source of the hormone. Thus, persistent Cushing's syndrome and elevated ACTH concentrations following complete hypophysectomy are indicative of an ectopic source of ACTH. Similarly, the failure of the ACTH concentrations to fall following large doses of dexamethasone in a patient without a pituitary neoplasm is strongly suggestive of ectopic ACTH production. Third, there should be a greater concentration of hormone in the tumor than in the surrounding tissue. In addition, histochemical or immunochemical localization of the hormone in the tumor, but not in the adjacent normal tissue, suggests that the hormone is produced by the tumor. Fourth, if the tumor produces a form of the hormone qualitatively different from that occurring under physiologic circumstances, a presumptive diagnosis of ectopic hormone production can be made. Again, using the ectopic ACTH syndrome as an example, the finding that the majority of the circulating immunoreactive ACTH is in fact pro-ACTH (''big'' ACTH) favors the diagnosis of tumor production of ACTH. The fifth criterion is the finding of an arteriovenous hormone concentration gradient across the tumor. If it can be shown that there is a greater concentration of the hormone in the venous drainage of the tumor than in the arterial blood supplying the tumor, one of the most rigid criteria for ectopic hormone production will have been met. Finally, the most reliable criterion for ectopic hormone secretion is the finding of continued production of the hormone by the cells maintained in *in vitro* culture. The continued secretion of the hormone into the culture medium or the incorporation of radiolabeled essential amino acids or carbohydrates into the hormone under culture conditions provides unequivocal demonstration of ectopic hormone production.

Spectrum of Ectopic Hormones

The spectrum of ectopic hormone production, the clinical syndromes that may be associated with overproduction of these hormones, and the tumor types most frequently associated with the syndromes are shown in Table 2. The table also illustrates the interesting fact that all the hormones that have been demonstrated to be produced ectopically are proteins or polypeptides. Although tumors may metabolize thyronines and steroids, no example of the ectopic production of thyroid, adrenal, or gonadal hormones has been documented. The reasons for this are unclear but may be related to the observations that the capability for producing proteins is present in the cytoplasm of every cell and only requires RNA to serve as a template for protein production, while the thyroid and steroid hormones require orderly enzymatic steps for synthesis which are lacking in tumors not of thyroid, adrenal, or gonadal origin.

One of the paradoxes seen in cancer patients is that ectopic hormone production appears to be quite common, while ectopic hormone syndromes are relatively uncommon. For instance, excessive serum concentrations of immunoreactive ACTH have been found in over 80% of patients with lung carcinoma. Yet, fewer than 3% of patients with lung carcinoma have clinical Cushing's syndrome. There are several explanations for this discrepancy. First, the quantities of hormone secreted may be only slightly greater than normal and insufficient to lead to a clinical syndrome. Second, it has been well documented that some tumors secrete hormones intermittently. Third, some tumors produce immunologically active but biologically inactive forms of hormones. For example, it appears that the majority of patients with lung cancer have ectopic production of ACTH precursors that have very little biologic activity. In addition to the production of immunologically active but biologically inactive hormone precursor molecules, many tumors have been found to synthesize subunits of hormones as well as fragments of hormones that are detected by hormone radioimmunoassays.

Table 2 **Spectrum of Hormones Produced Ectopically, Clinical Syndromes, and Tumors Most Frequently Associated with the Syndromes**

Hormone	*Syndrome*	*Tumors*
ACTH lipotropins	Cushing's syndrome, hyperpigmentation	Lung, thymus, thyroid (medullary cancer), pancreatic islets
Parathyroid hormone	Hypercalcemia	Lung, kidney, liver
Antidiuretic hormone (ADH)	Hyponatremia (SIADH)	Lung, pancreas, duodenum
Insulin-like growth factor	Hypoglycemia	Mesenchymal, liver, adrenal
Hypophosphatemia-producing factor	Oncogenic osteomalacia	Mesenchymal
Chorionic gonadotropin	Gynecomastia, precocious puberty	Lung, kidney, liver
Erythropoietin	Polycythemia	Kidney, liver, cerebellar hemangioblastoma
Prolactin?	Galactorrhea	Lung, kidney
Gastrin	Zollinger-Ellison syndrome?	Ovary, lung
Growth Hormone?	Hypertrophic osteoarthropathy?	Lung, uterus
Glucagon	Hyperglycemia	Lung, liver, kidney
Vasoactive intestinal peptide	Watery diarrhea	Lung, pheochromocytoma
Calcitonin	None usually, rare hypocalcemia	Lung, breast, colon, pancreas, liver
Placental lactogen	None	Lung, liver
Oxytocin	None	Same as ADH
Releasing or inhibiting factors		
Growth hormone-releasing factor	Acromegaly	Lung, bronchial carcinoid
Corticotropin-releasing factor	Cushing's syndrome	Lung, carcinoid, thymus
Somatostatin	None	Lung

Etiology

Several etiologic mechanisms have been proposed to explain ectopic hormone production. These include de novo synthesis, derepression, blocked ontogenesis, and the endocrine cell theory.

De Novo Synthesis

If, during the process of neoplasia, a variety of new proteins are formed and by chance one or more proteins are made that have biologic activity, it is conceivable that excessive expression of this biologic activity would lead to a syndrome. If the biologic activity is hormonal in nature, then an ectopic hormone syndrome may become apparent. However, two observations cannot be explained by this particular theory. First is the finding that ectopic hormone production is not a random phenomenon. Thus, almost 80% of the tumors associated with ectopic ACTH production are located within the chest, involving either the lung or thymic tissue. Similarly, squamous cell carcinoma of the lung and renal cell carcinomas of the kidney account for the majority of tumors associated with nonmetastatic hypercalcemia. If neoproteins with hormonal activity were produced by cancers, one would expect that a wide variety of neoplasms would be associated with such proteins rather than a restricted group. The second observation that cannot be explained by this hypothesis is the finding that ectopically produced hormones are structurally identical to eutopically produced hormones. Thus the ACTH precursors produced by lung tumors appear to be structurally identical to the small amounts of ACTH precursors produced by the normal pituitary. Although incomplete hormone fragments may be secreted, the molecules produced appear to be structurally identical to homologous regions on the normally occurring hormones.

Derepression

Every somatic cell in the body contains the same genetic material, and during the process of tissue and organ specialization, totipotential stem cells differentiate into specialized adult cells. This process of differentiation includes the repression of areas of the genome that are not necessary for expression in the adult state. It is then assumed that during neoplastic transformation some of the repressed areas may become derepressed and are allowed to express their gene products. For example, during the transition of a lung cell from the undifferentiated to the adult state, the genes responsible for ACTH production become repressed. Neoplastic transformation of such a cell may result in derepression of this area of the gene, allowing the cell to begin producing ACTH.

Blocked Ontogenesis

A third theory proposed to explain the ectopic hormone syndromes suggests that cancers actually arise from stem or renewal cells that are present in every organ and that have not fully differentiated into adult cells. It is proposed that these cells have areas of the genome that have never been repressed and that tumors arising from such cells may thus be able to express all unrepressed gene products, including hormones.

Endocrine Cells

The endocrine cell hypothesis states that ectopic hormone production occurs in cells that embryologically are related to the precursors of normal endocrine glands and tissues. One such type of common endocrine cell is that of the APUD series (*a*mine *p*recursor *u*ptake and *d*ecarboxylation). Some of these cells are of neural crest origin and are widely distributed throughout the body. Tumors derived from cells of the APUD series may secrete a number of vasoactive peptides and amines as well as proteins such as ACTH, antidiuretic hormone (ADH), oxytocin, and neurophysin. Although this is an attractive hypothesis, it cannot account for the spectrum of tumors that produce hormones ectopically and are not derived from neural crest tissue and do not have APUD characteristics. A variation of this hypothesis is the hybridization theory in which it is proposed that neoplasia involves the hybridization of a nonendocrine cell with an endocrine cell such as an APUD cell, and that this combination can then express the production of hormones. There is a dearth of experimental data supporting this concept.

Therapy

Before considering specific syndromes and their therapy it is appropriate to review some of the general concepts concerning therapy. There are essentially four approaches to therapy for ectopic hormone secretion. The first is to remove the tumor. If successful, there should be a rapid decrease in the elevated hormone levels and a reversal of the endocrine syndrome. Similarly, effective chemotherapy or radiation therapy directed at the primary neoplasm may give the same result. A second approach is to remove the target organ of the ectopically produced hormone. In the ectopic ACTH syndrome, the major metabolic derangements are due to excessive stimulation of glucocorticoid production. Bilateral adrenalectomy will remove the source of the glucocorticoids and result in a reversal of the metabolic abnormalities, even though large amounts of ACTH are persistently produced by the primary tumor. A third approach is to block the peripheral effects of the ectopically produced hormone. Again, using the ectopic ACTH syndrome as an example, inhibitors of glucocorticoid synthesis such as aminoglutethimide and metyrapone may block production of the glucocorticoids and reverse the syndrome. A final approach is to inhibit the production of the hormone selectively. Indeed, this is probably what happens in many patients who receive chemotherapeutic agents. Such agents may interfere with protein synthesis and the cellular machinery needed for production of hormones. In some instances such therapy may be effective in reducing or eliminating a clone of the cells within the tumor that produce the hormones. Destruction of such a cell line or interference with the biosynthesis of the ectopic hormone may lead to a discordance between the hormone level and tumor growth. The hormone level may decrease, while the bulk of the tumor increases. Such a discordance has been noted for many ectopically produced hormones as well as other tumor proteins.

CLINICALLY IMPORTANT SYNDROMES

Ectopic ACTH Syndrome

Clinical Features

The ectopic production of ACTH is generally associated with the rapid appearance of proximal muscle weakness, edema, hypertension, glucose intolerance, and hypochloremic alkalosis. Because of the rapidity of the onset and the high levels of glucocorticoids, there tends to be little or no development of Cushingoid fat distribution. Hyperpigmentation is found in approximately one-quarter of patients, and many have anorexia and cachexia. Central nervous system manifestations include personality changes, impaired mentation, and coma.

Pathophysiology

The relationships among the hypothalamus, pituitary, and adrenal glands in normal individuals, as well as in patients with Cushing's syndrome caused by excessive production of ACTH by the pituitary (Cushing's disease), primary adrenal tumors, and the ectopic ACTH syndrome are illustrated in Figure 1. In normal individuals, cortisol produced by the adrenals

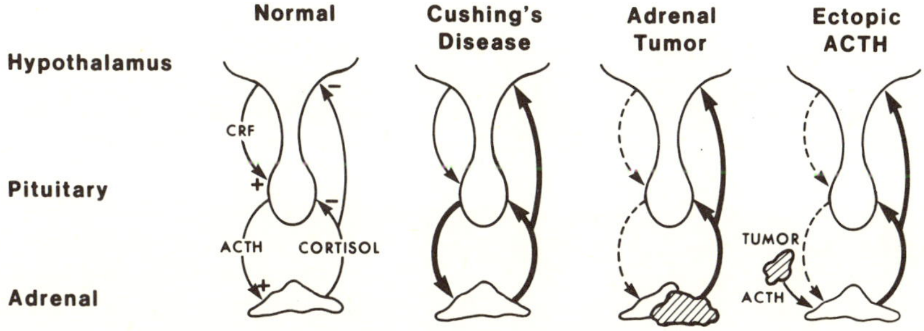

Figure 1. Hypothalamic-pituitary-adrenal relationships in normal individuals and in patients with Cushing's syndrome of various etiologies.

inhibits the secretion of ACTH from the pituitary. In patients with Cushing's disease, the set point for feedback inhibition of the pituitary by cortisol is increased. In this situation, supranormal amounts of cortisol are required to inhibit the pituitary production of ACTH. Because this is a primary hypothalamic or pituitary disorder, the individuals have elevated ACTH concentrations in respect to the circulating levels of cortisol. Nevertheless, in most instances, the pituitary ACTH production can be suppressed with pharmacologic amounts of exogenous glucocorticoids. Patients with primary adrenal neoplasms, whether adrenal cortical carcinoma or adrenal adenoma, have excessive adrenal production of cortisol as the primary disturbance. Because the pituitary and hypothalamus are normally responsive to the feedback inhibition by cortisol, ACTH concentrations are low. In the ectopic ACTH syndrome, excessive concentrations of ACTH produced by tumors stimulate both adrenals to become hyperplastic. There is a marked increase in the secretion of cortisol, as well as of mineralocorticoids and adrenal androgen precursors. The excessive quantities of cortisol inhibit the production of ACTH by the pituitary.

The marked increase in glucocorticoids leads to extensive protein catabolism, followed by breakdown of muscle proteins with the release of amino acids which are converted by the liver into glucose through the process of gluconeogenesis. This combination of effects results in the extensive muscle weakness and hyperglycemia seen in the syndrome. The excessive production of mineralocorticoids by the adrenals produces hypokalemic alkalosis, salt and water retention, and hypertension and edema. For reasons that are not clear, the renal escape phenomenon seen in other conditions of mineralocorticoid excess does not occur in patients with the ectopic ACTH syndrome. The hypoalbuminemia often seen in this condition may contribute to the edema. The hypokalemia may also contribute to the extensive proximal muscle weakness. Overproduction of adrenal androgens and androgen precursors generally do not result in clinical manifestations in males, but in females may lead to hirsutism and virilization.

In the pituitary, ACTH is initially synthesized as a high-molecular-weight (31,000) protein termed pro-opiomelanocortin. This molecule contains not only the 39 amino acids that comprise ACTH but also β-lipotropin, a 91-amino-acid protein. Within the pro-opiomelanocortin molecule are several amino acid sequences which contain melanocyte-stimulating activity. In addition, the opioid peptides, endorphins and enkephalins, have amino acid sequences identical to areas in the β-lipotropin molecule. In situations where excessive ACTH production by the pituitary takes place, parallel increases in the production of β-lipotropin and other fragments of pro-opiomelanocortin have also been found. The same phenomenon is also seen in many patients with the ectopic ACTH syndrome. Thus the hyperpigmentation seen in the ectopic ACTH syndrome may be due in part to the concomitant excessive production of melanotropic fragments of pro-opiomelanocortin. Similarly, some of the psychologic aberrations found in the syndrome may be the result of the excessive production of opioid peptides. Of course, elevated glucocorticoids per se may lead to psychological abnormalities (steroid psychosis).

The predominant molecular form of ACTH found in the circulation of patients with the clinical ectopic ACTH syndrome is the biologically active, 39-amino-acid molecule. However, many patients with cancer, especially lung tumors, have been found to have elevated plasma concentrations of immunoreactive ACTH and yet do not have the ectopic ACTH syndrome. As noted above, large precursor forms of ACTH that have little or no biologic activity but retain immunologic activity are the predominent circulating species of ACTH in such patients.

The overwhelming majority (approximately 80%) of tumors associated with the clinical syndrome are located in the chest and neck. These include carcinomas of the lung, especially of the oat cell variety, thymic neoplasms, bronchial adenomas, and medullary carcinoma of the thyroid. The remaining patients reported with the syndrome have had a variety of other neoplasms including islet cell carcinoma of the pancreas, ovarian tumors, prostatic carcinoma, renal cell carcinoma, pheochromocytomas, and other tumors of neural crest origin. Rare causes of the syndrome include carcinomas of the breast, esophagus, uterus, colon, and gallbladder.

Diagnosis

The scheme outline in Chapter 8 can be used to diagnose the ectopic ACTH syndrome. Although this scheme will suffice to allow the correct diagnosis in the majority of cases involving the ectopic ACTH syndrome, some patients with the syndrome (especially those with bronchial carcinoids) will suppress ACTH levels after the administration of 8 mg of dexamethasone given for 2 days. Conversely, some patients with pituitary-dependent Cushing's disease will not suppress ACTH levels with high doses of dexamethasone. In such patients with confusing dexamethasone suppression test results and elevations in the plasma concentration of ACTH, it has been found useful in some cases to obtain multiple venous blood samples from different areas of the body. Especially important is catheterization of the petrosal veins which contain blood that has drained from the pituitary gland. The finding of an elevated ACTH concentration in the petrosal veins relative to the peripheral veins is indicative of pituitary production of ACTH. If the concentration of ACTH in the petrosal veins is less than that found in the peripheral venous blood, an ectopic source of ACTH is present. By obtaining multiple samples from different areas of the body, localization of the tumor may be accomplished.

Treatment

Survival is generally less than 1 month from the time of diagnosis for patients with untreated clinically apparent ectopic ACTH syndrome. Most patients die from the metabolic complications of the disease. Several treatments are available for the condition. Surgical removal of the tumor is successful in approximately 10% of such patients. Radiation therapy or chemotherapy may also alleviate the clinical manifestations of the syndrome. If these therapies are unsuccessful, adrenal steroid production can be inhibited by aminoglutethimide (Cytadren). Daily doses of 1–2 g of the drug may lead to a rapid decrease in glucocorticoid, mineralocorticoid, and adrenal androgen secretion. The side effects of the drug are frequent and include skin rashes, somnolence, and gastrointestinal disturbances. Adrenal insufficiency may occur quite rapidly, and such patients should be given maintenance doses of hydrocortisone and fludrocortisone (Florinef). Another inhibitor of adrenal steroid biosynthesis is metyrapone (Metopirone). This drug inhibits the 11-hydroxylation step in glucocorticoid synthesis and leads to a reduction in cortisol concentrations. This drug may cause gastrointestinal disturbances and also result in the appearance of adrenal insufficiency. As with aminoglutethimide, glucocorticoid replacement therapy should be given in physiologic doses.

The peripheral effects of the mineralocorticoids can be antagonized to some extent by the administration of spironolactone (Aldactone). Very large doses of this drug may be required in order to reverse the hypokalemic alkalosis. Rarely, bilateral adrenalectomy may be performed to alleviate the syndrome. This mode of therapy should be considered only as a last resort after the other modalities have failed. Patients with the ectopic ACTH syndrome are extremely poor surgical risks, heal poorly, and tend to develop infections.

Tumor Hypercalcemia

Clinical Features

Hypercalcemia occurs in 10–20% of all patients with malignancies. The clinical manifestations are due in part to the underlying etiology (e.g., metastasis to bone), the rapidity of the rise in the serum calcium level, and the actual level of the calcium. There are marked individual differences in the response of a patient to hypercalcemia. The clinical features include weakness, anorexia, nausea, vomiting, abdominal pain, constipation, polyuria or oliguria, dehydration, increased thirst, and a variety of central nervous system disturbances including confusion, personality disturbances, obtundation, and coma.

Pathophysiology

The most common cause of hypercalcemia in patients with malignancies is the local lysis of bone due to bone metastasis. Over 80% of patients with hypercalcemia associated with a neoplasm have bone metastases. Such metastases stimulate osteoclastic bone resorption in the adjacent bone and result in the release of calcium and hydroxyproline into the circulation. It has been suggested that stimulation of the osteoclasts by malignant tumors may be due to the local production of prostaglandins or osteoclast-activating factor (OAF) (see below). The most common malignancies associated with bone metastases are disseminated breast carcinoma in women and carcinoma of the lung in men.

In patients without bone metastases, several humoral factors have been identified that can result in hypercalcemia. These include parathyroid hormone (PTH) produced ectopically, prostaglandins, OAF, and a recently described nephrogenous cyclic-AMP (cAMP)-stimulating factor.

The ectopic production of PTH has been described in over 300 patients with hypercalcemia of malignancy. Close to 90% of the reported patients have been males. The most frequent associated tumors are clear-cell carcinomas of the kidney and ovary, hepatocellular carcinoma and cholangiocarcinoma, pheochromocytoma, and squamous cell carcinoma of the lung, head, neck, esophagus, and genitourinary tract. In most instances, the diagnosis of ectopic PTH production was made by finding hypercalcemia associated with carcinoma and elevated levels of PTH. Very few of the reports have demonstrated unequivocal evidence of ectopic PTH production by the tumors by demonstrating either arterio-venous differences in PTH across the tumors or *in vitro* production of PTH by the tumor cells. In addition, there have been major discrepancies in analysis of the molecular forms of PTH in the circulation and tumor tissue of such patients. As would be anticipated, patients with ectopic PTH production have evidence of increased osteoclastic bone resorption. For reasons that are not clear, such patients tend to have hypochloremic alkalosis, in contrast to patients with primary hyperparathyroidism who demonstrate hyperchloremic acidosis.

Prostaglandin E_2 is widely distributed in cells throughout the body. In several animal models, as well as in humans, it has been demonstrated that a variety of solid tumors associated with hypercalcemia without bone metastasis have increased circulating levels of prostaglandin E_2. *In vitro* studies have shown that prostaglandin E_2 stimulates osteoclastic bone resorption, releasing calcium into the medium. As noted above, the local production of prostaglandins by metastatic deposits in the bone may be responsible for the hypercalcemia seen with such metastases. It has also been suggested that excessive prostaglandin production by tumors distant from the bone may result in bone resorption either from the secreted prostaglandin or a circulating metabolite. Indeed, it has been found that the concentration of the major urinary metabolite of the E prostaglandins, 7α-hydroxy-5,11-diketotetranorprostane-1,16-dioic acid (PGE-M), is elevated in patients with nonmetastatic hypercalcemia of cancer. In such patients, the immunoreactive PTH concentrations are low in serum, and the urinary nephrogenous cAMP levels are normal. Inhibition of prostaglandin synthesis by indomethacin or aspirin suppresses urinary PGE-M excretion and results in a parallel decrease in serum calcium concentrations.

OAF is a polypeptide that stimulates osteoclastic bone resorption. It is distinct from PTH, vitamin D or its metabolites, and the prostaglandins. This substance is produced by normal leukocytes stimulated *in vitro* by phytohemagglutinin. It has also been found to be spontaneously produced by tumor cells in patients with multiple myeloma, malignant lymphomas, and some leukemias.

Recent studies on patients with cancer-associated hypercalcemia have shown that 60–80% of patients have increased nephrogenous cyclic AMP, reduced tubular reabsorption of phosphorus, normal or low levels of PTH, and reduced serum concentrations of 1,25-dihydroxyvitamin D. Patients with primary hyperparathyroidism also demonstrate an elevation of the nephrogenous cAMP level and reduced tubular readsorption of phosphate, but in contrast have elevated serum PTH and 1,25-dihydroxyvitamin D concentrations. These studies suggest that many patients with cancer-associated hypercalcemia have a circulating renotropic factor that stimulates proximal tubular adenylate cyclase and inhibits proximal tubular phosphate reabsorption in a fashion similar to PTH, but which differs from PTH by its relative inability to stimulate distal tubular calcium reabsorption and to stimulate the renal 1α-hydroxylase enzyme responsible for converting 25-hydroxyvitamin D to 1,25-dihydroxyvitamin D.

Finally, it should be noted that hyperparathyroidism and cancer coexist with greater than chance frequency. It has been estimated that 5% or more of patients with cancer and hypercalcemia have coexisting primary hyperparathyroidism responsible for the hypercalcemia and that over 30% of patients with parathyroid adenomas have, have had, or will develop a carcinoma. It is unclear whether hyperparathyroidism per se predisposes an individual to the development of a neoplasm. It is unlikely that the tumors directly produce a parathyrotropic factor, since single parathyroid adenomas are usually found in cancer patients with coexisting primary hyperparathyroidism. It would be anticipated that a parathyrotropic factor produced by tumors would result in parathyroid hyperplasia rather than a single adenoma.

Diagnosis

In order to determine the underlying mechanism of hypercalcemia in a patient with cancer the scheme outlined in Chapter 6 can be followed. Additionally, a bone scan should be performed in cancer patients, since it is a more sensitive indicator of skeletal lesions than bone roentgenograms. The finding of an elevated serum PTH concentration is indicative of the presence of either primary hyperparathyroidism or, rarely, the ectopic production of PTH. The differentiation of these two disorders may be made by performing a venous catheterization study in which blood is obtained from the thyroidal veins that drain the parathyroid glands and from the venous drainage of the neoplasm. Concurrently, a peripheral venous blood sample should be obtained. If the concentration of PTH found in the thyroidal veins is greater than that found in the peripheral venous circulation or in the venous drainage from the tumor, the diagnosis of primary hyperparathyroidism is established. Conversely, if the greatest concentration of serum PTH is found in the veins draining the tumor, a diagnosis of ectopic PTH production is established. This procedure is rarely necessary, however, since nearly all hypercalcemic cancer patients with elevated serum PTH levels will prove to have hyperparathyroidism.

Therapy

Therapy for hypercalcemia of cancer is outlined in Chapter 6.

Syndrome of Inappropriate Secretion of Antidiuretic Hormone

The signs and symptoms of the syndrome of inappropriate secretion of antidiuretic hormone (SIADH) are due to water intoxication and the rate of fall of the serum sodium concentration. The clinical features generally do not become apparent until the sodium concentration falls below 120–125 mEq/liter. They include anorexia, nausea, vomiting, abdominal pain, bloating, ileus, restlessness, confusion, withdrawal, hostility, headache, muscle weakness, and myoclonus. Severe water intoxication may be seen when the serum sodium concentration falls below 110 mEq/liter and is characterized by muscle weakness, hemiparesis, ataxia, stupor, convulsions, and coma. A more detailed discussion of SIADH and its treatment is given in Chapter 3.

Tumor Hypoglycemia

Clinical Features

The signs and symptoms of hypoglycemia are due to two factors: the rate of fall of the blood sugar level and the actual serum glucose concentration. A rapid decrease in the blood glucose level activates the sympathetic nervous system, resulting in an increase in the secretion of norepinephrine and epinephrine. The resulting symptoms are those that would be anticipated from excessive concentrations of catecholamines. These include tremulousness, anxiety, tachycardia, diaphoresis, piloerection, and a feeling of impending doom.

The other major symptoms are those due to neuroglucopenia and are the result of a deficient supply of glucose to the central nervous system. These manifestations are generally seen when the plasma glucose concentration is below 45 mg/dl (blood glucose less than 40 mg/dl). Thus headache, confusion, disorientation, ataxia, focal neurologic disorders, seizures, and coma may be seen. In patients with tumor hypoglycemia, the latter neuroglucopenic symptoms predominate, since most of the patients have chronic hypoglycemia which has developed insidiously rather than abruptly. The hypoglycemic symptoms predominate in the fasting state and thus are most apparent in the early morning hours and in the late afternoon.

Pathophysiology

Approximately half of the tumors associated with hypoglycemia are of mesenchymal origin and include fibrosarcomas, liposarcomas, leiomyosarcomas, neurofibromas, rhabdomyosarcomas, mesotheliomas, and hemangiopericytomas. The tumors are generally located in the retroperitoneal or intrathoracic areas and range in size from several hundred grams to 10–20 kg. Hepatocellular carcinoma accounts for approximately one-quarter of patients with tumor hypoglycemia, and approximately 10% of patients have adrenocortical carcinoma. Hypoglycemia has also been noted with a variety of non-islet cell gastrointestinal tract tumors, as well as in patients with lymphomas and leukemias.

The pathogenesis of tumor hypoglycemia has not been fully clarified. In approximately 40% of patients with tumor-associated hypoglycemia elevated serum concentrations of low-molecular-weight insulin-like peptides have been detected. In patients with tumor hypoglycemia, insulin-like growth factor II is the substance most consistently found to be at an elevated level in the serum. It is unknown whether the tumors secrete insulin-like growth factor II or whether the liver or other potential normal sites of synthesis are responsible for elaboration of the material.

Another proposed mechanism for hypoglycemia seen with some tumors, especially those that are quite large, is overutilization of glucose by the tumor itself. It is possible that over a long period of time the capacity of the liver to compensate for extreme glucose utilization by tumors can be overcome, resulting in hypoglycemia.

Diagnosis

The cardinal feature of tumor hypoglycemia is the finding of a low plasma glucose level (less than 45 mg/dl) and a suppressed serum immunoreactive insulin concentration ($<10\ \mu U/ml$) in a patient with a neoplasm. Other causes of fasting hypoglycemia with suppressed insulin concentrations must be ruled out. Thus severe hepatic insufficiency, thyroid insufficiency, adrenocortical insufficiency, pituitary disease, and drug-induced hypoglycemia should be considered. Liver function tests, a determination of the free thyroxine index, a Cortrosyn stimulation test for cortisol secretion, and evaluation of pituitary function are necessary. Chapter 16 provides further details of the investigation of patients with hypoglycemia.

Treatment

Unfortunately, the results of treatment of tumor-associated hypoglycemia are generally poor. Successful resection of the tumor or effective chemotherapy or radiotherapy is the treatment of choice for the disorder. There are no specific agents available that are uniformly effective in antagonizing tumor-induced hypoglycemia. Frequent feedings throughout the day and night may decrease the symptoms. Occasionally the administration of glucocorticoids, growth hormone, or glucagon have relieved symptoms early in the course of the disease but do not usually result in complete amelioration of the hypoglycemia. As would be anticipated, diazoxide is ineffective in this disorder, since its major mode of action is to inhibit the secretion of insulin, a hormone that is already suppressed in patients with this condition.

Oncogenic Osteomalacia

Clinical Features

Oncogenic osteomalacia has been found in both children and adults with a history of severe bone pain, pathologic fractures, muscular weakness, and fatigue. Severe osteopenia is present on bone radiographs, and bone biopsy specimens demonstrate osteomalacia. Biochemically the patients have hypophosphatemia, normocalcemia, hyperphosphaturia, elevated levels of serum alkaline phosphatase, and occasionally renal tubular defects such as glycosuria and aminoaciduria.

Pathophysiology

This syndrome is associated with tumors of mesenchymal origin, both benign and malignant, that arise in bone and soft tissues. The tumor types include osteoid osteomas, giant-cell reparative granulomas, giant-cell tumors, sclerosing hemangiomas, pleomorphic sarcomas, fibromas, and hemangiopericytomas. The humoral factor responsible for this syndrome has not been identified, but extensive metabolic studies carried out in a few patients have suggested that a factor elaborated by the tumor inhibits the renal 1α-hydroxylation enzyme responsible for the conversion of 25-hydroxyvitamin D to the active metabolite 1,25-dihydroxyvitamin D. The resulting deficiency of 1,25-dihydroxyvitamin D appears to be the direct cause of the severe osteomalacia.

Diagnosis

The diagnostic criteria of oncogenic osteomalacia are the finding of hypophosphatemia, hyperphosphaturia, normocalcemia, normal serum levels of PTH and 25-hydroxyvitamin D, and low serum concentrations of 1,25-dihydroxyvitamin D. Other causes of severe osteomalacia such as malabsorption, hypophosphatasia, fluorosis, acidosis, renal disease, and exposure to drugs known to alter the metabolism of vitamin D (e.g., phenobarbital and diphenylhydantoin) must be excluded on the basis of history and appropriate biochemical testing.

Treatment

In most of the patients who have been studied, removal of the tumors has been associated with a reversal of the syndrome. Patients with unresectable neoplasms may be treated with physiologic amounts of 1,25-dihydroxyvitamin D (Rocaltrol) in doses ranging from 0.04 to 0.08 μg/kg body weight orally per day.

Ectopic Human Chorionic Gonadotropin Secretion

Clinical Features

Although 15–20% of patients with cancer have detectable levels of human chorionic gonadotropin (hCG) in their blood, very few develop clinical manifestations of hCG excess. Rarely, prepubertal boys with hepatoblastomas may develop isosexual precocious puberty. The clinical manifestations include accelerated skeletal growth, enlargement of the testicles and penis, the appearance of axillary and pubic hair, acne, and malordorous perspiration. An enlarging abdominal mass is usually also present, and several patients have been noted to have hemihypertrophy of the limbs and clubbing of the fingers. It would be anticipated that girls would also demonstrate isosexual precocious puberty, but to date no female child with the ectopic production of hCG by a nontrophoblastic neoplasm has been reported.

Adult women with tumors that produce hCG ectopically do not develop signs or symptoms referable to the hormonal production. Men with hCG-secreting tumors may develop gynecomastia, decreased libido, and hypertrophic osteoarthropathy. However, the majority of men with such tumors do not develop any symptoms.

Pathophysiology

In male children with hCG-secreting tumors, the gonadotropin stimulates testosterone production by the testicular Leydig cells. The elevated testosterone leads to the virilization and accelerated linear growth. In adult males with gynecomastia from hCG-secreting tumors, elevated levels of serum estrogens are present and are responsible for the stimulation of breast glandular growth. There are two sources of the excessive estrogens in these patients. First, chronic stimulation of the testicular Leydig cells by high concentrations of hCG may lead to excessive testicular production of estrogens relative to androgen secretion. Second, it has been shown that many of the tumors associated with gynecomastia contain the enzymes capable of aromatizing androgens or androgen precursors from the adrenal and testes to estrogens. The etiology of the clubbing noted in many of these patients is unknown. The tumors most commonly associated with the ectopic hCG syndrome in adults are large-cell carcinomas of the lung, renal cell carcinomas, hepatomas, and gastric carcinomas.

Diagnosis

The diagnosis rests on the demonstration of elevated concentrations of immunoreactive hCG in the circulation of a patient with the clinical syndrome. In addition to production of the intact hCG molecule, many patients will have excessive production of one of the subunits of hCG. Elevations of serum estradiol and estrone are also commonly found. As noted above, as many as 20% of patients with various malignancies may have immunoreactive hCG in their circulation. Most of these patients do not have any clinical manifestations of the hCG excess primarily because the concentrations of the molecule are too low to stimulate the Leydig cells. Generally one does not see clinical manifestations until the hCG concentration is above 200 mIU/ml of serum. Most of the patients with ectopic hCG production but without the clinical syndrome have hCG concentrations between 5 and 20 mIU/ml of serum.

Therapy

Treatment of the underlying tumor is the therapy of choice for the clinical syndrome. If painful gynecomastia persists, reduction mammoplasty or other measures outlined in Chapter 14 should be considered.

DISCUSSION CASES

Case 1

Description

A 58-year-old male with a 45-pack-year history of smoking reported a 3-month history of a cough productive of blood-streaked sputum, a 6-lb weight loss, and 1 month of tender breasts. He was not taking any medicine nor did he admit to heavy marihuana use. Physical examination revealed scattered wheezes in the left upper posterior chest and bilateral tender gynecomastia. Both testicles were of normal size, shape, and consistency. The remainder of the physical examination was unremarkable.

Laboratory tests included normal CBC, electrolytes, liver function tests, BUN, creatinine, calcium, phosphorus, thyroid function tests, and PRL. A urinary pregnancy test was negative, but the serum hCG was 600 mIU/ml by the beta-subunit method (normal less than 5 mIU/ml). Serum estradiol was 70 pg/ml (normal less than 50 pg/ml). A chest roentgenogram revealed a large mass in the left upper lobe of the lung and enlargement of the left hilar region.

Questions

1. What is the most likely diagnosis for this patient?

Answer

Given the presence of a lung mass, elevated serum hCG and estrogen concentrations, and gynecomastia, the major differential diagnosis is between an hCG-secreting germ cell neoplasm of the testes with lung metastases and a nontrophoblastic hCG-secreting malignancy. Over two-thirds of patients with nonseminomatous germ cell neoplasms of the testes have immunoreactive hCG in their circulation derived from trophoblastic giant cells or embryonal cells in the neoplasms. In these patients, the hCG production is eutopic rather than ectopic, since these tumors often contain trophoblastic elements. The common ectopic hCG-producing tumors associated with this clinical syndrome are giant cell carcinomas of the lung, renal cell carcinomas, hepatomas, and gastric carcinomas. The most likely diagnosis in this patient who has a single pulmonary lesion with hilar adenopathy is a primary lung carcinoma, although the other tumors cannot be totally ruled out with the information given. Other laboratory studies that would be of use include measurement of the serum α-fetoprotein level which is elevated in over two-thirds of patients with germ cell tumors of the testes but is not elevated in patients with ectopic hCG-producing neoplasms unless there are substantial hepatic metastases. An upper gastrointestinal tract series and an intravenous pyelogram would be useful ancillary studies. Of course, the most direct approach would be a biopsy of the lung lesion.

Question

2. Why was the urinary pregnancy test negative while the serum hCG level by radioimmunoassy was elevated?

Answer

Urinary pregnancy tests utilize antisera against the intact hCG molecule. Such antisera recognize both hCG and luteinizing hormone (LH). In order to avoid detecting the midcycle peak of LH found in menstruating women or the high levels found in postmenopausal women, the manufacturers of urinary pregnancy tests have adjusted the sensitivity of their assays in such a way as to avoid detecting less than 1,000–2,000 mIU/ml of hCG. It would be anticipated that this patient had approximately 600 mIU/ml of hCG in his urine, which is below the limit of sensitivity of the pregnancy test. The serum hCG was measured by a beta-subunit radioimmunoassay. This assay uses an antiserum raised against the isolated beta subunit of hCG that has immunologic determinants not shared by LH. Thus this assay is capable of detecting small amounts of hCG in the serum in the presence of physiologic concentrations of LH. It has a sensitivity of 5 mIU/ml which is 200 to 400 times greater then the sensitivity of the urinary pregnancy test. It is apparent that, in a patient with a neoplasm and gynecomastia, the most sensitive test for detecting the ectopic production of hCG is the serum hCG measurement performed by the beta-subunit radioimmunoassay.

Question

3. How should therapy for this lesion be monitored?

Answer

In addition to repeated chest roentgenograms and tomograms, serial measurements of serum hCG concentrations would be quite useful in monitoring the effects of therapy directed toward the neoplasm. Effective surgery, chemotherapy, or radiotherapy will reduce the hCG concentrations in the serum. The serum hCG levels may rise weeks to months before other objective evidence of tumor recurrence becomes apparent.

Case 2

Description

A 64-year-old male was admitted to a psychiatric hospital because of bizarre behavior of rather sudden onset. He was not ingesting any medications or using illicit drugs before his admission but had a 60-pack-year history of cigarette smoking. Physical examination at the psychiatric institution demonstrated a blood pressure of 180/110, a pulse rate of 110, marked agitation, mild cardiomegaly, moderate hepatomegaly, and bilateral pedal edema. Laboratory studies at the institution revealed a negative toxicology screen, mild normochromic normocytic anemia, an elevated concentration of alkaline phosphatase, mild hypoalbuminemia, and normal calcium, phosphorus, BUN, and creatinine levels. He had an elevated fasting glucose level of 160 mg/dl and hypokalemic alkalosis (potassium 3.2 mEq/liter, HCO_3 30 mEq/liter).

The patient was transferred to a medical institution where additional workup included a chest roentgenogram that demonstrated a right upper lobe mass lesion and several small lesions in the right lower and left upper lobes, a liver scan showing multiple filling defects, and a bone scan demonstrating numerous lytic lesions throughout the skeleton.

Question

1. What paraneoplastic endocrine syndrome is likely in this patient? What are the differential diagnostic considerations?

Answer

The constellation of a male smoker with a lung mass and obvious metastatic disease in the liver and spine associated with hypertension, peripheral edema, hyperglycemia, hypokalemic alkalosis, and neuropsychiatric symtpoms is most compatible with the ectopic production of biologically active ACTH from a lung tumor. Neuropsychiatric symptoms are relatively common with the ectopic ATCH syndrome and run the gamut from psychiatric disturbances (steroid psychosis) to confusion, disorientation, and coma. The differential diagnosis must include the possibility of metastatic disease in the central nervous system, as well as other paraneoplastic central nervous system syndromes and other causes of hypokalemia.

Question

2. What laboratory tests should be carried out to confirm the diagnosis?

Answer

The patient should have a measurement of the urinary free cortisol level and a formal dexamethasone suppression test. If the patient does not suppress his serum and urine cortisol concentrations appropriately following 8 mg of dexamethasone a day given for 2 days, then measurement of the serum ACTH concentration should be performed. The combination of nonsuppressible adrenal glucocorticoid production with an elevated ACTH level is most likely due to the ectopic ACTH syndrome. Rarely, pituitary-dependent Cushing's disease may not be appropriately suppressed with dexamethasone. However, such cases do not show evidence of a widely metastatic neoplasm.

Question

3. What therapeutic approaches could be used to treat this patient's metabolic syndrome?

Answer

Of course, the therapy of choice would be to treat the tumor effectively by chemotherapy. However, it is unlikely that such therapy will significantly alter the excessive production of ACTH, since the disease is diffusely metastatic. Adrenalectomy will cure the metabolic abnormality, although one generally does not like to perform a major surgical procedure in a patient who is moribund from cancer. There are several drugs that should be considered as an alternative to adrenalectomy. These include *o,p*-DDD (mitotane), metyrapone (Metopirone), and aminogluthetimide (Cytadren). Of these, aminogluthetimide therapy results in the most rapid reduction in glucocorticoid secretion and should be used before the other are considered. Peripheral antagonism of the mineralocorticoids produced in the syndrome may be accomplished through the use of spirolactone (Aldactone).

SUGGESTED READING

Abe K: Endocrinology and cancer. *Clin Endocrinol Metab* 9:209–360, 1980.

Baylin SB, Mendelsohn E: Ectopic (inappropriate) hormone production by tumors: Mechanisms involved and the biological and clinical implications. *Endocrinol Rev* 1:45–77, 1980.

Drezner MK, Feinglos MN: Osteomalacia due to 1α,25-dihydroxycholecaliferol deficiency: Association with a giant cell tumor of bone. *J Clin Invest* 60: 1046–1053, 1977.

Hall TC: Paraneoplastic syndromes. *Ann NY Acad Sci* 230:1–577, 1974.

Imura H, Matsurkura S, Yamamoto H, Hirata Y, Nakai Y, Endo J, Tanaka A, Nakamura M: Studies on ectopic ACTH-producing tumors. II. Clinical and biochemical features of 30 cases. *Cancer* 35:1430–1437, 1975.

Rees LH, Ratcliffe JG: Ectopic hormone production by non-endocrine tumors. Clin Endocrinol 3:263–299, 1974.

Shnider BI, Manalo A: Paraneoplastic syndromes: Unusual manifestations of malignant disease. DM. 5:1–60, 1979.

Singer W, Kovacs K, Ryan N, Horvath E: Ectopic ACTH syndrome: Clinical pathological correlations. *J Clin Pathol* 31:591–598, 1978.

Singer FR, Sharp CF Jr, Rude RK: Pathogenesis of hypercalcemia in malignancy. *Mineral Electrolyte Metab* 2:161–178, 1979.

Skrabanek P, McPartlin J, Powel D: Tumor hypercalcemia and "ectopic hyperparathyroidism." *Medicine* 59:262–282, 1980.

Skrabanek P, Powell D: Ectopic insulin and Occam's razor: Reappraisal of the riddle of tumor hypoglycemia. *Clin Endocrinol* 9:141–154, 1978.

Stewart AF, Horst R, Deftos LJ, Cadman EC, Lang R, Broadus AE: Biochemical evaluation of patients with cancer-associated hypercalcemia: Evidence for humoral and non-humoral groups. *N Engl J Med* 303:1377–1383, 1980.

Stolinsky DC: Paraneoplastic syndromes (medical progress). West J Med 132:189–208, 1980.

Vorherr H: Para-endocrine tumor activity with emphasis on ectopic ADH secretion: Genetic, diagnostic, prognostic and therapeutic aspects. *Oncology* 29:382–416, 1974.

12 DAVID R. MELDRUM

Female Gonadal Disorders

NORMAL GONADAL FUNCTION

Clinical Manifestations

Breast Development

The first sign of ovarian estrogen secretion is the beginning of breast development. Onset before age 8 or lack of initiation by age 14 is abnormal and warrants investigation. Relatively little estrogen (less than that required for menstruation) is necessary for breast development and maintenance.

Menstruation

Onset before age 8 or delay beyond age 16 should be considered abnormal. During the first 2 years menses are often anovulatory and may be very heavy. Irregularity is common until the third decade. Menses are considered regular if the interval is between 21 and 35 days. The mean interval steadily drops throughout reproductive life until 2–3 years before the menopause, when anovulation is again common.

Sexual Hair

The onset of pubic and axillary hair is termed *adrenarche,* since an increase in adrenal androgens provides the main stimulus. Androgen secretion by the ovary also increases at puberty and augments the amount of sexual hair. Scattered coarse, pigmented hairs are normal around the areolae of the breasts and in the lower midline of the abdomen.

Endocrine Physiology

The Menstrual Cycle

Normal menstruation occurs as a result of the rapid fall in estrogen and progesterone levels as the corpus luteum undergoes regression. In the normal female, the remaining sources of estrogen (e.g., peripheral conversion of androgens and secretion elsewhere in the ovaries) are limited at this time. The resulting nadir of circulating estrogen levels initiates a rise in gonadotropin levels and follicular development. Local processes within the follicle then result in accelerated development relatively independent of circulating levels of gonadotropins. Follicle-stimulating hormone (FSH) results in the proliferation of granulosa cells that contain FSH receptors. FSH stimulates receptors for luteinizing hormone (LH), which makes cholesterol available for steroidogenesis. LH stimulates the theca surrounding the follicle to produce androstenedione (A) and testosterone (T). FSH is required to convert these androgens to estrogen in the granulosa cells by stimulating aromatase. Estrogen in turn promotes mitotic activity of the granulosa cells and, indirectly, an increase in the total number of FSH receptors. The rapid rise in circulating estradiol that accompanies follicular development then stimulates a surge of LH by a positive feedback effect on the pituitary gonadotrophs and probably also at the hypothalamus to induce increased release of gonadotropin-releasing hormone (GnRH) and gonadotropins. The LH surge causes follicular rupture, luteinization of the granulosa cells, and formation of the corpus luteum.

CHRONIC ANOVULATION

General Considerations

Transient delays in ovulation are common and are often due to stress. These episodes are usually self-limited. They are more common at the extremes of menstrual life, after pregnancy, and after cessation of oral contraception. Chronic anovulation may be associated with amenorrhea, irregular bleeding, infertility, or signs of increased androgen production. Episodes of anovulation may be interrupted periodically by luteal activity that is often inadequate and of short duration. Anovulation may be the first sign of thyroid or adrenal disease or of a pituitary tumor. For the purposes of this discussion, the term *chronic anovulation* will be used to refer to acyclic function of the hypothalamic-pituitary-ovarian axis with activity at each level and normal circulating levels of estrogen. The term *hypogonadism* will be used to describe conditions due to failure of function at one of these levels, resulting in a hypoestrogenic state.

Categorization

Thyroid Disease

Anovulation is common in both hyperthyroidism and hypothyroidism, which have complex effects on the metabolism and serum binding of estradiol. Women with excess thyroid hormone have high circulating levels of estrogen because of increased concentrations of sex hormone-binding globulin (SHBG). Both FSH and LH levels may be elevated, perhaps secondary to lower levels of free estrogen. Decreased or absent menstruation predominates. In hypothyroidism, the opposite changes occur, with excess bleeding being common. An elevation of the LH level may be observed, the pathogenesis possibly being similar to that of polycystic ovarian disease (PCO) described below.

Adrenal Disease

Cushing's syndrome may be associated with anovulatory bleeding, which may also be associated with hirsutism and obesity. This disease commonly simulates PCO. Whenever suspected, it must be ruled out.

Polycystic Ovarian Disease

Most women with chronic anovulation have variations of this disease entity. Although each unit of the hypothalamic-pituitary-ovarian axis is functioning and responsive, there is abnormal integration among the feedback signals that normally result in ovulation. In normal women, the major feedback signal, estradiol, is predominantly ovarian in origin. In PCO the source of estradiol from extraglandular tissues is increased. Chronic estrogen stimulation of the gonadotrophs results in aberrant gonadotropin release. Gonadotropins exist within the pituitary cells in two pools, a readily releasable form (pool 1) and a storage pool that requires activation (pool 2). Estrogen stimulates synthesis (pool 2) and has a permissive role in its activation. Estrogen also has an effect in impeding the release of gonadotropins, particularly FSH, from the gonadotrophs. The overall effect of chronic estrogen stimulation on circulating levels of gonadotropins results in elevated levels and pulsations of LH and decreased levels of FSH, in comparison with the early follicular phase. The levels of non-SHBG-bound estradiol correlate directly with the LH/FSH ratio. The increased levels of LH result in excess stimulation of the ovarian stroma and theca and increased production of androstenedione (A) and testosterone (T). The lower levels of FSH result in decreased conversion of these androgens to estrogen within the follicle. Increased androgen concentrations within the ovary further decrease its response to FSH. The increased production rate of T by the ovary decreases the production of SHBG by the liver, resulting in further augmentation of the levels of non-SHBG-bound T, which stimulates increased sexual hair growth (hirsutism). Increased production of A results in increased peripheral conversion to estrone (E_1) and in turn to estradiol (E_2). Many patients with this condition are obese, which increases the rate of conversion of A to E_1 and, by an unknown mechanism, decreases the circulating levels of SHBG. All these factors combine to result in constant high levels of non-SHBG-bound E_2, which alters gonadotropin secretion as previously outlined. A vicious cycle is thus set up, which is self-perpetuating (Fig. 1).

Over 90% of women with PCO have a history of obesity at the time of puberty. Before and during puberty obese girls have higher circulating levels of dehydroepiandrosterone and A, suggesting exaggerated adrenarche. Obesity at puberty therefore would be expected to result in a chronic elevation of the level of non-SHBG-bound E_2, by all the mechanisms outlined above, and is probably a major underlying cause of PCO. Weight loss does not reverse the elevated conversion rate of A to E_1 but does increase the level of SHBG. Although marked weight gain can cause clinical PCO in previously normal women, and the disease has been observed to improve with weight loss in some women, the role of weight reduction in the treatment of this disease has not been defined.

Dysfunctional Uterine Bleeding

In some instances chronic anovulation can occur in the absence of the above diseases and may result in frequent, irregular bleeding episodes. When such bleeding occurs in the absence

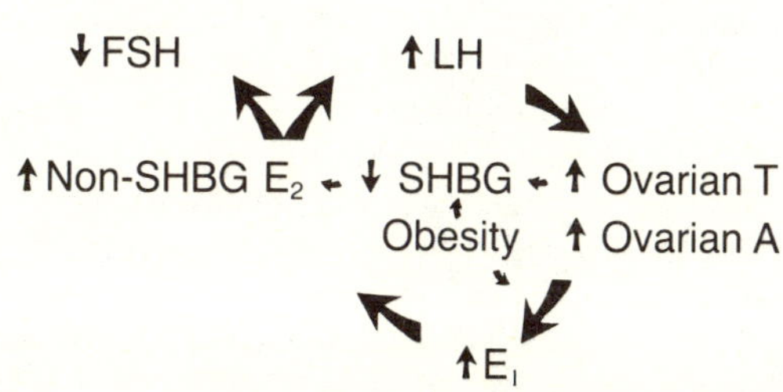

Figure 1. The self-perpetuating cycle of polycystic ovarian disease.

of pathologic lesions and is presumed to be due to anovulation, it is commonly termed *dysfunctional uterine bleeding*. Study of this condition has revealed normal levels of gonadotropins, fluctuating levels of E_2 indicating intermittent follicular development, but no sign of ovulation. Bleeding often occurs coincident with a drop in E_2 concentration. The positive feedback response of LH to exogenous estradiol is absent. This abnormality often appears to be secondary to stress and in some women recurs intermittently with intervening normal cycles. The first 1–2 years after puberty is a characteristic time when the disorder can occur, since positive feedback is the last maturational event in the evolution of normal ovulatory function.

Diagnosis

Underlying Disorder

Appropriate screening tests should be performed if thyroid or adrenal disease is suspected. The serum prolactin level should be measured, since 10–20% of patients with PCO have elevated levels and a pituitary adenoma may present in this manner. Measurement of gonadotropin or estrogen concentrations is not necessary unless the patient has amenorrhea. PCO is largely a clinical diagnosis. Most typically menstruation has been irregular since menarche. At the time of diagnosis 40% of patients are obese. Hirsutism usually becomes evident to the patient in the late teens, although a history of excess hair growth at the time of puberty has been elicited from over 90% of parents. Progression is gradual. Virilization is infrequent and mild. The ovaries are often bilaterally enlarged (most often 3–5 cm in greatest diameter). An atypical history with delayed or sudden onset, rapid progression, or marked virilization should suggest the possibility of diseases other than PCO.

Endometrial Pathology

In any woman with abnormal bleeding, the need for sampling of the endometrium should be considered. Although there is no real consensus as to when this should be done, some generalizations can be made. Most agree that this is unnecessary in young teenagers, and most agree that all women over 30–35 should have assessment of endometrial histology before treatment. Women between these extremes who have abnormal bleeding and chronic anovulation also require investigation.

Hirsutism

The presence of hair growth in excess of that which is usual in the patient's ethnic group generally indicates increased production of androgens. This sign is present in 70% of patients with PCO. The total level of circulating T is elevated in only 50% of women with hirsutism, whereas virtually all have increased testosterone production rates and increased free T levels. With current assay techniques, a level of T greater than 200 ng % is rare in the absence of an androgen-producing tumor. Measurement of the 24-hour urinary excretion of 17 ketosteroids (17-KS) or the circulating level of dehydroepiandrosterone sulfate (DS) is helpful in excluding the possibility of an androgen-producing adrenal tumor, which is generally associated with elevations over 50 mg/24 hr or 8,000 ng/ml, respectively. The levels of 17-KS and DS may be mildly to moderately elevated in women with PCO, suggesting that many of these women continue to show evidence of increased adrenal androgen production. Recent investigation suggests that approximately 20% of women with a clinical diagnosis of PCO have evidence of adrenal 21-hydroxylase deficiency. After the administration of 1 mg of dexamethasone at 11:00 PM, 0.25 mg of cosyntropin (synthetic ACTH) given as an i.v. bolus at 8:00 AM caused a rise in the 17-hydroxyprogesterone level after 60 minutes to very high levels in these women. Further experience with this test will be necessary to define the appropriate level indicating an enzyme defect, and whether chronic suppression with glucocorticoid is a preferred method of treatment. Various methods have been used in an attempt to define the source of excess androgen production in individual patients by suppression or stimulation of the ovary or adrenal. No accurate and practical means has emerged from these investigations.

Treatment

Underlying Disorder

Since no treatment is available to reverse the pathophysiologic abnormality in chronic anovulation, treatment is designed to affect the specific manifestations that are of concern.

Endometrial Pathology

If anovulation persists for long periods of time, endometrial proliferation may be sufficient to result in heavy bleeding or evolution to endometrial cancer. The cyclic progestin effect on the endometrium may be restored by ovulation induction, by treatment with a combination oral contraceptive, or by the cyclic administration of a synthetic progestin for 10 days every 1–2 months.

Hirsutism

The overproduction of ovarian androgens may be reduced by the suppression of gonadotropins with a combination oral contraceptive. A suitable preparation should be chosen that contains a nonandrogenic progestin. It is also preferable to limit the dose of estrogen to 50 μg to reduce the chance of thromboembolism. The combination of 50 μg of ethinyl estradiol and 1 mg of ethynodiol diacetate satisfies these criteria and is commercially available (Demulen). Excess adrenal androgen secretion may be decreased by the administration of a small dose of glucocorticoid (0.5 mg dexamethasone, 5 mg prednisone) each evening before bedtime. This method of administration reduces the nighttime surge of ACTH and achieves a maximal effect with the lowest amount of medication. Adrenal suppression may be indicated in women with adult manifestations of congenital adrenal hyperplasia or to accomplish a greater overall suppression of androgens in women with PCO who fail to have improvement of hirsutism on ovarian suppression alone. Local treatment is generally required in addition to hormonal suppression. Electrolysis is the ideal method but is time-consuming, expensive, and involves some discomfort. Shaving, plucking, and depilatory creams are more commonly utilized. Future advances will probably include the use of compounds that block the effect of androgens at the hair follicle. Spironolactone, currently used as a diuretic, is receiving considerable attention since it decreases circulating androgens, as well as having an end-organ effect, and produces a clinical response. Cimetidine also acts as an antiandrogen and may find some use in the treatment of hirsute females.

Anovulation

As outlined above, the etiology of the aberrant gonadotropin secretion in chronic anovulation is most often an abnormal increase in biologically available E_2 of extragonadal origin. It is therefore not surprising that an antiestrogen, clomiphene citrate (Clomid), is highly effective in inducing ovulation in women with this condition. The dose required shows a positive correlation with body weight (and therefore also with circulating estrogen concentrations), although individual variability precludes a prediction of the minimum effective dose. Clomiphene, a weak estrogen, blocks the negative feedback effect of endogenous estrogen, resulting in a rise in gonadotropins. Increased levels of FSH promote follicular development. Positive feedback is generally intact, resulting in spontaneous ovulation about 8 days after the standard 5-day course of clomiphene (day 13 of the clomiphene cycle). The daily dose is increased successively from 50 mg to a maximum of 250 mg until ovulation is detected by occurrence of the luteal shift of the basal body temperature (BBT) and a normal menstrual period. Occasionally, ovulation and normal menses may occur in the absence of a biphasic BBT. Measurement of the serum level of progesterone on approximately day 21 of the clomiphene cycle will verify whether ovulation is occurring. Before each cycle the patient should be examined to exclude an increase in ovarian size and to be sure that pregnancy has not occurred. Return of the BBT to preovulatory levels, disappearance of premenstrual symptoms, and occurrence of a normal period are reliable clinical criteria for excluding pregnancy. When no ovulation is evident, and before initiating clomiphene treatment, induction of menses with 100 mg of progesterone in oil intramuscularly will also help to exclude pregnancy. Alternatively, the presence of watery estrogenic cervical mucus, or a negative result in a sufficiently sensitive radioimmunoassay of serum beta-human chorionic gonadotropin (hCG) will also suffice. Occasionally, women failing to ovulate after the maximum dose of clomiphene will ovulate when an injection of hCG, 10,000 units i.m., is given on day 13 as an LH surrogate. Such a response indicates that a mature follicle is present but positive feedback is not normal.

Clomiphene with or without the addition of hCG will cause ovulation in over 90% of women with chronic anovulation. If all other infertility factors are excluded, almost 90% will conceive. Twinning is increased from the normal rate of about 1% to 6–8% of births. About 1% of conceptions are in excess of twins. Ovarian cyst formation is rarely of clinical significance provided the subsequent course of clomiphene is not given until the cystic enlargement has resolved. Of those failing to ovulate with clomiphene, most will ovulate with clomiphene–human menopausal gonadotropin–hCG and 60% will conceive.

HYPOGONADISM

General Considerations

If the level of function is insufficient at a hypothalamic, pituitary, or ovarian level, a hypoestrogenic state will ensue and the patient will develop amenorrhea (lack of bleeding for more than 6 months). This can be distinguished from the amenorrhea of chronic anovulation by measuring circulating E_2 or by testing for a withdrawal response to intramuscular progesterone (100 mg in oil). Estrogen is required for the induction of endometrial progesterone receptors. A positive response (i.e., withdrawal bleeding) indicates the presence of a circulating level of E_2 within the normal premenopausal range.

Categorization

Hypothalamic Amenorrhea

In order for normal gonadal function to occur, pulsatile release of GnRH and consequently of gonadotropins is necessary. In hypothalamic amenorrhea gonadotropin levels are low-normal to low and the normal pulsatile variation is absent. Circulating estradiol is decreased, often to the range seen in postmenopausal women. The response of gonadotropins to exogenous GnRH may be increased, normal, or decreased, depending on the extent and chronicity of the endogenous GnRH deficiency. The hypothalamic defect may be congenital, as in Kallmann's syndrome in which hypoplasia of the hypothalamus coexists with anosmia or hyposmia. An acquired deficiency is most often due to emotional stress or nutritional deficiency. Current investigation of this dysfunction implicates a heightened activity of dopaminergic neurons which inhibit gonadotropin secretion. Other endocrine changes observed in nutritional deficiency are elevated basal levels of growth hormone and cortisol, decreased levels of triiodothyronine (T_3), and increased levels of serum carotene. Anorexia nervosa is the most severe form of nutritional deficiency and is associated with a morbid fear of losing control over dietary intake, an obsessive pursuit of thinness, and an altered self-image. It is potentially life threatening because of electrolyte disturbances. Lowered levels of thyroxine (T_4) and T_3 are common and may be a homeostatic adjustment to the very low level of energy substrate. The onset of amenorrhea and restoration of normal function often do not correspond precisely to weight loss and gain, possibly reflecting the common coexisting psychogenic factor.

Pituitary Insufficiency

Inadequate function of the pituitary may occur because of encroachment by intrasellar tumors, granulomatous disease such as sarcoidosis, postpartum necrosis due to hemorrhagic shock (Sheehan's syndrome), and occasionally in association with the empty sella syndrome. Rarely, congenital deficits of pituitary gonadotroph function can occur (Prader-Willi, Laurence-Moon-Biedl, isolated gonadotropin deficiency).

Hyperprolactinemia (Amenorrhea–Galactorrhea)

Out of all women with amenorrhea, 15–20% have elevated circulating levels of prolactin. In women with amenorrhea and galactorrhea, 70% have hyperprolactinemia. Why galactorrhea occurs in some women with normal levels of prolactin is not understood. Usually there is a history of a condition or medication resulting in previous stimulation of the lactotrophs. Hypothyroidism can cause hyperprolactinemia. Some pituitary adenomas produce prolactin. A large number of drugs are capable of altering the control of prolactin secretion (estrogen, reserpine, α-methyldopa, phenothiazines, haloperidol, and narcotics are the most common etiologic agents). Galactorrhea may accompany acromegaly and Cushing's syndrome. A small proportion (10–20%) of women with PCO have hyperprolactinemia, perhaps due to chronic unopposed estrogen stimulation of the lactotrophs.

The mechanism of hypogonadism in the presence of hyperprolactinemia is not clear. A hypothalamic mechanism has been proposed, since the gonadotropin response to exogenous GnRH is normal or exaggerated, yet the positive feedback response to estrogen is impaired. Accumulated evidence suggests that there is a feedback effect of prolactin on hypothalamic dopaminergic neurons. Increased pituitary prolactin secretion thus leads to increased hypothalamic dopamine release, which inhibits GnRH neurons and, indirectly, pituitary gonadotropin release. A direct action on the ovary has also been postulated, impairing both folliculogenesis and luteal function. These ovarian effects are likely to be of minimal significance in hypogonadal women with hyperprolactinemia, since both exogenous GnRH and exogenous gonadotropins induce rises in E_2 levels similar to those seen in the absence of hyperprolactinemia.

Ovarian Failure

Gradual oocyte depletion occurs throughout life as a result of the process of atresia. During the several years preceding the menopause there is a rise in circulating FSH levels, yet follicular maturation and luteal activity continue. As the menopause approaches, periods of anovulation ensue and serum levels of both gonadotropins may be elevated, but still occasional ovulation occurs, with its attendant possibility of fertility. Finally, follicular activity ceases and the circulating E_2 level drops to the postmenopausal range. Ovarian failure occurring before age 40 is termed premature. Premature ovarian failure may be due to gonadal dysgenesis, autoimmune disease, gonadotropin resistance, radiation, chemotherapy, or simply early oocyte depletion (premature menopause). Gonadal dysgenesis is discussed later under Disorders of Sexual Development.

Autoimmune ovarian failure sometimes occurs in conjunction with autoimmune deficiencies of thyroid or adrenal function. Less commonly the ovary may be the first gland affected. The presence of antibodies to thyroid or adrenal tissue may signal the possibility of future hormone deficiencies.

An uncommon disorder is occasionally found wherein the ovary contains numerous oocytes lacking development beyond the antral stage. The low levels of circulating estradiol in spite of high levels of gonadotropins indicate that these oocytes are resistant to gonadotropins. Ovarian biopsy is necessary to make the diagnosis but is difficult to justify outside of an investigative protocol, since pregnancy has not been reported even with massive doses of exogenous gonadotropins.

Either radiation or chemotherapy may be accompanied by ovarian failure. Attempts may be made in patients with Hodgkin's disease to move the ovaries out of the field of irradiation at the time of staging laparotomy, although this may not prove successful. In about half of the cases occurring with chemotherapy, normal ovarian function will eventually recover.

Diagnosis

Amenorrhea will invariably be present. Lack of breast development in itself indicates that the breast has not been exposed to premenopausal levels of estrogen. The sense of smell must be tested with nonirritating odors of graded strength, since the patient often is unaware of a decrease in or even a lack of the sensation of smell. Sexual hair may be markedly decreased with pituitary insufficiency because of a decrease in both adrenal and ovarian androgen secretion. In the case of nutritional deficiency bradycardia and a delayed return phase of the Achilles reflex coexist paradoxically with low body weight and mental alertness, and often the patient unexpectedly shows little concern about her markedly thin habitus. Complaints of hot flashes and night sweats may be present if ovarian failure is preceded by exposure to endogenous or exogenous estrogen. The breasts should be expressed in the sitting position to elicit subclinical galactorrhea. Measurement of E_2 is the most direct method of detecting hypogonadism. With most assays the lower limit for normal ovarian function is approximately 30 pg/ml. Lack of withdrawal bleeding following progesterone injection is less accurate in identifying hypogonadism, since this may occur when the E_2 level is in the low-normal range (30–50 pg/ml). Conversely, some women with clear hypogonadism may have withdrawal bleeding due to obesity (resulting from elevated androgen conversion to estrogen in adipose tissue) and chronic stimulation of the endometrium.

If hypogonadism is present, further evaluation is necessary to indicate whether the patient has hypothalamic, pituitary, or ovarian failure. Measurement of serum FSH clearly differentiates women with ovarian failure from those with a central abnormality. Women with ovarian failure (elevated FSH) who are under 25 years of age may have gonadal dysgenesis and should have a karyotype determination to rule out the presence of a Y chromosome, in which case gonadectomy would be indicated. In the case of a central cause of hypogonadism the levels of gonadotropins may be normal or low. Measurement of the LH level may add additional information. Elevation of the serum LH level in the presence of an elevated FSH level may reinforce the diagnosis of ovarian failure; an increased LH level in association with a normal or low FSH concentration may indicate PCO; a low LH level with a normal FSH concentration is commonly observed in hypothalamic amenorrhea. Differentiation of hypothalamic versus pituitary causes of hypogonadism is seldom absolute. A hypothalamic etiology is often the diagnosis of exclusion.

Some radiologic evaluation of the sella is necessary in all women with amenorrhea–galactorrhea, hyperprolactinemia, or hypogonadism (with the exception of ovarian failure). The appropriate extent of radiologic evaluation of the sella depends on the clinical setting in regard to the level of suspicion of a pituitary or, more rarely, a suprasellar tumor. Cone-down views of the sella are sufficient to rule out a macroadenoma (a pituitary tumor over 1 cm in diameter). In combination with formal visual field testing, conditions that pose an immediate threat to health can be generally excluded. Sella tomograms are more likely to detect subtle alterations in the symmetry or contour of the sella or minor thinning or erosion of adjacent bone. However, the extent of anatomic variation in the sella is extremely great. A recent autopsy study showed a very high level of both false negative and false positive tomograms in the presence and absence of histologically confirmed adenomas. Computerized axial tomography (CAT), using fourth-generation technology, is currently the most reliable technique for identifying even very small adenomas and for ruling out suprasellar extension or suprasellar tumors. Because of the expense of this procedure, the main clinical decision in each case is whether to rely solely on cone-down views or to obtain this definitive test. Factors suggesting the need for a CAT scan are (1) substantial elevations of prolactin levels (over 200 ng/ml), (2) sellar changes suggesting a macroadenoma, (3) marked symptoms of headache or any visual defect, (4) a plan for inducing fertility in the presence of sellar changes or hyperprolactinemia. Formal visual field testing should be done when galactorrhea or hyperprolactinemia accompanies amenorrhea, when an abnormality of the sella is present, or when the CAT scan reveals suprasellar extension.

Testing of the pituitary response to perturbation has been of relatively little value in establishing the diagnosis of microadenoma in patients with hyperprolactinemia. The gonadotropin response to exogenous GnRH may be decreased, normal, or increased with both functional and neoplastic conditions. The extent of rise in the prolactin level after exogenous thyrotropin-releasing hormone is of some limited value. A blunted prolactin response is commonly seen when a prolactinoma is present, whereas a doubling of the level of prolactin is highly reassuring that a pituitary prolactin-producing adenoma is not present. Testing of the pituitary reserve is of greater value in clinical settings where pituitary insufficiency is of concern, as in the presence of radiologic signs of a macroadenoma, frankly low levels of gonadotropins, or signs suggesting thyroid or adrenal insufficiency.

Pituitary adenomas are notoriously slow growing and may not become manifest for as long as 10–15 years or more. Generally, yearly sella cone-down views (with visual fields as indicated) are sufficient for surveillance. If hyperprolactinemia is present, the measurement of prolactin every 6–12 months will add additional information to monitor tumor growth.

Treatment

Underlying Condition

Hypothalamic amenorrhea is the most potentially treatable condition. If it is due to weight loss, function will generally be restored following weight gain. If it is due to stress, simply the passage of time is often sufficient provided the stressful environment is altered. Function will be restored in a high proportion (60–70%) of patients after transsphenoidal excision of a prolactin-producing adenoma. This effect, however, is probably due to removal of the inhibiting effect of prolactin on hypothalamic function, rather than to the local effect of removal of the lesion. A similar effect can be produced with a dopamine agonist, bromocriptine. Very recent reports indicate that at least some prolactin-producing tumors may diminish in size with bromocriptine.

Anovulation

Elevated secretion of prolactin, whether due to a functional or neoplastic cause responds effectively to administration of the potent dopamine agonist bromocriptine. Ovulation is restored in approximately 70% of patients, and pregnancy occurs in most of these women if attempted. No adverse fetal or maternal effects of the drug have been noted in very large numbers of pregnancies. Pregnancy can have serious effects on a pituitary prolactinoma, however. The lactotrophs undergo marked hyperplasia as a result of high maternal levels of estrogen. If a macroadenoma is present, particularly with preexisting suprasellar extension, the tumor can grow sufficiently to compromise vision. The high-resolution (fourth-generation) CAT scan, a non–invasive technique, may be used routinely to rule out suprasellar extension before inducing ovulation. The risk of pregnancy in women with a microadenoma confined to the sella appears to be minimal. It must be realized that, although bromocriptine is being widely used to induce ovulation in women with microadenomas, its use is officially sanctioned only in the absence of a demonstrable pituitary tumor. If this treatment is utilized, a thorough informed consent should be undertaken. During pregnancy, formal visual field testing should be conducted monthly. If visual defects appear, surgery can be carried out during pregnancy. Bromocriptine has also been reported to be effective in isolated case reports. The use of this drug during pregnancy has not been associated with any deleterious effects.

In women with hypogonadism due to hypothalamic or pituitary failure, clomiphene is seldom effective. Because an occasional patient responds to clomiphene, however, a trial is usually given. If no ovulation occurs, substitution of pituitary gonadotropins is necessary. Purified FSH and LH are available in a concentration of 75 units each per ampul. It is given by daily injection in a steadily increasing dose. Response is monitored by pelvic exam and measurements of serum or urinary estrogen levels. This treatment is very expensive and hazardous (ovarian hyperstimulation, multiple pregnancy) and should be given only by someone experienced in its use.

Hormonal Deficiency

General Comments

Since hypothalamic failure is often reversible and women with this condition are exquisitely sensitive to the suppressive effects of estrogen, we prefer to avoid exogenous sex steroid therapy in this group unless the condition is expected to be prolonged or irreversible. In the case of permanent hypogonadism, hormone replacement may be considered. The use of long-term replacement of gonadal function requires careful consideration of the risks of hormone deficiency and the risks of treatment in each individual patient. This therapeutic decision is most often encountered in postmenopausal women but is of even greater importance in younger women who will have a much longer duration of either hormone deficiency or treatment. A full appreciation of this question necessitates an understanding of hormonal function in women lacking ovarian function and the effects of hormone deficiency on various body tissues.

Extragonadal Sources of Estrogen

When the ovary stops producing significant amounts of estrogen, both estrone (E_1) and estradiol (E_2) continue to be produced. Essentially all the E_1 produced by the postmenopausal woman can be accounted for by the conversion of A of adrenal origin in nonglandular tissues. Since the bulk of this conversion occurs in adipose and muscle tissue, the rate of conversion varies directly with body weight, particularly relative to height. Although the actual rate of E_1 to E_2 conversion is unclear, this is probably the major source of E_2. Circulating concentrations of both E_1 and E_2 correlate directly with body weight. It has been suggested that age is a further factor that may affect A-to-E_1 conversion. However, in a recent study on a large number of postmenopausal women, age was shown to have no effect on the circulating levels of E_1 and E_2. Enhanced conversion is observed in the presence of liver disease and hyperthyroidism.

The biologic action of circulating estradiol is further influenced by the concentration of SHBG, which is produced by the liver. The level of SHBG varies inversely with body weight by an unknown mechanism. Thus obesity leads to increased levels of biologically active circulating estrogen by its dual action on E_2 production and binding. Conversely, in the thin woman, estrogen deficiency becomes exaggerated. Changes in body weight do influence the SHBG concentration, presumably through an effect on hepatic function.

Effects of "Unopposed" Estrogen

When follicular activity is no longer present, luteal progesterone secretion will also not occur. Progesterone has marked antimitogenic effects on the responses of the endometrium and breast to estrogen stimulation. Progesterone depletes the intracellular receptor protein that binds E_2 and initiates estrogen action. Progesterone also stimulates an enzyme, 17β-hydroxysteroid dehydrogenase, which converts E_2 to E_1 within the target cell. These two mechanisms result in decreased nuclear binding and action of E_2 and thereby keep in check the marked stimulation of these tissues by estrogen. Chronic unopposed estrogen stimulation may be sufficient in some women to promote malignant evolution of breast and endometrial tissue. This effect is probably responsible for the sixfold increase in endometrial cancer and the twofold increase in breast cancer observed in postmenopausal women who are obese.

Central Nervous System Effects of Estrogen Deficiency

The loss of steroid feedback (estrogens and progestogens) from the ovary leads to an open-loop circuit with increased activity of hypothalamic centers responsible for the release of gonadotropin-releasing hormone (GnRH). The gonadotrophs within the pituitary become more prominent and synthesize increased amounts of FSH and LH. Circulating levels of both gonadotropins are elevated but, in contrast to the situation in premenopausal women, FSH exceeds LH. The reasons for this reversal are that FSH has a longer half-life, is released more readily from the gonadotroph when circulating estrogen levels are low, and may no longer be under negative feedback control of ovarian inhibin (a putative FSH-suppressing hormone produced by the maturing follicle). With hypothalamic failure, function at both the hypothalamic and pituitary levels is decreased. With pituitary failure, heightened hypothalamic activity would still be expected.

Women with increased hypothalamic activity due to ovarian or pituitary failure may experience hot flashes. After natural menopause or surgical castration three-quarters of all women develop this disturbance. In one-quarter they last for more than 5 years. They are characterized by sudden episodes of flushing and perspiration, which last a few minutes and occur as often as every 45 minutes. These changes can be objectively measured as discrete rises in skin temperature (flushing) and falls in skin resistance (perspiration). Recent research has indicated that the disturbance is caused by a sudden activation of the thermoregulatory mechanism initiating heat loss. A striking temporal relationship has been shown between LH pulses and the occurrence of each hot flash. It appears that neurotransmitter changes within the hypothalamus, resulting from the open-loop feedback system described above, trigger augmented release of GnRH and simultaneously affect adjacent neuroeffector pathways causing heat loss. The nature of the link between the hypothalamic centers controlling gonadal function and thermoregulation has not been defined.

It has been observed clinically that it is usually the thin or normal-weight woman who is most likely to seek treatment for hot flashes. It has been recently found that women having frequent marked episodes have lower levels of total E_2, E_1, and non-SHBG-bound E_2 than asymptomatic women. The significantly lower relative body weight found in the women with hot flashes is most likely the major factor influencing the levels of biologically available estrogen through its dual effects on peripheral aromatization and SHBG concentration.

Until recently, no controlled studies were available to indicate whether estrogen replacement therapy specifically relieves the emotional problems common at the time of the menopause. Because there are many situational stresses at this time of life, it has been commonly said that the loss of ovarian function is only incidental. Investigators have recently studied the effects of estrogen treatment in a large group of postmenopausal women with severe symptoms, using a randomized double-blind design, and have shown significant reductions in hot flashes, insomnia, irritability, headaches, and anxiety, and improvement in memory. Improvement in sleep quality has been noted by other investigators with decreased sleep latency, and increased REM sleep and duration and depth of sleep. It has been suggested that the other improvements in affective or cognitive function noted above may be due to relief from a chronic sleep disturbance and also that relief from hot flashes may underlie the improvement of insomnia. A close temporal relationship has recently been reported between objective parameters of hot flashes and the occurrence of waking episodes. Decreases in both waking episodes and hot flashes were noted with estrogen treatment.

Estrogen is the most effective treatment of hot flashes and diminishes or abolishes both the subjective and objective disturbances. Empirically the estrogen dose can often be gradually tapered and eventually discontinued if the occurrence of hot flashes is the sole indication for treatment. Progestins have also been shown to treat hot flashes effectively (medroxyprogesterone acetate, 20 mg daily, or megestrol acetate, 40 mg daily), presumably through action at the hypothalamus. Progestins also have a synergistic effect on hypothalamic function when given in combination with estrogen. Theoretically, the cyclic use of progestin in postmenopausal women taking estrogen will aid in providing more effective treatment of hot flashes at lower estrogen doses. Other agents noted to relieve hot flashes are Bellergal (a combination of a sedative, belladona, and ergot alkaloids) and clonidine, an α-adrenergic agonist–antagonist used for hypertension. The latter medication may have this additional benefit in hypertensive women complaining of hot flashes.

Osteoporosis

Chronic estrogen deficiency from any cause may lead to osteoporosis and its attendant fractures of the vertebrae, wrist, and hip, due to increased bone resorption. The disease is less common in obese women and is rare in black women. The fasting excretion of calcium is inversely proportional to body weight and circulating E_1 and E_2. A recent study on postmenopausal women who had sustained a hip fracture showed that they were of lower body weight and had lower levels of free E_2 and free T than age-matched controls. Estrogen treatment prevents objective bone loss, and a history of past estrogen use has recently been reported to be associated with a decreased risk of wrist and hip fractures.

Loss of bone density is greatest over the 4 years immediately following the menopause (approximately 2.5% per year) and then becomes more gradual over the remaining years of life (0.75% per year). A similar period of accelerated loss follows the cessation of estrogen treatment. Therefore, the greatest degree of protection will be realized when estrogen treatment is initiated soon after menopause and long-term replacement is used. Fasting calcium and hydroxyproline excretion is returned to the premenopausal range with 0.625 mg of conjugated estrogens or 10 μg of ethinyl estradiol daily. Studies on bone density and actual fracture prevention with these lower estrogen doses are not yet available. Calcium supplementation at bedtime (2.5 g of calcium carbonate) has been shown to retard bone loss significantly.

In regard to death, disability, and health care cost, osteoporosis is the most significant problem related to the menopause. Almost one-third of all women eventually sustain a hip fracture, one-sixth of these will die of ensuing complications, and many of the remainder are permanently disabled. The cost for acute care of hip fractures annually in the United States is estimated at $1 billion.

Cardiovascular Disease

Although older information disputed any protective effect of ovarian function on the cardiovascular system, a recently reported prospective study (the Framingham study) shows an increased incidence of heart disease related to the menopause rather than to age alone. In addition, early castration was found to increase the incidence of heart disease. Although there is a minor increase in cholesterol, particularly low-density lipoprotein cholesterol, with the menopause, this does not appear to be sufficient to explain this change in cardiovascular risk.

Skin

The skin contains specific estrogen receptors, thins following castration, and thickens with estrogen therapy. Whether these effects are of importance, even cosmetically, is uncertain.

Reproductive Organs

The epithelium of the vagina becomes thinner with less superficial cornification. These changes may lead to dyspareunia, dryness, increased susceptibility to infections, or occasionally vaginal bleeding. Local application of estrogen cream provides a greater local effect with less systemic effect than treatment by the oral route. After a satisfactory effect has been achieved, administration once to twice weekly is often sufficient to relieve symptoms. This problem is much less often seen in young women, perhaps because of a greater frequency of coitus.

The endometrium may become overstimulated by endogenous estrogen, since luteal activity no longer occurs. Obese postmenopausal women, who have increased levels of E_1, E_2, and particularly non-SHBG-bound E_2, have a six-fold increase in the incidence of endometrial cancer. The increased levels of biologically active estrogens in women with endometrial cancer appear to be entirely accounted for by excess body size, since no differences are present when compared with weight-matched controls. Although mean levels of non-SHBG-bound E_2 are markedly increased in women with endometrial cancer, they are lower than those in ovulatory premenopausal women who rarely develop this tumor. The most significant defect in these women is the lack of progesterone effect on the endometrium. Recently it has been suggested that postmenopausal women, particularly those who are overweight, should be periodically tested with a progestin. The occurrence of withdrawal bleeding indicates significant endometrial stimulation by endogenous estrogens. Cyclic administration of the progestin would be expected to protect against the development of endometrial cancer in the same way that it does with exogenous estrogen administration.

Risks of Estrogen Therapy

General Comments

Logically, if estrogen replacement could be provided in a manner identical to premenopausal ovarian secretion, with cyclic progestin provided for a duration comparable to luteal function, risks would not be expected. In fact, accumulating evidence suggests that risks are due to unphysiologic methods of administration. A single oral dose of an estrogen preparation is not comparable to the continuous secretion of estradiol by the ovary into the systemic circulation. Orally administered drugs pass via the portal circulation to the liver before being distributed to the systemic circulation, allowing hepatic cells more opportunity for exposure to the material, particularly at the time of peak absorption. Several metabolic functions of the liver are estrogen-sensitive (renin substrate, clotting factors, and lipoprotein and lipid metabolism). The risks of estrogen therapy can be conceptually divided into two categories—those due to unopposed estrogen and those due to pharmacologic effects on the liver.

Risks of "Unopposed" Estrogen

Endometrial cancer occurs three to eight times more frequently in postmenopausal women using estrogen (unaccompanied by a progestin) when compared with women not using hormones. Risk is related to the dose and duration of treatment. Both progesterone and synthetic progestins decrease the concentration of endometrial estrogen receptors and decrease the intracellular concentration of E_2 by stimulating 17β-hydroxysteroid dehydrogenase activity. The use of cyclic progestin in conjunction with estrogen decreases the risk of endometrial cancer to the normal risk. In one large study the use of a progestin was associated with a rate of endometrial cancer significantly lower than that in women not using any hormones. Endometrial biopsies taken during various treatment regimens indicate that the lowest incidence of abnormal endometrial proliferation occurs with the use of a progestin for 10 days or more.

Three recent studies on postmenopausal estrogen replacement have found a two- to threefold increased risk of breast cancer. Two of these studies found that the risk was not increased in oophorectomized women. Since early oophorectomy reduces the risk of breast cancer by 70%, it may be that in such women low-dose estrogen replacement only partially reverses this protective effect. In one study, women with biopsy-proven cystic mastitis were at markedly increased risk (fivefold) when replacement therapy was administered. One 10-year prospective randomized study found a significantly lower risk of breast cancer in women taking 2.5 mg of conjugated estrogens with cyclic medroxyprogesterone acetate than in women taking a placebo. Other unpublished data appear to confirm this protective effect of cyclic progestin.

Risks Due to Pharmacologic Effects on the Liver

The mean blood pressure and the mean level of triglycerides increase with estrogen treatment. Gallbladder disease is increased 2.5 times. Studies on the effect of estrogen replacement on cardiovascular disease are conflicting, with some studies showing no effects, one study showing a twofold increase in angina, and a recent case-control study showing a reduction in cardiovascular sequellae by one-half. Replacement doses of estrogen have been shown to have pharmacologic effects on liver proteins, including renin substrate. Progestins do not counteract these metabolic effects. In fact, the choice of progestin appears to be important, since 19-nortestosterone derivatives have been shown to reduce high-density lipoprotein cholesterol significantly, whereas the C-21 progestin medroxyprogesterone acetate did not have this adverse effect. Newer methods of estrogen administration that avoid excessive exposure to the liver (vaginal, transcutaneous) may potentially obviate this group of risks.

The blood pressure should be routinely checked before and during estrogen use. Although elevated blood pressure is not an absolute contraindication to estrogen use, the risk/benefit ratio should be carefully reassessed and alternative methods of treating the patient's particular menopausal problems should be considered.

The Treatment Regimen

Our current recommendation is 0.625 mg of conjugated equine estrogens daily, since the greatest amount of information has been gathered on this preparation in regard to both risks and benefits. It should be given for 25 days (conveniently days 1–25 of each calendar month) with the addition of medroxyprogesterone acetate, 10 mg on days 16–25. The majority of women will have withdrawal bleeding. Provided that bleeding occurs at the expected time, there should be no concern of endometrial abnormality. If bleeding occurs at other times, endometrial biopsy should be considered.

DISORDERS OF SEXUAL DEVELOPMENT

Gonadal Dysgenesis

General Comments

A variety of chromosome anomalies and single-gene defects can result in a lack of normal gonadal development with accelerated oocyte atresia and either primary (premenarche) or secondary (postmenarche) ovarian failure. In the absence of testosterone secretion from the gonad, the external genitalia of the fetus develop along female lines, while the Wolffian structures fail to develop into the vas deferens and epididymis. The absence of another testicular product, Müllerian inhibiting factor, results in development of the fallopian tubes, uterus, and upper vagina. The rate of oocyte atresia varies. Some patients may have menstrual function or even pregnancy before ovarian failure ensues. Occasionally, evidence of androgen secretion is present (ambiguous genitalia, hirsutism, or clitoromegaly). This may be due to the presence of actual testicular tissue (mixed gonadal dysgenesis), to an androgen-producing ovarian tumor, or to hilus cell hyperplasia secondary to elevated circulating gonadotropins.

Diagnosis

Gonadal dysgenesis should be suspected in any patient with primary ovarian failure, particularly without breast development, and in women with the onset of secondary ovarian failure before age 25. The most common form of gonadal dysgenesis, Turner's syndrome (absence of the second X chromosome), is also associated with variable somatic anomalies that include short stature, cubitus valgus, low posterior hairline, high arched palate, ptosis, multiple skin nevi, wide-spaced nipples, and coarctation of the aorta. In addition, autoimmune thyroid disease, essential hypertension, and decreased glucose tolerance are more common in these patients. Gonadal dysgenesis in the absence of somatic anomalies is termed *pure gonadal dysgenesis*.

Lack of secondary sexual characteristics and a eunuchoid habitus are present if oocyte atresia is completed before any ovarian activity occurs. Lack of withdrawal following progesterone injection and an elevated serum FSH level are sufficient to establish a diagnosis of ovarian failure. A karyotype determination is necessary to rule out the presence of an XY cell line. If the karyotype is abnormal (X0, XY, or mosaic), then gonadal dysgenesis is most likely present. If the karyotype is XX, pure gonadal dysgenesis may be present due to a single-gene defect, or ovarian failure may be due to another cause.

Treatment

If an XY cell line is present, the gonads should be removed, since the incidence of germ cell tumors increases from the time of normal puberty to a plateau of approximately 25–30% by the middle of the third decade. Hormonal replacement should be provided to all patients as outlined in the discussion of ovarian failure.

Defects of Androgen Synthesis or Action

General Comments

In the presence of a testis, phenotypic development in certain instances may develop along female lines or development may be ambiguous. Androgen exposure in utero may cause partial or complete male differentiation of the external genitalia, whereas exposure after birth leads to hirsutism or virilization. Such absent or partial differentiation of the genetic male may occur as a result of enzyme defects in the synthesis of androgens or a defect in the intracellular processing of T by the end organ.

Diagnosis and Treatment

The production of Müllerian inhibiting factor by the testes results in absence of the upper vagina, uterus, and fallopian tubes. Individuals with a complete defect in the cellular receptor protein for testosterone (testicular feminization) will have entirely normal female external genitalia. Their low circulating levels of estrogen, in the absence of an opposing androgen effect, result in prominent breast development and feminine contours. Sexual hair is scant. The testes are either intraabdominal or in the inguinal canals. The gonads are generally removed following puberty, since tumor incidence begins to rise in the latter part of the second decade and steadily rises to a cumulative incidence of 40% by age 60. The defect in the T receptor may be incomplete, resulting in ambiguous genitalia, or the occurrence of hirsutism and clitoromegaly at puberty. Less commonly, the cellular defect may be in the enzyme 5α-reductase, which converts T to the more potent intracellular effector, dihydrotestosterone. In this abnormality, referred to as *pseudovaginal perineoscrotal hypospadias*, the genitalia are ambiguous at birth but more closely resemble female in development. At puberty the phallus enlarges and the voice deepens as a result of increased T production, although the beard, which is dependent on dihydrotestosterone, does not develop. Defects in enzymes necessary for androgen synthesis (3β-hydroxysteroid dehydrogenase, 17,20-desmolase, and 17β-hydroxysteroid dehydrogenase) can also result in incomplete masculinization of the male.

The diagnosis of these disorders is made by a combination of clinical criteria, measurement of serum T, and a karyotype determination. In the case of testicular feminization the phenotype is so distinct that the finding of a T level in the male range is sufficient.

True Hermaphroditism

When both testicular tissue and ovarian tissue coexist, phenotypic development externally most often resembles the male. Presumably since the amount of testicular tissue is decreased, male differentiation is usually incomplete and variable Müllerian development occurs. Breast development is generally noted at puberty, and in two-thirds menstruation occurs. In 60–70% the karyotype is XX, and in the remainder XY or XX/XY mosaicism is found. The gonads should be removed because of their tumor potential.

Congenital Defects of the Reproductive Tract

Müllerian agenesis is the most common defect observed. Rarely, the uterus is present with only the vagina being absent, in which case cyclic lower abdominal discomfort may be observed. Pelvic sonography may be used to detect the presence of a uterus. Approximately one-third of patients with vaginal atresia have coexistent renal anomalies. Treatment is by progressive dilation or by surgical reconstruction using a split-thickness skin graft. Occasionally, an imperforate hymen can simulate this diagnosis. Cyclic abdominal discomfort is present in such cases, and rectal examination reveals a vaginal mass due to accumulation of secretions and blood. Treatment is simply by incision of the hymen.

SEX STEROID-PRODUCING OVARIAN TUMORS

A hormone-producing neoplasm is suspected as a result of either hirsutism and virilization or clinical signs of estrogen stimulation when not normally expected (before puberty or after menopause) or excessive (endometrial hyperplasia). Androgen-producing ovarian tumors (arrhenoblastoma, lipoid cell tumors, hilus cell adenoma, gonadoblastoma) are almost invariably associated with virilization (clitoromegaly, deepening of the voice, temporal balding, or male body habitus). Circulating levels of T exceed 200 ng % in 85–90% of cases. In some cases these tumors may also be accompanied by signs of excess estrogen stimulation (endometrial hyperplasia). This is most often due to peripheral aromatization of A to estrogen and is a common finding in hilus cell adenomas. Pure estrogen-secreting tumors (granulosa cell tumors) are also seen. Circulating estrogen levels are generally not above the normal premenopausal range. Retrograde venous catheterization may be helpful in differentiating these conditions from functional disturbances and in localizing small tumors.

DISCUSSION CASES

Case 1

Description

An 18-year-old female came to the UCLA gynecologic endocrinology clinic complaining of lack of menstruation. Menarche had occurred at age 13, but only two periods were noted over the following year and none since. Breast development began at age 12 and proceeded satisfactorily. On examination she was of normal height. The breasts, sexual hair, and pelvic structures were normal with the exception that the uterine fundus was very small. No withdrawal bleeding occurred following an injection of 100 mg of progesterone in oil. The level of FSH was 60 mIU/ml (normal 5–15 mIU/ml).

Question

1. Name four conditions that could cause her disease.

Answer

Gonadal dysgenesis, autoimmune disease, premature menopause, gonadotropin-resistant ovary syndrome.

Question

2. What further test is necessary and why?

Answer

A karyotype determination. Gonadectomy is necessary if an XY cell line is present, since gonadal tumors are more common in such individuals.

Question

3. What treatment would you begin?

Answer

Conjugated estrogens, 0.625 mg on days 1–25, each month with medroxyprogesterone acetate, 10 mg on days 16–25.

Case 2

Description

A 28-year-old nulliparous female was referred to the UCLA gynecologic endocrinology clinic for evaluation of amenorrhea. Her last menstrual period had occurred 14 months previously, after discontinuing a 3-year course of oral contraception. She had attempted to conceive since that time without success. On examination the only abnormality detected was the presence of bilateral expressible milky breast secretion. No withdrawal bleeding occurred following intramuscular progesterone. The serum prolactin level was 80 ng/ml (upper normal 20 ng/ml); the serum FSH level was 7 mIU/ml (normal 5–15 mIU/ml). Sellar cone-down views and formal visual field examinations were normal.

Question

1. What factor(s) may be responsible for her galactorrhea?

Answer

Estrogen stimulation during oral contraceptive treatment predisposes to galactorrhea. Amenorrhea occurring after oral sex steroids is often accompanied by hyperprolactinemia. A prolactin-producing pituitary adenoma may also be present.

Question

2. Would you order any further tests?

Answer

A fourth-generation CAT scan is helpful in diagnosing a pituitary tumor and in ruling out suprasellar extension before consideration of ovulation induction. In this case, an 8-mm tumor without suprasellar extension was visualized.

Question

3. Would you advise ovulation induction? What agent would you choose?

Answer

Observation over 1 year's time with repeat prolactin measurement and evaluation of the sella would give reassurance that a fast-growing lesion is not present. More commonly the patient would be advised of the very small likelihood of problems during pregnancy and ovulation induction would be offered without delay. Bromocriptine is the agent of choice either with careful informed consent or within a research protocol.

Question

4. What follow-up would you recommend?

Answer

Prolactin levels should be obtained every 6 months, with sella cone-down views and visual fields yearly. If pregnancy occurs, visual fields should be obtained monthly.

SUGGESTED READING

Hammond CB, et al: Effects of long-term estrogen replacement therapy. I. Metabolic effects. II. Neoplasia. *Am J Obstet Gynecol* 133:525–547, 1979.

Jaffe RB: Disorders of sexual development, in Yen SSC, Jaffe RB (eds): *Reproductive Endocrinology.* Philadelphia, WB Saunders, 1978, pp 271–296.

Judd HL, et al: Estrogen replacement therapy. *Obstet Gynecol* 58:267–275, 1981.

Kletsky OA, Davajan V: Galactorrhea, in Mishell DR, Davajan V (eds): *Reproductive Endocrinology, Infertility and Contraception.* Philadelphia, FA Davis, 1979, pp 249–268.

March CM: Dysfunctional uterine bleeding, in Mishell DR, Davajan V (eds): *Reproductive Endocrinology, Infertility and Contraception.* Philadelphia, FA Davis, 1979, pp 299–309.

Speroff L, Glass RH, Kase NG: Amenorrhea, in Speroff L, Glass RH, Kase NG (eds): *Clinical Gynecologic Endocrinology and Infertility.* Baltimore, Williams & Wilkins, 1978, pp 93–122.

Yen SSC: The human menstrual cycle, in Yen SSC, Jaffe RB (eds): *Reproductive Endocrinology.* Philadelphia, WB Saunders, 1978, pp 126–151.

13

RONALD S. SWERDLOFF
DAVID HEBER

Modern Management of Male Hypogonadism

The testes are dual organs consisting of two related functional compartments: (1) the endocrine cells (Leydig or interstitial cells, and Sertoli cells) and (2) the germ cells (spermatozoa and sperm precursors). The Leydig, Sertoli, and germ cells serve as an anatomically and functionally integrated unit resulting in normal reproductive function.

The Leydig cells, located in the peritubular space, are the source of the vast majority of circulating testosterone (T) and its metabolites responsible for male sexual differentiation and maturation, normal potency and ejaculatory capability, spermatogenic maturation, and semen fluid consistency. The Sertoli cells and germinal cells are located within the tubular compartment and are separated from the Leydig cells by the tubular basement membrane. While the function of the Sertoli cells is incompletely understood, they are in close proximity to the germ cells and are believed to be the mediators of hormonal regulation of spermatogenesis. The Sertoli cells are the source of androgen binding protein (ABP), the tubular contribution to the seminal fluid, Müllerian inhibiting hormone, and inhibin. The germ cells, by the process of spermatogenesis, differentiate into spermatozoa which provide the male genetic contribution for fertilization of the egg and embryonic development. Testicular function is regulated by a series of closed-loop feedback systems involving the central nervous system (hypothalamus), the pituitary gland, and testicular products and hormones.

For the purposes of this review, we will subdivide hypogonadism into disorders of: (1) androgen production or action (underandrogenization), (2) sperm production or function (infertility), and (3) combined androgen and germ cell dysfunction (panhypogonadism).

NORMAL MALE REPRODUCTIVE PHYSIOLOGY

Figure 1 depicts the normal male reproductive hormonal axis. This subject has been reviewed in detail elsewhere. Briefly, the hypothalamus is the integrating center of central nervous system (CNS) regulation of gonadotropin-releasing hormone (GnRH). Extrahypothalamic CNS input has both inhibitory and stimulatory influences on GnRH secretion. The GnRH-secreting neurons have androgen and estrogen receptors and are modulated by the circulating

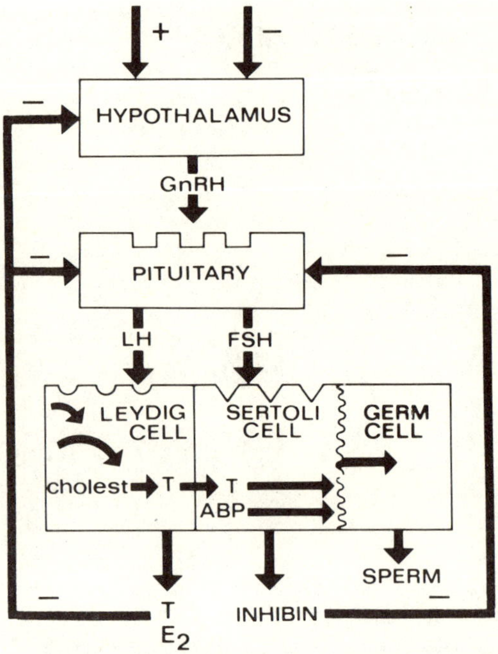

Figure 1. The normal male reproductive hormonal axis. T, testosterone; E_2, estradiol; ABP, androgen-binding protein.

levels of these steroids. Neurotransmitters such as norepinephrine, dopamine, endorphin, and melatonin serve as regulators of GnRH synthesis and pulsatile release into the hypophyseal portal blood system. At the pituitary gland, GnRH stimulates the synthesis and release of two gonadotropic hormones, luteinizing hormone (LH) and follicle-stimulating hormone (FSH). LH serves as the primary stimulus for Leydig cell sex steroid secretion, while FSH acts on the Sertoli cells, providing a favorable milieu for spermatogenic development.

Spermatogenesis, the process of maturation of primitive spermatogonia to mature spermatozoa, requires approximately 74 days in humans. Hormonal regulation of germ cell maturation is a complex process requiring both adequate local concentrations of testosterone (LH-stimulated) and Sertoli cell function (FSH- and testosterone-stimulated).

Testosterone circulates in the blood bound to several proteins, the most important of which is sex hormone-binding globulin (SHBG). The bound hormone is in equilibrium with a very small amount of free or biologically available hormone (<2%). Testosterone and its 5α reduced metabolite (dihydrotestosterone, DHT) act on specific receptors for androgen action. Table 1 is a list of the major androgen-sensitive tissues.

Four relatively distinct phases of testosterone secretion exist: (1) fetal, which results in differentiation and development of the male genital tract; (2) postnatal, occurring between the second and sixth months of life, the action of which is poorly understood; (3) pubertal and adult, commencing from 11–13 years of age and resulting in masculinization and fertility; and (4) senescent, resulting in a gradual but significant decline in testosterone secretion and declining sexual function in many men after age 60.

Estradiol (E_2) is also secreted by the testis, but most of the circulating E_2 is the product of peripheral conversion of precursors such as testosterone and androstenedione.

Table 1 **Examples of Androgen-Sensitive Tissue in Humans**

Testicular tubules
Sex accessories (prostate, seminal vesicles)
Skeletal muscles
Skeletal system
Larynx
Skin, hair follicles, sebaceous glands
Hematopoietic system
Central nervous system

Testicular secretory products also serve as important closed-loop feedback regulators of gonadotropin secretion. Testosterone and E_2 appear to be the major inhibitors of LH secretion, thereby modulating Leydig cell function. These steroids appear to act both at the hypothalamic and pituitary sites and influence pulse frequency and amplitude of LH secretion. FSH secretion is also negatively influenced by testicular hormones, although a putative Sertoli cell product, inhibin, is believed to be a second inhibitory factor. Knowledge of feedback regulation of gonadotropins is of practical value, since depressed serum testosterone levels in the presence of elevated gonadotropins indicate primary testicular damage, while depressed gonadotropin levels indicate a hypothalamic or pituitary disorder. Isolated increases in serum levels of FSH (normal testosterone and LH) suggest diminished Sertoli cell and germ cell function.

CLINICAL MANIFESTATIONS OF ANDROGEN DEFICIENCY

The time of onset of androgen deficiency influences the clinical features.

Fetal Onset

Differentiation of the genitalia along male lines is an androgen-dependent process occurring in the first trimester of gestation. Testosterone deficiency or end-organ unresponsiveness during this critical developmental period results in pseudohermaphroditism. The degree of the sexual ambiguity is determined by the extent of the androgen deficiency and may range from normal female external genitalia (with a short vagina) to hypospadias. If androgen secretion or action is diminished before birth but after the genitalia have differentiated along male lines, a small but anatomically intact phallus may be seen.

Prepubertal Onset

If androgen deficiency begins after fetal development but before the completion of puberty, the clinical presentation will be that of eunuchoidism. The lack of testosterone and its metabolite, E_2, results in a failure to stimulate epiphyseal closure. Growth of long bones thus continues, and the patient develops eunuchoid proportions (arm span >3 in. more than the height).

Postpubertal Onset

Since these patients have proceeded through normal pubertal maturation, they have normal body measurements, normal voice, and normal male scalp hair distribution. The commonest complaints are decreased libido, impotence, and infertility. These symptoms may be associated with decreased facial, pubic, and body hair, decreased muscle strength, and small, soft testes. Gynecomastia may occur as a result of an imbalance of serum testosterone and E_2 (a decreased T/E_2 ratio).

In assessing testosterone-responsive body hair, the clinician must take into account the patient's genetic and racial background. Whereas Caucasian men may need to shave several times a day, blacks, Asians, and American Indians may normally shave every third day. Many normal black, Asian, and American Indian men have body hair limited to the axillary, pubic, and sternal areas, while many Caucasian men have additional pectoral, back, and flank hair. The absence of chest hair, a sparseness of pubic hair, and a female escutcheon suggest severe, long-standing hypogonadism. Less severe defects produce more subtle changes in body hair and a decreased need to shave. It is often helpful to ask the patient to compare the status of his facial and body hair to that of other male members of his family.

DIAGNOSIS OF UNDERANDROGENIZATION

Clinical suspicion of low testosterone secretion can be confirmed by measuring the serum testosterone level. Since testosterone may be secreted in a pulsatile fashion, a more accurate measurement of serum testosterone levels may be obtained by pooling three blood samples taken approximately 20 minutes apart. If the serum testosterone concentration is low (in the absence of impaired production of the binding protein, SHBG), the diagnosis of hypogonadism is confirmed and the evaluation proceeds to identification of the anatomic level of the defect. If underandrogenization exists in the absence of lower serum testosterone levels, then androgen resistance is suspected. Low serum testosterone concentrations may be seen in the absence of clinical manifestations and suggest a low SHBG level. SHBG deficiency may be either a congenital or acquired defect. An example of an acquired deficiency of SHBG production and associated low levels of measured total serum testosterone is severe obesity. A free testosterone measurement (normal) will be helpful in such cases.

ANATOMIC LOCALIZATION OF AN UNDERANDROGENIZATION DEFECT

A classification of underandrogenization according to the site of major primary organ impairment is provided in Table 2.

PRIMARY TESTICULAR INSUFFICIENCY

Primary testicular insufficiency is characterized by low serum testosterone levels accompanied by elevated serum concentrations of LH and FSH. The disorder may result from a long list of conditions which include Klinefelter's syndrome (47,XXY), untreated or poorly managed cryptorchidism, bilateral torsion of the testes, and anorchia. The androgen deficiency is usually accompanied by damage to the seminiferous tubules, resulting in azoospermia and infertility.

Table 2 **Classification of Hypogonadism (Underandrogenization)**

Abnormalities in hypothalamic-pituitary function
- Panhypopituitarism (congenital or acquired)
- Hypothalamic syndromes (congenital or acquired)
  - Prader-Willi syndrome
  - Lawrence-Moon-Biedl syndrome
- Isolated LH and/or FSH deficiency (may be associated with anosmia)
  - Kallman's syndrome
  - Functional defects secondary to malnutrition, anorexia nervosa, hyperprolactinemia, and drugs

Primary gonadal abnormalities
- Acquired (irradiation, orchitis, castration, cancer chemotherapy)
- Chromosomal
  - Klinefelter's syndrome and variants
  - True hermaphroditism
- Defective androgen synthesis
  - 20α-Hydroxylase deficiency
  - 17,20-Desmolase deficiency
  - 20α-Hydroxysteroid dehydrogenase deficiency
  - 17α-Ketoreductase deficiency
  - 5α-Reductase deficiency
- Testicular agenesis
- Selective seminiferous tubular disease
- Miscellaneous
  - Noonan's syndrome
  - Streak gonads
  - Myotonia dystrophica
  - Cystic fibrosis
- Chronic disease (hepatic, renal)
- Drugs (e.g., alcohol)

Defects in androgen action (pseudohermaphroditism)
- Complete androgen insensitivity (also called testicular feminization)
- Incomplete androgen sensitivity
  - Type I (testosterone receptor and postreceptor defects)
  - Type II (5α-reductase deficiency)

SECONDARY TESTICULAR FAILURE

Secondary testicular failure (hypogonadotropic hypogonadism) is characterized by low serum testosterone levels accompanied by low serum concentrations of LH and FSH. In turn, low gonadotropin secretion may result from impaired hypothalamic secretion of GnRH or as a result of direct pituitary gland dysfunction. Hyperprolactinemia of any cause may produce hypogonadotropic hypogonadism, primarily by suppressing LH secretion.

The distinction between hypothalamic and pituitary causes may be suggested if androgen deficiency is accompanied by anosmia or diabetes insipidus (hypothalamic) or bitemporal upper-quadrant visual field defects (pituitary). Further resolution will usually require radiographs of the pituitary fossa and computerized tomography (CT) scans, which may be combined with angiography or pneumoencephalography to determine the extent of lesions. Laboratory confirmation sometimes requires stimulation tests, since the distinction between subnormal and low-normal levels of FSH and LH is difficult using some radioimmunoassays. An absent or subnormal response of FSH and LH (less than a doubling) to clomiphene citrate (100 mg/day for 7–10 days) confirms an impaired hypothalamohypophyseal gonadotropic secretory reserve. Since both hypothalamic and pituitary disease may result in a blunted or absent response of LH and FSH to an acute bolus of GnRH, this test is not of use in distinguishing these two pathologic anatomic sites. Recent studies have suggested that multiple, properly spaced injections of GnRH will result in stimulation of LH secretion in patients with hypothalamic GnRH deficiency and could be of value in separating such patients from those with pituitary disease.

END-ORGAN RESISTANCE

End-organ resistance to testosterone may occur as a result of failure of the enzyme 5α-reductase to convert testosterone to dihydrotestosterone, or may be due to the absence of testosterone receptors or failure of receptor-bound testosterone to influence DNA-dependent RNA synthesis.

Androgen receptor defects appear to be the most common cause of testosterone resistance and to have a characteristic hormonal pattern of elevated serum testosterone and LH levels. Such patients often have clinical manifestations of pseudohermaphroditism. Gynecomastia is common and is due to excessive production of estradiol, from both aromatization of circulating testosterone and direct hypersecretion by the testis.

A summary of the laboratory changes in underandrogenization according to anatomic site is provided in Table 3.

TREATMENT OF ANDROGEN INSUFFICIENCY

General

If the hypogonadism is caused by extratesticular factors, attempts should be made to correct them. If this fails, libido and potency can be restored by androgen replacement therapy.

Patients with hypothalamic or pituitary lesions causing secondary hypogonadism should be treated with FSH and LH, or GnRH replacement therapy if restored fertility is required. If it is not, androgen replacement therapy can be instituted.

Primary Testicular Failure

The majority of testicular conditions causing androgen deficiency are irreversible, and consequently treatment consists of androgen replacement therapy. It is important to emphasize that the gradual decline in testosterone secretion can lead to the insidious onset of symptoms such as loss of libido and potency, tiredness, lack of ambition and drive, hot flushes, and depression. Many of these symptoms can be attributed to other causes, hence it is important to establish the diagnosis by the measurement of testosterone levels. It is equally important to realize that a patient who has never had adequate testosterone secretion may claim that the libido and potency he experiences are normal, since he does not have a normal comparison.

Table 3 **Summary of Hormone Levels and Treatment in Major Diagnostic Categories of Hypogonadism**

	FSH	*LH*	*T*[a]	*Treatment*
Hypogonadotropic hypogonadism	↓[b]	↓	↓	hCG or testosterone to virilize, hCG and hMG for fertility
Primary testicular insufficiency	↑[c]	↑	↓	Testosterone to virilize only
Isolated germinal cell damage	↑–N[d]	N	N	Testosterone rebound or clomiphene for fertility
Testosterone resistance	N–↓	↑–N	↑–N	None

[a]T, testosterone.
[b]↓, decreased.
[c]↑, increased.
[d]N, normal.

Both oral and parenteral preparations of androgens are available, but adequate replacement therapy can be achieved only by parenteral administration, though it involves some discomfort for the patient. Treatment commences with intramuscular injections of a long-acting ester (e.g., enanthate or cypionate) of testosterone in doses of 150–250 mg given every 10 days for 1 month. Once the patient has experienced the effect of the androgens, the interval between injections is increased until he experiences symptoms of androgen withdrawal (tiredness, loss of libido, irritability, mood swings, and occasionally hot flushes). The next injection is then given, and thereafter the interval is slightly shortened to prevent these symptoms from recurring. The patient is then encouraged to administer his own injections.

The optimum time interval for injections varies considerably, but 14–17 days is usual, except in patients with Klinefelter's syndrome, who tend to require more frequent injections (10–14 days). Occasionally, patients respond to these doses by an increased red cell mass and may become symptomatically polycythemic—hence it is important to measure the hematocrit at intervals of 3–6 months. Other side effects are rare, though fluid retention may sometimes occur.

The criteria of successful therapy are (1) development of normal secondary sexual characteristics, (2) increased frequency of shaving, (3) restoration of libido and potency, (4) increased muscle mass, and (5) decreased tiredness. Synthetic oral androgens such as methyltestosterone, fluoxymesterone, and oxymetholone are available, but are not recommended since they usually produce only partial androgenization and have been associated with several hepatic disorders including cholestatic jaundice, liver cell carcinoma, and a rare vascular disorder, peliosis hepatis.

Secondary (Pituitary-Hypothalamic) Hypogonadism

Secondary hypogonadism varies in presentation according to the age and sexual maturity of the individual. For example, if it occurs before puberty, the presentation is that of failure of sexual maturation.

The initial aim in management is always to exclude tumors of the pituitary or hypothalamus by the appropriate investigations. In the adult, subsequent management involves replacement therapy with FSH and LH (according to the scheme outlined below) if fertility is required; otherwise, androgens are administered.

The presence of isolated gonadotropin deficiencies will require replacement therapy with FSH- and LH-like hormones to restore fertility. Testosterone injections are given to achieve masculinization in prepubertal males and can be administered without concern about irreversible compromise of testicular function. When fertility is desired, testosterone is withdrawn and injections of human chorionic gonadotropin (hCG, which acts like LH), 3,000 IU, are given weekly for a period of approximately 6 months. If semen analyses show that sperm production has not commenced, FSH as human menopausal gonadotropin (hMG) in a dose of 75 IU three times a week is added to the hCG regimen. Combined therapy is often needed for 12–15 months.

End-Organ Resistance

There is no known effective therapy for the eunuchoidism resulting from androgen resistance. Patients with male phenotypes and gynecomastia usually require cosmetic surgery to remove the breast tissue.

INFERTILITY

Abnormalities in sperm production and function frequently result in couples seeking medical assistance. Infertility is defined as a lack of conception after 1 year of unprotected coitus. An abnormality in the male partner appears to be a causative factor in 30–50% of infertile couples. All evaluations for infertility must include a thorough assessment of both the male and the female; in many cases abnormalities of reproductive function exist in both partners.

An algorithmic approach to the evaluation of a man for infertility has recently been recommended by the author. A proposed workup for the infertile male is presented in Figs. 2–6.

Semen Analysis

The semen sample should be collected in a standardized manner. A sexual abstinence period of 2–4 days is recommended before collection of the specimen in a clean container; the semen specimen should be kept warm (as close to body temperature as possible) during transport. Since there is considerable variation in the characteristics of semen specimens obtained from a given patient, multiple assessments should be obtained. Characterization of three to six samples at least 10 days apart is optimal for semen analysis.

Evaluation of the semen specimen includes the assessment of:

1. Coagulation and liquifaction: Freshly ejaculated semen is a coagulum. Liquefaction occurs in 3–25 minutes.
2. Viscosity: Viscosity is a reflection of the enzymatic function of the prostate and seminal vesicles. Semen should flow freely when poured.
3. Volume: The normal volume varies, depending on the abstinence interval, with a range of 1–6 ml.
4. pH: The normal range of pH is 7–8. A low pH suggests occlusion of the ejaculatory ducts or contamination of the specimen with urine. An alkaline pH raises the question of acute diseases of the secondary sex glands.
5. Sperm count: Liquified semen is pipetted onto a standard blood cell-counting chamber.

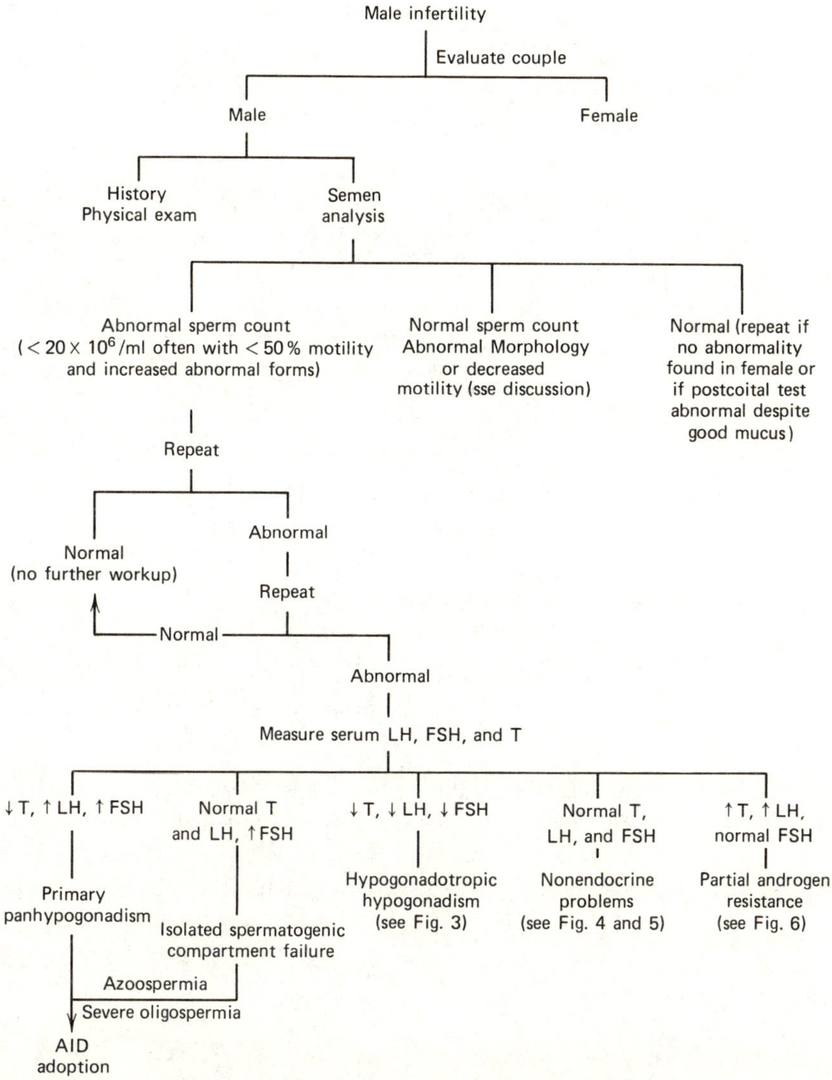

Figure 2. An algorithmic approach to the workup of the infertile male. T, testosterone; LH, luteinizing hormone; FSH, follicle-stimulating hormone; AID, artificial insemination with donor semen.

Oligospermia is defined as a count of less than 20 million /ml of semen. Fertility with lower sperm counts is not uncommon. Azoospermia is the complete absence of sperm.

6. Sperm motility: A drop of semen is evaluated microscopically within 2 hours of collection. A determination is made of the percent of motile and nonmotile cells, and the motion of the sperm is graded on a scale of 0 to 4: 0, no motility; 1, sluggish activity; 2, poor to fair motility; 3, good motility; 4, excellent forward progression.
7. Sperm morphology: The normal morphologic pattern of a semen sample should contain more than 60% normal oval forms, less than 6% tapering forms, less than 0.5% immature forms,

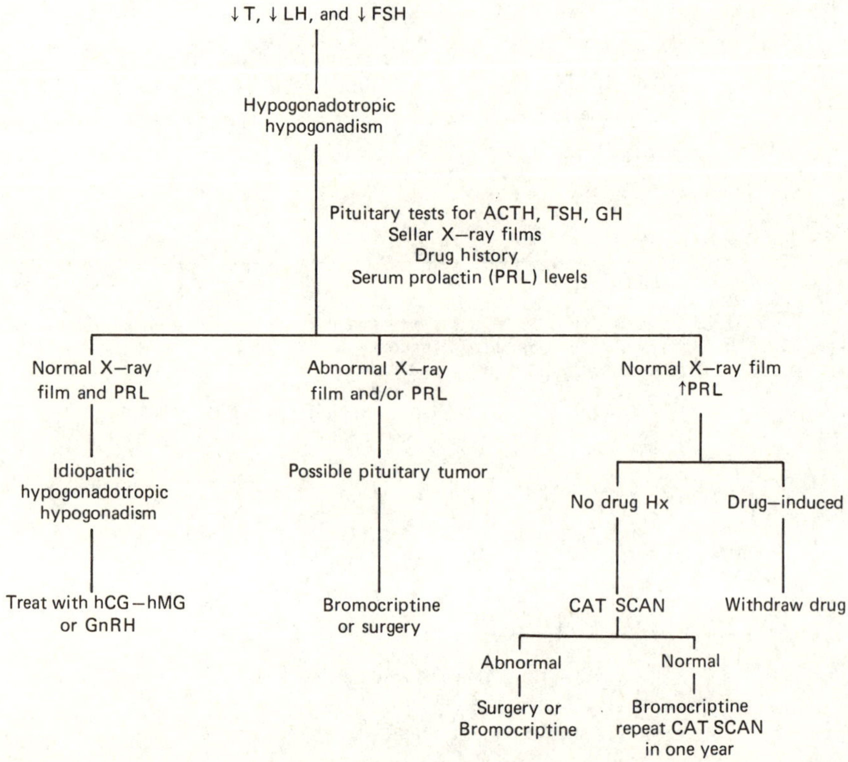

Figure 3. An algorithmic approach to the workup of the infertile male. T, testosterone; hCG, human chorionic gonadotropin; hMG, human menopausal gonadotropin.

and less than 8.6% amorphous forms. It is frequently difficult to distinguish immature spermatogenic cells from leukocytes, and special staining may be required.

Hormonal Assessment

All patients with abnormal semen analyses should have measurements of serum LH, FSH, and testosterone levels performed (Fig. 2). The evaluation and management of patients with primary or secondary Leydig cell dysfunction or end-organ resistance to androgen have been discussed in the section on androgen insufficiency. Patients with isolated FSH elevations have severe damage to the Sertoli cell germinal compartment and respond poorly to any therapy.

Patients with oligospermia, azoospermia, or impaired morphology and motility despite normal serum LH, FSH, and testosterone (Figs. 4 and 5) will be discussed below.

Azoospermia with Normal Serum Testosterone, LH, and FSH

These patients have either retrograde ejaculation or an obstruction of the ejaculatory system (Fig. 4). Retrograde ejaculation is suspected by the presence of autonomic neuropathy and is

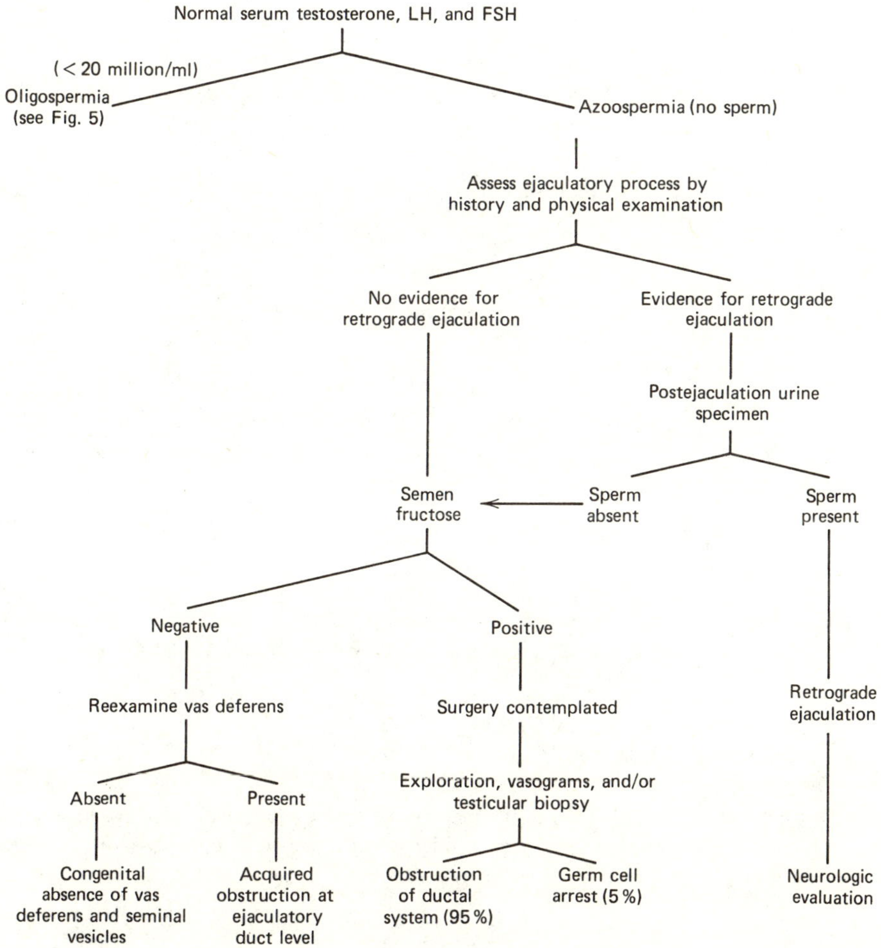

Figure 4. An algorithmic approach to the workup of the infertile male.

most frequently seen in patients with diabetes mellitus. The presence of large numbers of sperm in postejaculation urine specimens confirms the diagnosis. Recognition of obstructive disorders is important, as therapy must be directed toward surgical correction of the disorder. Fructose is normally produced by the seminal vesicles and transported into the vas deferens by the ejaculatory ducts. The absence of seminal fructose usually indicates a congenital absence of the vas deferens and seminal vesicles. The absence of the vas deferens can be observed in most instances by palpation of the scrotal contents. Patients with azoospermia, normal serum FSH, and a normal semen fructose concentration will, in greater than 95% of cases, prove to have an obstruction of the ductal system, proximal to the entry of the ejaculatory ducts. The finding of normal-sized testes with or without palpable enlargement of the caput epididymis almost certainly indicates obstructive disease. If surgery is contemplated, exploration with a testicular biopsy and vasograms may be required to define the nature of an obstructive defect.

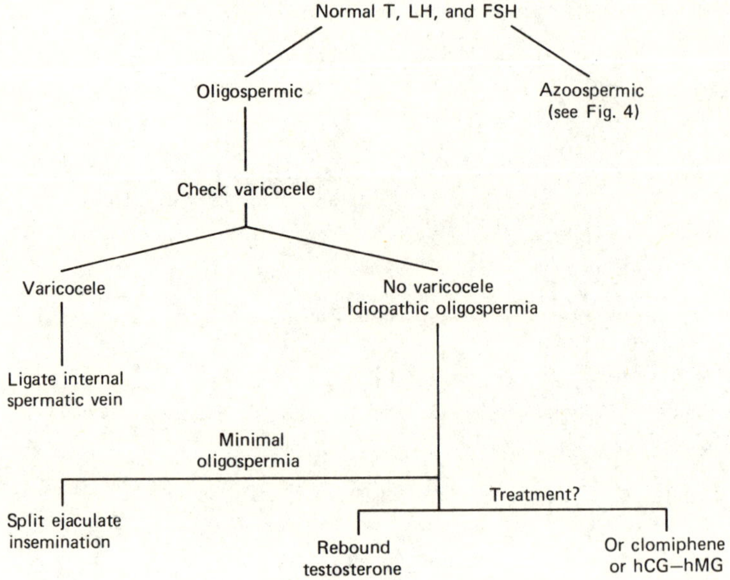

Figure 5. An algorithmic approach to the workup of the infertile male. T, testosterone; hCG, human chorionic gonadotropin; hMG, human menopausal gonadotropin.

Oligospermia with Normal Serum Testosterone, LH, and FSH

This hormonal pattern is seen in the majority of oligospermic patients (Fig. 5). Patients with varicoceles make up one subcategory of oligospermic men with normal hormonal profiles. The pathogenic mechanism for impaired spermatogenesis in these patients remains elusive, and

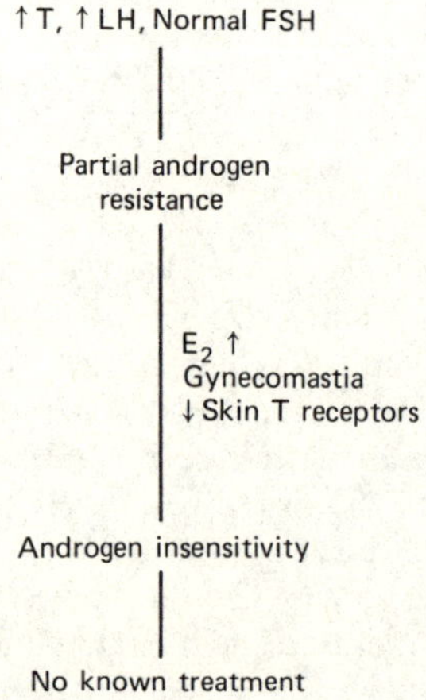

Figure 6. An algorithmic approach to the workup of the infertile male. T, testosterone; E_2, estradiol.

the appropriate therapeutic approach is controversial. Despite a lack of uniformity of data supporting its efficacy, most experts in the field have advocated ligation of the internal spermatic vein on the side of the varicocele. The remainder of patients with oligospermia and normal hormonal profile are categorized as having idiopathic oligospermia; several forms of therapy have been proposed. These include insemination with the first portion of a split ejaculate, rebound treatment with testosterone, and treatment with clomiphene or with hCG-hMG. None of these treatments have been shown to be unequivocally beneficial in carefully controlled studies. If one of these therapies is instituted, a time limit should be invoked after which the options of artificial insemination with donor semen or adoption should be discussed. When the male has oligospermia, the female should be evaluated to ensure that subfertility does not exist in both members of the couple. Frequently, correction of anovulation in the female partner of an oligospermic male will result in pregnancy, despite the low sperm count.

Normal Sperm Count, but Impaired Sperm Morphology or Motility

Necrospermia

Dead sperm can be identified with supravital stains. While no treatment is available for necrospermia, recent discovery of abnormal sperm metabolism in several patients may presage a period of specific therapies.

Abnormal Sperm Motility or Morphology

This is usually seen in oligospermic specimens but can occur in men with normal counts (Fig. 2). Abnormal forms indicate impaired spermatogenesis. Decreased motility may occur with structural or metabolic sperm defects or may represent a hostile semen environment. Specific defects of cilia structure in both the respiratory and reproductive tracts have been identified, resulting in infertility associated with a severe reduction in sperm motility ($<10\%$ motility). The presence of inflammatory cells suggests genital tract infection, indicating the need for appropriate culture and antibiotic treatment.

Agglutination may indicate the presence of antisperm antibodies. The level of serum sperm-agglutinating antibodies can be measured, although a causal relationship between serum sperm-agglutinating antibodies and male infertility has not been unequivocally established.

DISCUSSION CASES

Case 1

Description

An 18-year-old unmarried man was referred to an endocrinologist after failing to pass an induction physical examination for the army. He indicated that he had been slow in developing pubic, beard, and mustache hair and presently shaved only twice a week. He was of normal height during grammar school, but did not have the usual growth spurt in his midteens and is still growing at present. On questioning, he indicated that he had less than average strength.

He stated that he had only occasional nocturnal penile erections, rarely masturbated, and had not experienced sexual intercourse. He denied radiation or toxin exposure, had not had hernia or scrotal surgery or trauma, or testicular swelling. Physical examination revealed a young-appearing male. He was 5 ft 8 in. tall with an arm span of 5 ft 11 in. He had only slight temporal hair recession, a small amount of mustache hair, and minimal beard hair. He had bilateral palpable breast glandular tissue (3–4 cm in diameter). The penis was normal in appearance and measured 8 cm (stretched). The testes were small (8 cm^3 on the right and 6 cm^3 on left; normal adult >12 cm^3) and of normal consistency. Neurologic examination was normal, including the sense of smell.

Question

1. What tests would you order for the patient?

Answer

All patients with suspected hypogonadism should have LH, FSH, and testosterone levels measured in a pooled serum specimen. In this case, the serum testosterone level was 270 ng/dl (normal 300–1200 ng/dl), the serum LH level was 26 mIU/ml (normal 3–15 mIU/ml), and the serum FSH level was 34 (normal 3–15 mIU/ml).

Question

2. How would you interpret the results?

Answer

The pattern of low serum testosterone and elevated serum LH and FSH is characteristic of primary testicular insufficiency.

Question

3. What is the most common etiology of this testicular failure?

Answer

Primary testicular insufficiency in an 18-year-old male is likely to be the result of a sex chromosome abnormality. Klinefelter's syndrome (XXY) is most common, but mosaic variants might be found in the patient with only partial androgen insufficiency. His chromosome analysis revealed XXY/XY.

Question

4. How would you treat the patient?

Answer

The therapeutic approach is straightforward, in that the testicular hormones should be replaced. Testosterone enanthate, 150 mg i.m. every 14 days, resulted in normal beard, chest, and pubic hair; his voice deepened, and his muscle strength improved. He developed an increased sexual drive and normal heterosexual relationships.

Case 2

Description

A 32-year-old man and his 26-year-old wife presented with a complaint of infertility despite 4 years of unprotected coitus. The wife had been evaluated by her gynecologist and found to be ovulating normally (normal menstrual pattern, BBT, luteal phase progesterone values) with normal patent fallopian tubes (normal hysterosalpingograms and a laparoscopy). The husband's semen analysis revealed no sperm. His physical examination was normal, with adequate secondary sexual development (beard, chest, and pubic hair normal); his testes were 20 ml in volume bilaterally and the vas deferens were palpable on both sides.

Question

1. What tests were indicated?

Answer

The semen analysis needs to be repeated. Results are sufficiently variable that a single semen assessment is never adequate. Two additional sperm counts were zero. The semen fructose level was also assessed and found to be normal. This indicates that the seminal vesicles and ejaculatory ducts were functional and that congenital absence of the vas deferens was not the cause of the azoospermia (a finding already noted on the physical examination). Serum LH, FSH, and testosterone tests were also ordered. The serum LH and testosterone levels were normal, confirming the physical findings of normal-sized testes and secondary sexual development. The serum FSH concentration was 8 mIU/ml (normal 3–15 mIU/ml). The presence of a normal serum level of FSH in a patient with azoospermia is of extreme diagnostic importance and indicates a 95% likelihood of obstruction of the ejaculatory duct system. Since the vas deferens are palpable and the semen fructose is normal, the obstruction must be proximal to the ejaculatory ducts. Most often, the obstruction is in the epididymis. At the time of surgical exploration, intraoperative vasograms were performed and an epididymal obstruction demonstrated. Microsurgical reanastomosis was performed with only partial success. The sperm count increased to 2 million/ml 10 weeks after the surgery, but motility remained poor and the wife had not conceived 9 months after the operation.

SUGGESTED READING

1. Baker HWG, Bremner WJ, Burger HG, deKretser DM, Dalmanis A, Eddie LW, Hudson B, Keogh EJ, Lee VKW, Rennie DC: Testicular control of follicle stimulating hormone secretion. *Recent Prog Horm Res* 32:429, 1976.
2. deKretser DM, Swerdloff RS: Eunuchoidism. *Med Int* 1:308, 1981.
3. deZerega GS, Sherins RJ: Endocrine control of adult testicular function, in Burger H, deKretser D (eds): *The Testis*. New York, Raven Press, 1981, p 127.
4. Eliasson R, Massberg B, Camner P, Afzelius B: The immobile cilia syndrome. *N Engl J Med* 297:1, 1977.
5. Odell WD, Swerdloff RS: Abnormalities of gonadal function in men. *Clin Endocrinol* 8:149, 1978.
6. Ritzen EM, Hanson V, French FS: The Sertoli cell, in Burger H, deKretser D (eds): *The Testis*. New York, Raven Press, 1981.

7. Sherins RJ, Howards SS: Male infertility, in Harrison JH, Gittes RF, Perlmutter AD, Stamey TA, Walsh PC (eds): *Campbell's Urology*, ed 2. Philadelphia, WB Saunders Co, 1978, vol I, pp 715–778.

8. Sokol RZ, Palacios A, Campfield LA, Saul C, Swerdloff RS: Comparison of kinetics of injectable testosterone in eugonadal and hypogonadal men. *Fertil Steril* 37:425, 1982.

9. Swerdloff RS, Glass AR: Male reproductive abnormalities, in Hershman JM (ed): *Endocrine Pathophysiology: A Patient Oriented Approach,* ed 2. Philadelphia, Lea & Febiger, 1982, pp 157–170.

10. Swerdloff RS: Physiology of male reproduction: Hypothalamic-pituitary function: The hypothalamic-pituitary-gonadal axis, in Harrison JH, Gittes RF, Perlmutter AD, (eds): *Campbell's Urology,* ed 2. Philadelphia, WB Saunders Co, 1978, p 125.

11. Swerdloff RS, Heber D: Endocrine control of testicular function from birth to puberty, in Burger H, deKretser D (eds): *The Testis*. New York, Raven Press, 1981, p 107.

12. Swerdloff RS, Heber D: Effects of aging on male reproductive function, in Korenman S (ed): *The Endocrinology of Aging*. New York, Elsevier North Holland, 1981.

13. Swerdloff RS, Sokol RZ: Male reproductive abnormalities, in Hershman JM (ed): *Management of Endocrine Disorders*. Philadelphia, Lea & Febiger, 1980, pp 116–133.

14. Swerdloff RS, Boyers SP: Evaluation of the male partner of an infertile couple: An algorithmic approach. *J Am Med Assoc* 247:2418, 1982.

15. Swerdloff RS, deKretser DM: Endocrine evaluation of the infertile male, in Lipschultz L, Howards S (eds): *Infertility in the Male*. New York, Churchill Livingston, 1983.

14 HAROLD E. CARLSON

Gynecomastia

Gynecomastia, defined as enlargement of the male breast, is a common disorder. In recent years, clinical and pathologic advances have clarified the nature and significance of gynecomastia, while new findings in the fields of steroid and receptor biochemistry have provided a basis for an understanding of the molecular pathophysiology involved. This discussion will review these recent developments and suggest a reasonable approach to the clinical problems posed by the male patient with breast enlargement.

DETECTION OF GYNECOMASTIA

The definition of gynecomastia may be further restricted to include only palpable breast tissue, excluding simple adiposity. Careful physical examination is necessary to differentiate fat from glandular and ductular tissue. Gynecomastia may take the form of either a discrete subareolar plate of tissue, easily distinguished from adipose tissue, or a more diffuse mass which may resemble surrounding fat. Comparison of the breast with nearby subcutaneous tissue on the upper chest wall or the upper anterior axillary fold may allow a definitive diagnosis of gynecomastia to be made.

PATHOLOGY

Histologically, gynecomastia consists of a varying mixture of ductular epithelial elements, fat, and connective tissue. True acini, as occur in the female breast, are rarely seen in gynecomastia. Although early reports attempted to link specific causes of gynecomastia with unique histologic findings, later investigation has suggested that the duration of gynecomastia may be more important than the etiology in determining the histologic appearance: Shortly after onset, gynecomastia typically shows prominent ductules embedded in loose connective tissue, while gynecomastia of several years' duration usually exhibits inconspicuous ductular structures in a dense, hyalinized, and fibrous stroma.

PREVALENCE OF GYNECOMASTIA

Recent work has shown that palpable, asymptomatic gynecomastia is frequently found in normal men. Nuttall detected gynecomastia in 36% of 306 military reservists; the prevalence appeared to increase modestly with advancing age. We have recently confirmed these findings; in a study of 100 male veterans (50 consecutive inpatients on a general medical ward and 50 consecutive outpatients presenting to a triage clinic), we found an overall prevalence of palpable gynecomastia of 32% (30% in the inpatients and 34% in the outpatients). As in Nuttall's series, all our subjects denied breast pain or tenderness and had been unaware of breast enlargement. Both of these clinical studies agree well with an older autopsy series that found histologic evidence of gynecomastia in 40% of 477 men examined.

Taken together, these results clearly indicate that asymptomatic gynecomastia is remarkably common in normal men. This finding is of significance for two reasons: First, some previous reports linking gynecomastia to certain disease states or drugs have failed to take into account this high prevalence of breast enlargement in the general population, thus casting doubt on the purported association. Second, it appears that clinicians need not exhaustively investigate patients with chronic, asymptomatic gynecomastia who are otherwise healthy, since such patients are probably normal. Instead, diagnostic efforts should generally be reserved for patients with painful or tender breasts, or for those in whom the enlargement has clearly been recent.

CAUSES OF GYNECOMASTIA

There is strong evidence for a trophic and stimulatory effect of estrogens on mammary epithelial tissues and lesser support for an opposite and inhibitory action of androgens. Gynecomastia might therefore result from an alteration in the balance between these two influences, with a relative (or absolute) excess of circulating estrogens or a deficiency of circulating androgens leading to breast enlargement. Most causes of gynecomastia are believed to operate through the production of such an imbalance.

As might be expected, estrogen receptors have been demonstrated in some gynecomastic tissues. Whether increased numbers or sensitivity of estrogen receptors might also lead to enhanced estrogen action, hence to gynecomastia, has not been determined. Defective androgen receptors, as found in testicular feminization and related syndromes, may contribute to the emergence of gynecomastia by leading to a loss of inhibitory androgenic influences on breast development.

Although prolactin clearly promotes lactation, the role of lactogenic peptide hormones (prolactin and, possibly, growth hormone and placental lactogen) in the genesis of gynecomastia is unclear. Serum prolactin is normal in most patients with gynecomastia and, conversely, gynecomastia does not develop in most subjects with hyperprolactinemia. It is possible that prolactin may occasionally contribute to gynecomastia through indirect effects on gonadal and, possibly, adrenal function, leading to alterations in the ratio of circulating estrogens to circulating androgens.

CLINICAL CONDITIONS ASSOCIATED WITH GYNECOMASTIA

Puberty

Gynecomastia develops in 60–70% of normal boys during puberty; most are asymptomatic. Breast enlargement typically occurs at ages 12–15 but may take place at any time during the teenage years. The gynecomastia and tenderness (if present) usually regress spontaneously in 1–2 years. The onset of gynecomastia seems to coincide with increasing testicular steroid secretion, and a recent study found that serum estradiol was consistently high in relation to testosterone in boys with gynecomastia; this ratio returned toward lower, normal adult values as puberty progressed and the gynecomastia resolved. Much of the excess estrogen appears to be derived from peripheral conversion of testosterone and androstenedione. The diagnosis of pubertal gynecomastia is made by recognition of the clinical setting: onset of breast enlargement in an otherwise healthy pubertal male.

Advancing Age

The prevalence of gynecomastia appears to increase modestly with advancing age. In many men past age 65, testicular failure occurs to a varying degree, with a lowering of total and free serum testosterone levels, a rise in serum luteinizing hormone (LH) levels, and a maintenance of normal serum estradiol levels. Additionally, increasing adiposity with advancing years may enhance peripheral aromatization of androgens to estrogens. Together, these alterations lead to a predominant estrogen effect on the breast, with the emergence of gynecomastia.

Hypogonadism

Gynecomastia is said to occur more commonly with primary testicular failure but may also be seen in patients with secondary (i.e., pituitary-hypothalamic) hypogonadism. Any of numerous specific etiologies may be responsible for the hypogonadism (e.g., mumps orchitis, leprosy, orchiectomy, Kallman's syndrome, cancer chemotherapy). In all these situations, serum testosterone levels appear to be low or low-normal, while the levels of serum estrogens (principally estrone and estradiol) are usually normal or slightly elevated, thus resulting in an increased estrogen/androgen ratio. Normal estrogen levels may reflect unaltered peripheral conversion of circulating precursors (e.g., androstenedione and testosterone) to estrogens, as well as the disproportionate stimulation of direct testicular estradiol secretion by elevated serum LH in primary testicular failure. The diagnosis of hypogonadism-associated gynecomastia depends on the documentation of physical and hormonal features of hypogonadism.

Klinefelter's Syndrome

Gynecomastia occurs in the majority of patients with Klinefelter's syndrome; most are asymptomatic. In addition to the mechanisms operative in other men with primary hypogonadism (see above), patients with Klinefelter's syndrome may also be predisposed to the development of gynecomastia by the presence of a second X chromosome. This genetic factor may also be responsible for the increased incidence of breast carcinoma seen with Klinefelter's syndrome. Since the risk of breast cancer approaches that seen in normal women, it is prudent to provide periodic breast examinations for these men and to instruct them in the technique of breast self-examination.

The diagnosis of Klinefelter's syndrome is usually suspected on the basis of hypogonadism, infertility, and small, firm testes and may be confirmed with a buccal smear or blood and tissue karyotype analyses.

Adrenal Carcinoma

Feminizing adrenal tumors are rare; most are malignant. Nearly all patients with such tumors develop gynecomastia. The neoplasm may directly secrete estrogens or produce excessive amounts of estrogen precursors (e.g., androstenedione) which are converted to active estrogens in peripheral tissues. Half of patients with feminizing adrenal cancer have a large palpable abdominal mass at the time of diagnosis; two-thirds have elevations of urinary 17-ketosteroid levels.

Testicular Leydig Cell Tumors

Tumors of the Leydig cells of the testis are also rare; most are benign. Normal Leydig cells synthesize predominantly testosterone, with lesser amounts of androstenedione and estradiol being produced. Neoplastic Leydig cells, however, appear to make relatively more estradiol. This would in itself create an estrogen excess, while at the same time tending to suppress pituitary LH secretion, leading to deficient androgen secretion from normal Leydig cells; together these factors produce gynecomastia. Leydig cell tumors are readily detected when of sufficient size to be palpable; small tumors may require bilateral spermatic vein catheterization with measurement of serum estradiol levels for confirmation. Testicular thermography or radioisotopic scanning with cholesterol derivatives may also be useful in detecting occult testicular tumors.

Testicular Carcinomas

A variety of malignant neoplasms originating in the non-Leydig cell elements of the testis have been associated with gynecomastia. In many cases, such tumors produce human chorionic gonadotropin (hCG), often from chorionic elements in the tumor. Since hCG has LH-like actions, normal Leydig cells are stimulated to produce excessive amounts of estradiol, creating a relative estrogen excess and leading to gynecomastia; in accord with this action, chronic administration of hCG to normal men has resulted in the production of gynecomastia. Additionally, chorionic tumors have the ability (like normal placenta) to take up steroid hormone precursors (e.g., DHEA-sulfate) from the circulation and convert them to estrogens. Successful treatment of the tumor with a lowering of hCG levels often leads to a resolution of the gynecomastia. Gynecomastia may be the presenting symptom of testicular tumors, and detection of hCG in the serum or urine should initiate a thorough search for a testicular neoplasm.

Other Malignant Tumors

A wide variety of nontesticular tumors have been found to produce hCG. Such tumors presumably produce gynecomastia by hCG-mediated stimulation of testicular estradiol production. A few tumors may also have the capacity to produce estrogens by biotransformation of available circulating precursors, thereby leading to gynecomastia, as has been reported for hepatoma. Since nontesticular tumors usually secrete less hCG than testicular neoplasms, the use of the serum hCG radioimmunoassay (directed against the specific betasubunit) is absolutely essential for hormone detection because urine pregnancy tests, which also measure hCG, are not sufficiently sensitive (see Chapter 11).

Refeeding Gynecomastia

Shortly after World War II, it was noted that upon refeeding many former prisoners of war and concentration camp inmates developed transient, tender gynecomastia, which regressed within a few months to 2 years. This phenomenon, known as refeeding gynecomastia, may also occur upon recovery from any prolonged, severe illness, especially if associated with significant weight loss and gain. In a recent study of men with hypogonadism due to malnutrition, there was evidence for both Leydig cell and pituitary impairment. When weight is regained, gonadotropin secretion and gonadal function return to normal, producing, in effect, a "second puberty." Gynecomastia in this setting might therefore be analogous to pubertal gynecomastia, discussed above. Paraplegia-associated gynecomastia may also arise through refeeding mechanisms. The diagnosis of refeeding gynecomastia is typically made on the basis of the clinical setting; no specific tests are available to make this diagnosis definitively.

Dialysis

Patients on chronic hemodialysis for renal failure commonly develop gynecomastia within several weeks or months after beginning treatment; the breast enlargement usually regresses within a year. It is possible that refeeding gynecomastia plays a role in this situation; patients with renal failure are often anorectic and may be receiving restricted diets. Following initiation of dialysis, well-being and appetite improve, and the diet may be liberalized, perhaps producing a "refeeding" state. Alternatively, a variety of hormonal abnormalities have been described in uremia and dialysis patients. Most studies have demonstrated low serum testosterone levels in uremic men with elevated serum LH levels. Serum estrogen concentrations are normal or elevated, leading to an elevation of the estrogen/androgen ratio. Additionally, the serum prolactin level is modestly elevated in many patients with renal failure. Nonetheless, it has been difficult to demonstrate differences between dialyzed and nondialyzed patients to explain the occurrence of dialysis-associated gynecomastia.

Liver Disease

Gynecomastia is commonly observed in conjunction with hepatic disorders, especially alcoholic cirrhosis. Several mechanisms may operate to produce a relative estrogen excess. First, alcohol may act on both the testis and the hypothalamic-pituitary system to produce hypogonadism and lowered serum testosterone levels. Second, in cirrhosis there appears to be excessive production of estrogens from circulating precursors (e.g., androstenedione and testosterone). In addition, serum levels of sex-hormone-binding globulin are elevated, further reducing circulating free testosterone levels with lesser effects on free estrogen levels. All these abnormalities appear to be more severe in cirrhotic patients with gynecomastia. Contrary to previous hypotheses, clearance of estrogens does not appear to be altered in cirrhosis.

Hyperthyroidism

A modest but significant fraction (10–40%) of men with hyperthyroidism develop clinically evident gynecomastia coincident with their altered thyroid status; this usually regresses when euthyroidism is restored. Because of elevations in circulating sex-hormone-binding globulin, both serum testosterone and serum estradiol levels are increased in hyperthyroidism. However, since it is believed that estradiol is less completely bound to this carrier protein than testosterone, the elevation in sex-hormone-binding globulin levels results in an elevation in free (unbound) estradiol levels while free testosterone levels remain normal, thus creating a relative excess of free estrogen. Additionally, peripheral tissues appear to be overly active in producing estrogens by biotransformation of circulating precursors. The diagnosis of hyperthyroidism-associated gynecomastia is made by recognition of the clinical setting and documentation of the hyperthyroidism.

Pituitary Tumors

Although a few clinical reports have described the co-occurrence of pituitary tumors and gynecomastia, breast enlargement appears to be a relatively uncommon manifestation of pituitary neoplasms. When it occurs, it presumably is due to mechanisms operative in other cases of secondary hypogonadism (see above), with decreased testosterone production from the testes and relatively normal estrogen production, probably by peripheral conversion of circulating precursors. The role of prolactin in the direct stimulation of breast growth remains controversial; most investigators feel that hyperprolactinemia is more important in the genesis of galactorrhea and that it plays only a minor indirect role, if any, in the production of gynecomastia.

Male Breast Carcinoma

Enlargement of the breast in males with breast cancer is, of course, a reflection of a growing tumor mass. As in women, signs of a bloody nipple discharge, fixation, ulceration, unusual firmness, asymmetry, an eccentric location (other than subareolar), and adenopathy all support the diagnosis of malignancy. Biopsy provides a definitive diagnosis and should be performed on all suspicious masses. Mammography may also be helpful, but normal results should not preclude biopsy of otherwise worrisome lesions. Gynecomastia per se does not appear to predispose the male breast to the development of carcinoma; thus far, Klinefelter's syndrome is the only condition known to be associated with a clearly increased incidence of breast malignancy.

Drug-Induced Gynecomastia

A rather long list of medications has been associated with gynecomastia; some prior reports did not take into account the prevalence of breast enlargement in normal subjects and are thus suspect. Nevertheless, there remains a group of drugs for which a fairly clear relationship has been established (Table 1). Several mechanisms may account for the observed effects on the breast. Estrogens obviously are capable of direct stimulation of the breast. Testosterone administration may also be associated with gynecomastia, perhaps through conversion to estrogens; however, nonaromatizable androgens such as methyltestosterone have been reported to produce breast enlargement, suggesting that additional mechanisms may also be operative.

Spironolactone frequently produces gynecomastia and may do so by inhibiting testosterone synthesis, by increasing conversion of androgens to estrogens, and by competitively displacing dihydrotestosterone from its intracellular receptor. Cimetidine, an H_2 antihistamine, and tetrahydrocannabinol, the active ingredient in marijuana, occasionally produce breast enlargement; both may act as antiandrogens by occupying androgen receptors. Digitalis preparations may also result in gynecomastia; digitoxin appears to have inherent estrogen-like properties and is capable of binding to the intracellular estradiol receptor and simulating estrogen action. Digoxin, however, does not appear to act as an estrogen agonist; it, along with other digitalis preparations, may occasionally produce gynecomastia through a refeeding mechanism in debilitated men with congestive heart failure. Isoniazid may likewise act via a refeeding mechanism in men with tuberculosis.

Table 1 **Drug-Related Gynecomastia**

Estrogens	Reserpine
Androgens	α-Methyldopa
Human chorionic gonadotropin	Marijuana
Spironolactone	Tricyclic antidepressants
Cimetidine	Diazepam
Digitalis	Cytotoxic agents
Isoniazid	Busulfan
Phenothiazines	Vincristine
Amphetamines	Nitrosoureas
Diethylpropion	Combination chemotherapy

A wide variety of central nervous system (CNS)-active agents have been reported to cause gynecomastia; mechanisms are unknown, although several of these agents may raise serum prolactin and perhaps thus induce a secondary hypogonadal state. Additionally, reserpine and phenothiazines may bind to estrogen receptors and act as estrogen agonists. Cytotoxic agents used in cancer chemotherapy damage the testes, producing primary hypogonadism with elevated serum gonadotropin levels and, presumably, inordinate stimulation of testicular estradiol secretion.

Drug-related gynecomastia is usually diagnosed by associating the onset of gynecomastia with the recent use of one of these agents; there is usually at least partial regression of the breast enlargement and symptoms when the offending medication is discontinued.

INVESTIGATION OF THE PATIENT WITH GYNECOMASTIA

The first duty of the clinician evaluating a patient with gynecomastia is to exclude the presence of breast carcinoma; a clinical examination is usually sufficient, as discussed above. In the absence of findings suggestive of malignancy, mammography and breast biopsy are not warranted, since benign breast enlargement is so common. It should be noted that gynecomastia of any cause may be markedly asymmetric or even unilateral; the presence of unilateral gynecomastia does not in itself indicate a greater likelihood of breast cancer.

Following the breast examination, it should be determined whether the gynecomastia is of long or short duration and whether there is associated breast pain or tenderness. If the gynecomastia is of long or uncertain duration and is asymptomatic, it may usually be safely ignored in any otherwise healthy patient, since a large proportion of normal men have been found to have painless breast enlargement. Recent-onset or symptomatic gynecomastia is more likely to be of clinical significance, and further investigation should be undertaken. Of prime importance in this regard is a careful drug history. Likewise, evidence of other systemic illness should be sought (e.g., cirrhosis, hyperthyroidism, dialysis, recent weight loss and gain), and the testes examined carefully. In patients with no obvious cause, a variety of screening tests may be undertaken; these might include measurement of serum hCG levels to screen for a variety of carcinomas, urinary 17-ketosteroid or serum DHEA-sulfate levels to investigate adrenal carcinoma, serum testosterone and gonadotropin levels to diagnose hypogonadism and, possibly, serum prolactin levels to diagnose hyperprolactinemia and probable pituitary tumor. After these studies, the etiology of gynecomastia will remain undiagnosed in some patients.

TREATMENT OF GYNECOMASTIA

With some conditions (pubertal, refeeding, dialysis) gynecomastia is usually transient, and often only simple reassurance is indicated. In other cases, correction of an underlying disorder may lead to regression of the breast enlargement and symptoms (withdrawal of a drug, removal of a tumor, treatment of hyperthyroidism, improvement of liver disease). External radiotherapy has been used to prevent gynecomastia in prostate cancer patients scheduled to receive estrogen treatment. Testosterone administration may be used to produce regression of gynecomastia, presumably both by supplying androgen and by suppressing LH-mediated estradiol secretion from the testes; however, as noted, androgens may themselves cause gynecomastia, and their use should thus be limited to patients with hypogonadism. Antiestrogens (tamoxifen, clomiphene) and danazol (a weak androgen that suppresses gonadotropin secretion and lowers testicular steroid production) have been given to small numbers of gynecomastic patients with excellent results, but their long-term effects are unclear. At present, only short-term use (6 months or less) of these agents is recommended, unless long-term toxicity is not a concern (as in patients with incurable malignancies). Finally, plastic surgery (reduction mammoplasty) may be required in patients in whom gynecomastia is persistently tender, painful, or cosmetically or psychologically disabling.

DISCUSSION CASES

Case 1

Description

A 30-year-old man had a large left varicocele ligated at the age of 24. At age 28, he was treated for seminoma of the right testis with orchiectomy and radiotherapy. One year later, he noted the emergence of tender bilateral gynecomastia. On physical examination, he appeared healthy; bilateral gynecomastia was present. The remaining (left) testis was 3.5 cm in length (normal >3.5 cm) and soft.

Question

1. What are the possible causes of gynecomastia in this patient?

Answer

It is possible that this patient has a mixed testicular tumor, with chorionic elements present. Such tissue would probably produce hCG, which would stimulate estradiol production by normal Leydig cells, resulting in suppressed endogenous LH and follicle-stimulating hormone (FSH) secretion and decreased serum testosterone levels. Alternatively, it is possible that the patient's remaining testis was damaged by surgery or radiotherapy; a compensatory rise in LH and FSH secretion would occur, with disproportionate stimulation of estradiol secretion.

Question

2. How would you distinguish between these possibilities?

Answer

Serum gonadotropin and hCG levels should be measured. In this patient, hCG was undetectable (<10 mIU/ml), while the LH concentration was 33 mIU/ml (normal 4–20 mIU/ml) and the FSH level was 45 mIU/ml (normal 3–20 mIU/ml), confirming the diagnosis of primary hypogonadism. Note that, if the LH level alone had been elevated, one might have initially suspected hCG production by the neoplasm, since hCG cross-reacts completely in the LH, but not the FSH, assay.

Question

3. How should he be treated?

Answer

He was given synthetic androgen by mouth, with suppression of LH and FSH levels and disappearance of his gynecomastia over a 3-month period. There has been no evidence of recurrence of his testicular cancer.

Case 2

Description

A 22-year-old man complains of painful left gynecomastia of 3 weeks' duration. For the past 4 months, he has experienced a 25-pound weight loss despite a good appetite, and he has also noted heat intolerance, palpitations, and tremor. He has smoked marijuana heavily for 4 years but denies other drug use. On physical examination, he has tender left gynecomastia; a small amount of tissue is also palpable on the right. The thyroid is twice the normal size, and the skin fine and moist. The testes are normal, as is the remainder of the examination.

Question

1. What are the possible causes of this patient's gynecomastia?

Answer

Marijuana use has been associated with male breast enlargement, probably through a mechanism involving antagonism of endogenous androgen. The relatively recent onset of this man's breast enlargement, however, makes marijuana use an unlikely cause in this case. His history and physical findings suggest hyperthyroidism, the most likely cause. As a remote possibility, he could have a choriocarcinoma, with hyperthyroidism resulting from massive hCG production (in large amounts, hCG has thyroid-stimulating activity); the gynecomastia could then be related to either the hyperthyroidism or the choriocarcinoma.

Question

2. What further tests should be performed?

Answer

The serum thyroxine level was 18.4 μg/dl, the free thyroxine index 22, the serum T_3 level 864 ng/dl, and the serum hCG undetectable. These results confirm hyperthyroidism and virtually exclude choriocarcinoma.

Question

3. What treatment should be given?

Answer

When his hyperthyroidism was controlled with propylthiouracil, 300 mg/day, the gynecomastia gradually disappeared over a 6-week period.

SUGGESTED READING

Buckle R: Studies on the treatment of gynaecomastia with danazol (Danol). *J Intern Med Res* 5(suppl. 3):114–123, 1977.

Carlson HE: Gynecomastia. *N Engl J Med* 303:795–799, 1980.

Jefferys DB: Painful gynaecomastia treated with tamoxifen. *Br Med J* 1:1119–1120, 1979.

Large DM, Anderson DC: Twenty-four hour profiles of circulating androgens and oestrogens in male puberty with and without gynaecomastia. *Clin Endocrinol* 11:505–521, 1979.

Morley JE, Melmed S: Gonadal dysfunction in systemic disorders. *Metabolism* 28:1051–1073, 1979.

Nicolis GL, Modlinger RS, Gabrilove JL: A study of the histopathology of human gynecomastia. *J Clin Endocrinol Metab* 32:173–178, 1971.

Nuttall FQ: Gynecomastia as a physical finding in normal men. *J Clin Endocrinol Metab* 48:338–340, 1979.

Stepanas AV, Burnet RB, Harding PE, Wise PH: Clomiphene in the treatment of pubertal-adolescent gynecomastia: A preliminary report. *J Pediatr* 90:651–653, 1977.

Williams MJ: Gynecomastia: Its incidence, recognition and host characterization in 447 autopsy cases. *Am J Med* 34:103–112, 1963.

Wilson JD, Aiman J, Macdonald PC: The pathogenesis of gynecomastia. *Adv Intern Med* 25:1–32, 1980.

15 SEYMOUR R. LEVIN

Diabetes Mellitus

Diabetes is a generalized nutrient metabolic disorder that is the result of defective insulin secretion and/or action. As the disease continues, certain specific and nonspecific anatomic lesions develop.

Notice that the above definition does not include any mention of glucose. Although a hallmark of diabetes is hyperglycemia, there is evidence in diabetes of deranged fat and protein metabolism as well. The prototype for diabetes in which insulin secretion is markedly deficient is *type I diabetes*. Former names for this type of diabetes were ketoacidosis-prone and juvenile-type diabetes. The primary example of diabetes in which insulin action is defective is called *type II diabetes*. In this type of diabetes (formerly called maturity-onset or non-ketoacidosis-prone), there is often an association with obesity.

The anatomic defects that are specific for diabetes are retinopathy, nephropathy, and neuropathy. The nonspecific anatomic defects that result are macrovascular disease, such as advanced atherosclerosis of the coronary arteries, the aorta, and the peripheral arteriovascular tree.

LABORATORY TESTS

The plasma glucose level is the most helpful index in assessing carbohydrate metabolism in the diabetic patient. Patients should also regularly have fasting serum triglyceride, cholesterol, and creatinine levels measured. Urinalysis should be performed at regular intervals. Glycosylated hemoglobin reflects long-term hyperglycemia, that is, that which has been present over a period of weeks or months, so that its measurement may help to assess antecedent metabolic control. Diabetic patients need general medical evaluation and examination at regular intervals, as well.

Clinical diabetes mellitus is present when the fasting plasma glucose exceeds 140 mg/dl on more than one occasion. The present criteria set up by the National Diabetes Data Group also suggest that the diagnosis of diabetes mellitus can be made in a patient whose fasting plasma glucose is less than 140 mg/dl but whose plasma glucose, determined every 30 minutes for 2 hours, exceeds 200 mg/dl both 2 hours after the ingestion of 75 g of glucose and at some time point between 0 and 2 hours, using half-hourly collections.

In evaluating the glucose tolerance test the National Diabetes Data Group did not discuss who should and should not have a glucose tolerance test. I do not believe the test should be used as a routine screen in all patients. On the other hand, assessment of fasting and postprandial plasma glucose levels should be done in a pregnant patient regardless of her previous history of diabetes. This is because a patient with impaired glucose tolerance during pregnancy is more likely to have an abnormally large baby than a patient with normal glucose tolerance during pregnancy.

The diagnosis of impaired glucose tolerance should be made in patients whose fasting plasma glucose concentration is less than 140 mg/dl but whose 2-hour glucose level during the oral glucose tolerance test exceeds 200 and 140 mg/dl at 1 and 2 hours, respectively, after ingestion of 75 g of oral glucose. If a glucose tolerance test is performed, there should be normal activity for several days before the test. During the 3 days preceding the test, the subject should have ingested at least 150–200 g of carbohydrate per day. Abnormal glucose tolerance can be brought on by medication (e.g., phenytoin, diuretics, birth control pills, glucocorticoids, synthetic estrogens), starvation, or stress. For older patients, 10 mg/dl for each decade above 50 is added to the normal 2-hour postprandial value and is still considered normal. Thus a normal 2-hour postglucose value may be 180 mg/dl in an 80-year-old patient.

For practical purposes the diagnosis of diabetes is avoided unless fasting hyperglycemia is found to be present. This is because such a diagnosis may affect insurance premiums and job applications. While it is true that 30–50% of patients with impaired glucose tolerance will develop clinical diabetes after a 15-year observation period, it is impossible to tell which patients will degenerate to diabetes. Therefore, it is unfair to label the patient with impaired glucose tolerance as diabetic.

GENERAL PRINCIPLES OF TREATMENT

Physicians and allied medical personnel are becoming aware that patients have a multiplicity of physical, emotional, and socioeconomic needs that are influenced by having diabetes. Professional personnel should understand the special needs of diabetic patients in order to contribute to the teaching and care of diabetic patients. Self-care is fundamental to the management of diabetic patients. Education through effort by the physician and allied personnel and by local diabetes associations can be of great benefit.

THE TREATMENT OF DIABETES WITHOUT MEDICATION

Patients can be taught to practice dietary and exercise principles that may contribute greatly to developing and maintaining a more normal metabolic state.

Dietary Management

The objective for the lean diabetic patient who is usually receiving insulin is to keep weight stable and to prevent, as much as possible, wide excursions of plasma glucose levels from extremely high ranges to extremely low ranges. The objective for the obese diabetic patient is to reduce body weight to the ideal range.

The dietician is an essential member of the patient care team. The dietician teaches the patient about the exchange system and how to use it in daily meals. In essence, the exchange list instructs the patient about the six major types of foods; milk exchanges, vegetable exchanges, fruit exchanges, bread exchanges, meat exchanges, and fat exchanges. The dietician teaches the patient about the caloric value of each of these food types. Exchange lists can be obtained from local American Diabetes Association (ADA) affiliates or from the national ADA office, 2 Park Avenue, New York, New York 10016.

The diet is essentially a nutritionally complete diet. The current ADA exchange lists, however, do not give recommendations for controlling dietary fiber (see below).

Most important to the obese (type II) diabetic patient is a thorough knowledge of the caloric value of food. It is not necessary to weigh foods, but the patient who practices the exchange system will learn the caloric values of given amounts of food. Physicians and dieticians should spend some time asking patients about their estimate of the caloric content of their diet to test patient knowledge and compliance. Follow-up visits to the dietician are essential for this type of training. Moreover, the dietician is able to obtain some idea about patient compliance and discuss it with the physician. Bedtime snacks and food between meals are not indicated for the ADA diet as applied by the obese patient. Nor is the day-to-day consistency or time of eating critical. Extra food for unusual exercise is also not indicated in the obese diabetic.

In contrast, the nonobese, insulin-requiring diabetic (type I) requires a relatively consistent intake of calories and timing of eating is very important. After reasonable control with insulin, most insulin-requiring patients should use food to prevent hypoglycemia. This often necessitates between-meal snacks and a small meal at bedtime. Extra food (or reduced insulin) may be required with unusual exercise.

In our clinic about 25% of the patients are neither obese nor insulin-requiring. In such patients weight loss down to slimness and a program integrating exercise with diet is fundamental. Where indicated, oral hypoglycemic agents or insulin applies to the care of this group of patients. As with obese patients, between-meal snacks and timing of eating is not crucial to dietary management.

Specific Content of the Diabetic Diet

Major considerations in prescribing dietary content are total calories, percentage carbohydrate, percentage protein, percentage and characteristics of fat, and fiber.

Calculation of the total calories depends upon the ideal body weight of the patient, the activity of the patient, the body build of the patient, and whether it is desirable to change the body weight or to maintain it the initial level. Table 1 describes a method of calculating ideal body weight and total calories and deals with the other variables.

Table 1 **General Approach to Calculation of Caloric Needs**

Ideal body weight (IBW)

Men (medium frame): IBW = 106 lb per 5 ft of height *plus* 6 lb for each additional inch

Women (medium frame): IBW = 100 lb per 5 ft of height *plus* 5 lbs for each additional inch

Add 10% for wide frame; subtract 10% for small frame.

Caloric needs (cal) based upon IBW: cal = IBW (in pounds) × 10 Adjust for activity as follows:

sedentary, cal + (IBW × 3); moderately active, cal + (IBW × 5); very active, cal + (IBW × 10)

Carbohydrate Content

Current diabetic diets allow a higher carbohydrate content than those seen up to the late 1960s. Thus the total carbohydrate allowance has been increased to 45–55% of the day's caloric allowance. The previous ADA diet had indicated that total carbohydrates should be 35–40%. Simple sugars, for example, sucrose or table sugar (a disaccharide consisting of fructose and glucose) are limited to 5–15% of the total calories. Total carbohydrate content in the new ADA diet is equal to or somewhat above that in the typical American diet. Fructose is readily converted to glucose by enzyme systems in the liver if diabetes is poorly controlled. Thus fructose offers no advantage over glucose-containing carbohydrates. Other nutritive sweeteners, such as sorbitol and xylitol, can also be converted to glucose if the diabetes is not under control. However, since they have a greater sweetening effect per gram of sugar, in certain cases they may be considered advantageous. The difference in calories, however, is very minor.

The major form of carbohydrate should be the complex variety. This is because such carbohydrates are more slowly absorbed and allow more gradual elevation of the plasma glucose level. Examples of complex carbohydrates include potatoes, rice, wheat, and legumes.

One further advantage of a high-complex-carbohydrate diet is that the older, low-carbohydrate diet meant higher dietary fat content and thus probable deleterious, atherogenic effects on the macrovascular system.

If the patient requires nutritive sweeteners, they should be included in the daily simple-carbohydrate ration. Nonnutrient sweeteners such as saccharin and aspartame have no caloric value. The oncogenic properties of these latter substances in humans remain a topic of debate. At this time, if sweetening of food is desired, nutritive sweeteners seem satisfactory.

Protein Content

The typical American diet is higher in protein than the recommended 0.8 g/kg of ideal body weight. Approximately 17% of the calories ingested should be protein.

Fat Content

Current diabetic diets contain about 33% fat. It is recommended that the cholesterol intake not exceed 300 mg/day and that the ratio of unsaturated to saturated fat be 2 : 1. Of the unsaturated fat one-half should be monounsaturated and the other half should be polyunsaturated. About 11% of the total number of calories (one-third of dietary fat) will thus be saturated.

These guidelines are aimed at reducing the atherogenic effect of the typical American diet. While it has not been proven that this diet will reduce atherosclerotic problems in diabetic patients, it seems clinically reasonable to recommend such diets for diabetic patients. High triglyceride levels may play a role in macrovascular disease in diabetes. A complex-carbohydrate diet along with a high fiber content (see below) may actually reduce fasting and postprandial triglyceride levels. Thus it is the carbohydrate content of the diet, and not the fat content, that is related to triglyceride levels. Simple carbohydrates raise triglyceride levels, whereas complex carbohydrates appear to lower serum triglyceride levels.

Fiber Content of the Diabetic Diet

Fiber is the structural element of plants. In the diet fiber includes the husks and shells of food such as are found in bran or corn, as well as the structural elements, as in celery. Dietary fibers are not absorbed or metabolized by the small intestine. Total fiber is made up of cellulose, hemicellulose, pectin, gums, lignins, and storage polysaccharides.

Crude fiber is the fiber left after food is boiled in water or other reagents, whereas *total fiber* includes fibrous elements that are important in nutrition but may be removed by boiling.

Most current references no longer use the term crude fiber. However, roughly three to five times the crude fiber represents the total fiber in the diet, with a few exceptions.

Fiber reduces the postprandial glucose and insulin levels in both normal and diabetic subjects. It is not completely understood how fibers do this. Fibers, such as guar and pectin, absorb water and may slow the transit time through the gastrointestinal tract. This could influence the absorption of carbohydrates and other elements of the diet secondarily. Postprandial glucose levels are lowered by a high dietary fiber content in insulin-requiring diabetic patients as well.

It has been shown that careful adherence to a high-fiber diet can reduce the requirement for medication. Thus insulin and sulfonylurea doses have been reduced and, on occasion, these drugs have been eliminated for patients placed on a high-fiber diet. Patients receiving insulin who could eliminate injections of this hormone were taking less than 25 units/day before beginning the high-fiber diet.

In general, the typical American diet contains 6 g crude fiber or about 24 g of total fiber. Thus a high-fiber diet contains about 60–90 g total fiber.

The high-carbohydrate, high-fiber diet will lower triglyceride levels as well as reduce fasting and postprandial glucose levels. Although the causes of each of these effects are being investigated, these changes are considered beneficial for the diabetic patient.

Some patients have problems adhering to a high total fiber diet. There is an increase in fullness and gas and an increased frequency of bowel movements. Many patients stop their diet because of these gastrointestinal side effects. It is unlikely that high-fiber diets reduce the absorption of vitamins and minerals.

Vegetables that are especially high in fiber include broccoli, string beans, celery, cucumber, lettuce, radishes, summer squash, zucchini, kernel corn, peas, parsnips, and white potatoes. Fruits that are particularly high in fiber, considering the amount of carbohydrate contained in the fruit, are strawberries, blackberries, oranges, and apples. Breads, cereals, and beans that are high in fiber include kidney beans, bran, and rye bread. Fiber contents of food are not described in current ADA exchange lists. However, two excellent guides, "Plant Fiber in Foods" (for professionals) and "User's Guide to High Carbohydrate High Fiber (HCF) Diets," (for patients), can be obtained through Dr. James Anderson, (HCF Diabetes Foundation, 1872 Blairmore Road, Lexington, Kentucky).

Miscellaneous

Alcohol furnishes 7 calories/g. In terms of the volume of alcohol ingested the formula that can be used to calculate the total number of calories is 0.8 times "proof" times number of ounces. Percentage alcohol times 2 equals the "proof" of an alcoholic beverage. Up to 7% of total calories are allowed as alcohol in the ADA diet. A small amount of alcohol each evening may increase high-density lipoprotein (HDL) cholesterol. HDL is considered to be a protective factor against atherosclerosis. Alcohol may induce hypoglycemia in a patient who is fasting or taking insulin. It may also cause a flushing syndrome (the disulfiram or Antabuse effect) in patients taking alcohol or sulfonylurea drugs, especially chlorpropamide (Diabinese).

Vitamin and mineral supplements might be considered in patients who have had poor metabolic control for a long time. Although this has not been well studied, it is likely that the patient with poor metabolic control has lost a number of important substances. Zincuria has been reported, as well as magnesuria which is normalized with regulation of the fasting plasma glucose. Though red blood cell chromium deficiencies have been demonstrated in a group of diabetic patients, it is not known whether this is the result of poor metabolic control, and consequent loss of this mineral, or in some way causally related to the diabetes.

The ADA diet contains adequate amounts of vitamins and minerals. Thus with proper metabolic control the body content of these valuable elements should become normal.

EXERCISE IN DIABETES

Physicians have recommended exercise for their diabetic patients for years. Physiologic experiments done on both diabetic patients and on nondiabetic subjects have indicated that muscles utilize glucose and fatty acids. Caloric consumption during various forms of exercise has been assessed. Despite these short-term studies there has been no long-term controlled study on the effects, both bad and good, of exercise in diabetic patients. Nevertheless, an exercise prescription can be written for patients to assist in maintaining a sense of well-being, and possibly in inducing trends toward metabolic normalization of glucose and lipids, to be used along with a diet and any required medication. The intensity of the exercise prescribed for individual patients and the number of exercise periods a patient can tolerate are related to the patient's prior exercise history and the degree of prior conditioning. Table 2 describes how to assess the severity of exercise using the pulse and gives an example of an exercise prescription. Again, this must be individualized. If a patient has had a myocardial infarction or has cardiac failure, this program should not be utilized. In such cases, proper medication and possibly a cardiac rehabilitation exercise program may be indicated.

A 10-week course of moderate exercise, ½ hour each day, 4–5 days a week, can lead to lower serum triglyceride levels. Effects on the fasting and postprandial glucose levels in the various forms of diabetes over a long period of time have not been explored in detail.

Bedridden patients, for example, those with a foot ulcer, should be able to exercise in bed using the arms.

A degree of albuminuria occurs normally for a short time after exercise. However, in diabetics albuminuria may persist for a few hours. There is no evidence for or against the possibility that this reflects damage to the kidney.

Insulin-dependent patients whose metabolic control is very good may experience hypoglycemia during exercise. This is probably due to two factors: First, glucose is taken up by muscle at a faster rate than hepatic gluconeogenesis and glycogenolysis can provide this substrate to the circulation. Uptake of glucose by muscle versus provision of glucose to muscle is quite well balanced in the nondiabetic state, so that the plasma glucose in normal subjects remains rather constant during exercise. To deal with the imbalance that occurs in the well-controlled, insulin-treated patient, we advise the patient to take less insulin (one-third to one-half less)

Table 2 **Guidelines for Writing an Exercise Prescription**

1. Calculate theoretical maximal pulse (TMP). This is a theoretical number based upon the patient's age. TMP = 220 *minus* age (years). The number approximates the maximum work capacity
2. Teach patients with normal cardiovascular status[a] how to take their pulse
3. Have patient exercise at 0.60 TMP (jogging, rapid walking, swimming, bicycling on a stationary or moving bicycle). Pulse should be taken while exercising or within 1 minute after stopping the exercise.
   (a) Do this for 5–10 minutes/day for 2–3 weeks.
   (b) Then increase to 15 minutes/day for 2 weeks. Increase by 5-minutes increments weekly until 30 minutes of exercise is attained.
   (c) Exercise at 0.60–0.70 TMP (=moderate exercise) for 30 minutes 4–7 days/week.

[a] Some form of stress ECG is recommended before initiating the exercise program, though falsely negative and falsely positive results can occur.

before exercise. The patient can also eat a somewhat larger meal containing 10 or 15% more simple carbohydrate before the exercise. The third alternative is that the patient carry simple sugars, as contained in juices, during the exercise. Physicians should discuss the alternatives with their patients. This then can be individualized. The second reason for hypoglycemia during exercise is mobilization of insulin from injection sites. Since mobilization of injected insulin appears to be greatest from the limb that is exercising, it may also be helpful to inject into a location that is least exercised. Thus, with leg exercise, injection of insulin in the arms or abdomen may be helpful. Alternatively, with arm exercise, abdominal or thigh injection may slow down the rapid mobilization of insulin associated with exercise.

Diabetic patients with poor metabolic control may develop more severe hyperglycemia and ketonuria after exercise. This is because the counterinsulin hormones (glucagon, cortisol, epinephrine, and growth hormone), which increase during exercise, have effects that outbalance the effects of insulin in such patients. I prefer to utilize diet and insulin to control the plasma glucose level, applying the criteria for control as in the section discussing insulin treatment prior to beginning a full exercise program. However, for these patients a regimen of mild exercise such as walking can be used while gaining better metabolic control of the glycemia.

We ask our hospitalized, nonbedridden patients to walk on the ward as much as possible rather than allowing them to sit or lie in bed.

In summary, exercise is a traditional modality of treatment just recently being evaluated scientifically for its effects on metabolic control.

The effects on the anatomic complications of diabetes are also being examined. Meanwhile, it is reasonable to prescribe an exercise program and to follow renal function, retinal anatomy, and other anatomic parameters. If these worsen, then the intensity of the exercise program should be temporarily reduced or exercise should be suspended.

ORAL HYPOGLYCEMIC SULFONYLUREAS

These drugs act by enhancing insulin action and possibly by increasing insulin secretion with meals. Table 3 summarizes the characteristics of these drugs. Glyburide (Micronase) is one of the most widely prescribed hypoglycemic agents in Europe, but it is not yet available in the United States. On a weight basis it is 50 to 200 times more potent than the other sulfonylureas. Its duration of action is probably in the range of that of tolazamide or acetazolamide. I prescribe sulfonylureas for obese patients whose hyperglycemia persists on a diet and exercise program. I use insulin when medication is required in lean patients. Currently, the combined use of sulfonylureas and insulin in some patients is being studied. This combination is not prescribed at our hospital at this time.

The controversial University Group Diabetes Program (UGDP) study was first published in 1970. Today, over a decade later, volumes are written about this study, both for and against it. Briefly, patients taking tolbutamide were found to have almost $2\frac{1}{2}$ times more deaths from myocardial infarction than a group taking a placebo or those taking a constant or a variable insulin dose. Other studies on large populations have been performed and have not duplicated the findings of the UGDP study. As with the UGDP study, these studies have defects in design, statistics, and interpretation.

We tell our patients about the UGDP study when sulfonylureas drugs are initiated. We also tell them that, if they are able to adhere to a diet and exercise program with weight loss, we will attempt to discontinue these drugs.

The choice of which of these drugs to use is often arbitrary. I use chlorpropamide for patients with moderate to extreme obesity. This drug should not be used in patients with serum

Table 3 **Oral Hypoglycemic Sulfonylurea Drugs**

Drug	*Trade Name (U.S.)*	*Tablet Size*	*Maximum Daily Dose*	*Dosage Range*	*Duration (hours)*
Tolbutamide	Orinase	0.5 g	2–3 g	1.0–3.0 g	6–8
Chlorpropamide	Diabinese	100 and 250 mg	500 mg	100–500 mg	36
Acetohexamide	Dymelor	250 and 500 mg	1.5 g	0.25–1.5 g	10–24
Tolazamide	Tolinase	100, 250, and 500 mg	1.0 g	0.25–1.0 g	10–24
Glibenclamide (glyburide)	Micronase	5 mg	25 mg	2.5–25 mg	10–24

creatinine levels over 1.5 mg/dl. I use the other sulfonylureas in patients of medium build who have evidence of fat deposits which indicate the presence of endogenous insulin. Since chlorpropamide, tolazamide, and acetohexamide have circulating metabolites, some of which are excreted in the urine, these drugs should be used with caution in patients with reduced renal function. Since they are metabolized in the liver, the same caution should be applied with patients who have decreased hepatic function. Chlorpropamide can be given once a day because of its long half-life. Tolazamide and acetohexamide are usually given twice a day, and tolbutamide may require two to four doses per day.

All these drugs may have undesirable gastrointestinal side effects. Rashes and bone marrow suppression can also occur. Disulfiram effects with alcohol ingestion occur in patients who take chlorpropamide. However, this can be seen with any of the sulfonylureas.

Chlorpropamide especially can cause a syndrome that simulates excessive antidiuretic hormone (ADH) secretion or action. Patients, usually elderly, have severe hyponatremia with headache, lethargy, stupor, coma, and even seizures.

Potentially dangerous drug interactions, especially with drugs that are bound by albumin in the circulation, can occur. Especially important are interactions with sulfonamides, chloramphenicol, coumarin anticoagulants, phenylbutazone, and clofibrate. These drugs can accentuate the hypoglycemic effects of sulfonylureas. In turn, sulfonylureas can accentuate the effect of the previously mentioned drugs. Propranolol, used in combination with any hypoglycemic agent including insulin, can accentuate hypoglycemia by reducing certain normal defenses against hypoglycemia, such as glycogenolysis. Propranolol (Inderal) may also interfere with the perception of hypoglycemia, thus permitting more severe hypoglycemic reactions.

The goal of therapy with sulfonylureas is to attain a fasting plasma glucose level of no more than 150 mg/dl and the same level of plasma glucose 2 hours after a usual mixed meal, as well. In reality only the most compliant and selected patients attain these levels. *Primary failure* means that lowering of the fasting glucose level is not obtained with these drugs. *Secondary failure* means that reduction in the fasting glucose level is attained for a period of time but that the symptomatic hyperglycemia again supervenes. For either primary or secondary failure, rather than increase the sulfonylurea dosage even beyond the maximum, I again try a period of orientation to diet and exercise. If this fails, insulin is started.

In summary, sulfonylurea drugs can be used in patients who are non-ketosis-prone and in whom a diet and exercise program have not led to optimal control. Dosage should be as low as possible in elderly patients and, if compliance increases, attempts should be made to discontinue the drug.

INSULIN THERAPY

There is no question that the ketosis-prone, lean diabetic (type I) should be treated with insulin. This is because such a patient has near depletion of endogenous insulin and thus requires exogenous insulin. The lean, non-ketosis-prone patient whose fasting plasma glucose level becomes elevated over 150 mg/dl may be tried on either oral agents or on insulin, although I prefer the latter treatment for this type of patient. Because most obese patients have endogenous insulin, the use of exogenous insulin is theoretically not required. However, poor compliance to diet and exercise by the obese patient may lead to the use of insulin, especially if oral agents fail to be effective. There are circumstances in which I use insulin in obesity. Table 4 indicates what I believe are the indications for the use of this hormone for such patients.

Table 4 **When to Use Insulin in Hyperglycemic Obese Patients**[a]

Severe infection or stress
High doses of steroids
Surgery (pre-, intra-, and postoperatively)
To acutely lower very high plasma glucose (>400 mg/dl).
Pregnancy (if diet not effective)
When diet, exercise and, possibly, oral agents are not effective

[a] In other situations, a trial of diet or exercise should be conducted before starting any medication.

Table 5 **Insulin Preparations**[a]

Action (hours)[b]	*Trade Name*	*Retarding Agent*
Rapid (0.5:1–3:8)	Regular (crystalline) Iletin (Lilly) (improved single peak)	None
	Squibb insulin, regular	None
	Velosulin (Nordisk)	None
	Actrapid (Novo)	None
Less rapid (1–3:2–8:12–16)	Semi-Lente (Lilly)	Zinc
	Semitard (Novo)	Zinc
Intermediate (1.5:4–12:24)	NPH (Isophane)	
	Iletin (Lilly)	Protamine
	Squibb NPH insulin	Protamine
	Insulatard (Nordisk)	Protamine
	Protophane (Novo)	Protamine
	Lente	
	Iletin (Lilly)	Zinc
	Squibb Lente insulin	Zinc
	Monotard (Novo)	Zinc
	Lentard (Novo) (beef/pork)	Zinc
Long (4:10–30:36)	Ultra-Lente (Lilly)	Zinc
	Ultratard (Novo) (beef)	Zinc
	Protamine zinc (Lilly)	Protamine plus zinc
	Globin zinc (Squibb)	Globin plus zinc
Premixed	Mixtard (Nordisk) (Velosulin 30% Insulatard 70%)	Protamine

[a] Modern insulins are buffered with phosphate or acetate and are at neutral pH. American preparations are beef and/or pork (usually beef and pork), whereas Scandanavian preparations are pork (except for Lentard and Ultratard). Preservatives are *m*-cresol or methylparaben.
[b] Onset, peak, and duration are shown in parentheses.

PREPARATIONS AND PURITIES OF INSULIN

Table 5 describes the preparations of insulin. Since foreign insulin is now available in the United States (Novo or Nordisk), the terms for preparations analogous to the American preparations (Lilly or Squibb) are also given in this table.

Until 1974 commercial preparations of insulin contained 3–6% proinsulin, the precursor of insulin. In addition to proinsulin, its breakdown products, and the breakdown products of insulin, commercial preparations contained variable amounts of glucagon, somatostatin, pancreatic polypeptide, and vasoactive intestinal peptide (VIP). A high titer of antibodies to pancreatic polypeptide was found in 47% of 93 insulin-treated diabetic patients. Newer preparations, listed in Table 6 have lesser amounts of these contaminants.

PRACTICAL CONSIDERATIONS IN THE USE OF INSULIN

Most insulin preparations in the United States contain 100 units/ml (U100). Occasionally, a patient on small amounts of insulin can be given U40 so that a small dose can be measured more precisely.

In nondiabetic subjects plasma glucose levels reach nadirs of 70 mg/dl and, after mixed meals, go no higher than 130 mg/dl. Thus the term euglycemia or normoglycemia describes glucose oscillations within very narrow ranges. The goal of insulin therapy should be euglycemia without hypoglycemia. In reality, the plasma glucose of most patients who are completely insulin-dependent reaches very high levels and very low levels throughout the day. With present techniques I aim for the following response: avoidance of hyperglycemia (over 250 mg/dl) and hypoglycemia (under 50 mg/dl). I attempt to regulate fasting plasma glucose to less than 150 mg/dl and to attain a 4–5 PM plasma glucose in this range as well.

After long-term usage, commercial preparations of insulin have durations of activity that differ greatly from the expected duration as described in Table 4. This is probably related to the development of antibodies after long-term administration of insulin. Thus in some patients NPH insulin achieves its major activity between midnight and 6 AM, and in others this insulin achieves peak activity in the late morning or early afternoon. Excessive nocturnal insulin activity

Table 6 **Purity of Current Insulin Preparations**[a]

Manufacturer	*Trade Name*	*Proinsulin Content (ppm)*[b]
Lilly	(a) Iletin (improved single peak)	<50
	(b) Iletin II (purified)	<10
Nordisk	(c) All (see Table 5)	<10
Novo	(d) All (see Table 5)	<1

[a] Similar data not available for current Squibb insulin preparations. Squibb plans to distribute (between 1981 and mid-1982) new Improved insulin (<25 ppm proinsulin), which will also be monospecies (beef, except for porcine regular).

[b] Proinsulin content is considered to reflect peptide contaminants, including glucagon, pancreatic polypeptide, somatostatin, and vasoactive intestinal peptide. Indications for purer insulin (b–d) currently include insulin atrophy, hypertrophy, allergy, hypersensitivity, and short-term use (e.g., surgery, gestational diabetes).

can be determined by asking the patient whether he or she has night sweats or nightmares. On the other hand, if most glycosuria occurs with intermediate-acting insulin later in the day but the patient is free from early glycosuria, it is likely that early maximum insulin activity (first 12 hours after injection) is present. I estimate that about 10% of patients have insulin activity that is earlier than expected and that about 40% of patients who have been taking insulin more than a year have activity that is later than expected. Thus the classic peak activity is seen in approximately 50%. Splitting the insulin dosage (described below) is a way to deal with any of the variable durations of response to insulin, because it allows a more even spread of insulin action throughout the day.

For patients who take less than 30 units of intermediate-acting insulin or for patients who have maximum insulin activity at the classic peak time (i.e., during the eating hours), a single dose of insulin should be sufficient. However, most patients, especially after 3–5 years of administration of insulin, can obtain optimal control without deep nadirs and/or peaks of glucose levels by receiving insulin twice a day. One-half to two-thirds of NPH or Lente insulin is given in the morning, and one-half to one-third is given within $1\frac{1}{2}$ hour before the evening meal. If the metabolic criteria described above are met, then regular insulin is not required. Some patients require regular insulin with NPH or Lente insulin to metabolize breakfast and supper properly. Regular insulin is drawn up into the syringe before withdrawing the intermediate-acting insulin. Usually the dose of regular insulin given is half the intermediate-acting insulin dose. Thus, if the patient takes 20 units of NPH insulin in the morning, 10 units of regular insulin can be given along with the NPH insulin.

It is difficult to provide criteria for total insulin requirements. The lean nondiabetic subject secretes about 20–25 units of insulin per day. About two-thirds of this is secreted at mealtime. Thus, adult type I (ketoacidosis-prone) patients initially require 15–30 units of insulin per day. Requirements increase as time passes, probably as a result of antibody formation. Obese patients characteristically require increasing amounts of insulin over the years. Sometimes these doses become astronomical. I thus try to refrain from using insulin in obese patients, as discussed above. For some patients regular insulin in the morning will control the afternoon blood glucose. These patients are usually those in whom the insulin appears to have its maximum effect later than expected. In these patients 4–5 PM plasma glucose levels can best be regulated by morning regular insulin. Similarly, for patients with prolonged insulin action, evening regular insulin can be used to regulate nocturnal and morning plasma glucose levels. However, with most patients I use the afternoon intermediate-acting insulin to regulate the next morning's fasting glucose level, and the morning insulin to regulate the plasma glucose level for the day.

Rather than reduce insulin to avoid a mild hypoglycemic reaction between meals, I believe a between-meal snack can be quite helpful. Usually this is a carbohydrate exchange taken from the antecedent meal. A snack before bedtime is helpful to avoid mild nocturnal hypoglycemic reactions. Clearly, if hypoglycemic reactions are severe, insulin dosage must be reduced.

When the insulin is divided, one important precaution should be taken: The total insulin dosage should be reduced. Thus, for example, if a patient is taking 60 units of insulin as a single injection in the morning, a split dose of 25 units in the morning and 15 units in the afternoon should be initiated. Sometimes, after splitting the insulin dosage, a total dose of 40 units (e.g., 30 units in the morning and 10 units in the afternoon) results in smoother and more predictable control than 60 units given as a single injection.

Some patients refuse to take insulin twice a day and yet appear to require insulin later in the day. For these patients I often recommend Ultra-Lente insulin with or without a small amount of regular or Semi-Lente to increase the intensity of insulin action throughout the day.

Unless the patient has a urinary threshold problem, it is unnecessary to draw blood specimens for glucose testing until the urine is glucose-free throughout the day. Control of the afternoon glycosuria with insulin can be attained, as described above. When the prebreakfast urine is negative or shows only trace glucose, a fasting plasma glucose level can then be obtained. In the afternoon, plasma glucose can be drawn, for example, after work and before supper.

Renal or hepatic failure usually results in reduced insulin requirements, since the liver and the kidney are the major degraders of insulin.

DELIVERY OF INSULIN THROUGH PREPROGRAMMED, OPEN-LOOP INSULIN INFUSION PUMPS

Our patients have found it practical to use small insulin pumps and can obtain euglycemia with these portable instruments. Although at this writing they are still considered to be in the developmental stage, the physician should know the principles of their usage. Within the very near future increasing numbers of patients in the community will be using such instruments. *Open loop* means that there is no glucose-measuring system. *Preprogrammed* means that insulin is given based upon the patient's size, previous dosage, and a period of observation. This is in contrast to the currently more expensive *closed-loop* system which applies glucose sensing and delivery of insulin based upon the plasma glucose level. Quantities of insulin required with the mechanized methods often simulate those given by the usual injection route. However, with the mechanized methods, the timing of insulin administration is more physiologic. Meal-associated rapid injections are superimposed upon the constant basal rate.

For patients starting on the open-loop system, if the insulin has previously been given chronically, the principle of 20–25 units of insulin each day, two-thirds being secreted at mealtime, is reasonable to apply to the choice of initial dose. The application of these instruments is quite simple. A constant infusion of insulin during the noneating hours (approximately 0.8 units/hour in the 70-kg adult) is given. Ten to 30 minutes before a meal, the patient usually operates a device, such as a dial or a button, that increases the insulin infusion rate to six to eight times basal rate. The insulin is usually given via a cannula or a needle placed in the subcutaneous space. The instrument is usually attached to the belt. We usually admit patients for 3–6 days to determine individual needs and to ensure that the patient is receiving optimal control. Most of the patients perform home glucose monitoring (described below) using 1 or 2 typical days during the week. A variety of pumps will be commercially available by the time this book is published.

Home Blood Glucose Monitoring

Patients with type I diabetes and even many patients with type II diabetes can utilize a home blood glucose-monitoring program. With this system patients can measure their own fasting, postprandial, and between-meal glucose levels. The general principle is simple: The patient samples a small drop of blood, puts it on a strip, examines the plasma glucose level and, after discussion with a professional, uses insulin or meals to obtain more normal control of the plasma glucose level. For the type II diabetic the need for reduction in calories can be guided by the plasma glucose level.

Two options are used for sampling of blood glucose. The first is the hematology stylet used for blood counts. The disadvantage to this is that patients are often apprehensive and the aim of the stylet might be inaccurate. The second is a spring-operated stylet (Auto-Let). This apparatus is operated by a spring after pressing a button. It injects a very sharp needle into the finger at a depth regulated by the protrusion of the lateral part of the fingertip pad into a hole on a plastic platform. I have found the latter device most practical for home blood glucose monitoring.

There are two devices for measuring glucose from finger blood. The first is Dextro-Stix (Ames). This requires the careful application of a drop of blood on a strip; the blood remains there for exactly 1 minute, after which it is washed off. The patient can then visualize the degree of "blueness" on the stick to determine a general range of glucose. For more precision, the patient can also use an Ames Glucometer. The strip is inserted into this meter for measuring the plasma glucose level, giving a digital readout. The advantage of this meter is precise reading of the glucose level. The disadvantage is the expense: the Dextrometer (or the new Glucometer) costs between $200 and $300. The strips are costly as well. A second option is BG strips (Bio-Dynamics). With these strips, which are coated with a chemical that changes color depending on the plasma glucose level, the patient can visually detect the glucose level over a wide spectrum. The disadvantages are that some patients have difficulty discerning the precise color that describes the correct plasma glucose level. Advantages are that they do not have to buy an accompanying meter to read glucose measurements.

Some diabetologists ask patients to read the plasma glucose level several times daily with this monitoring device. We, however, ask our patients to monitor several times per day on two or three typical days during the week.

Urinary testing still has some value on occasion in these patients. For example, if a ketodacidosis-prone diabetic has hyperglycemia, and some nausea and vomiting, a urine test for acetone would be helpful in deciding whether frequent communication with the physician and possible consideration of hospitalization are indicated.

SPECIAL CIRCUMSTANCES IN MANAGEMENT OF THE DIABETIC PATIENT

Diabetic Emergencies

Table 7 describes the diabetic emergencies and the emergent conditions in which diabetic patients may be found. Patients with diabetes-specific emergencies are usually not in a coma at the time they are admitted. The death rate for ketoacidosis remains about 7–8%. This increases when the patient has a complication, such as myocardial infarction or severe infection. The death rate in the hyperosomolar nonketotic hyperglycemic state is 30–50%. This condition usually occurs in elderly patients. Lactic acidosis, which is rare in diabetics, has become even rarer since phenformin (DBI) was removed from the U.S. market. The death rate is greater than 90%.

Table 8 describes the clinical features of each of the diabetic emergencies, and Table 9 describes the treatment approaches. All diabetes-specific conditions require the availability of rapid bedside blood glucose measurements, dilutions of serum acetone using crushed Acetest tablets, and ECG rhythm strips. Hospital laboratories should be able to make reliable arterial blood gas measurements and reasonably rapid electrolyte and glucose determinations to confirm the bedside tests.

By the time the plasma glucose results arrive from most laboratories, the physician should have been treating the patient for an hour or more, based upon the bedside tests. Do not wait for the laboratory values to arrive in order to begin therapy. Fluid and electrolyte therapy should not be neglected. Replacement of these is as important as lowering of plasma glucose.

The use of insulin and glucose infusions in lactic acidosis, while not proven, is worth trying because of the very high death rate.

Table 7 **Diabetic Emergencies**

Emergent conditions not specific to diabetes. These include a wide range of vascular, traumatic, metabolic, and pharmacologic catastrophies that may be accompanied by or exacerbate hyperglycemia in diabetic patients. Some of these stresses (e.g., stroke) may be accompanied by hyperglycemia in a patient who previously did not have a diagnosis of diabetes

Metabolic emergencies in diabetic patients.
- Hypoglycemia
  - Due to sulfonylurea agents
    - Excessive dose
    - Impaired hepatic or renal function. (The latter is especially important with chlorpropamide)
    - Taking usual dose but not eating
  - Due to insulin
    - Excessive dose
    - Not eating adequately, yet taking insulin
- Hyponatremia secondary to chlorpropamide
- "Diabetes-Specific" conditions
  - Diabetic ketoacidosis
  - Hyperglycemic nonketotic hyperosmolar state
  - Lactic acidosis

The Diabetic Surgical Patient

The avoidance of severe hyperglycemia, which will result in losses of water and electrolytes during the postoperative period, as well as interfere with white cell function and subsequent healing, is a major goal. Even more important is the avoidance of hypoglycemia. This is because severe neurologic damage may result when the brain is exposed to prolonged glucose deprivation.

Table 8 **Diagnostic Features of Diabetes-Specific Emergencies: Ketoacidosis (DKA), Hyperglycemic, Hyperosmolar Nonketotic State (HHNK), and Lactic Acidosis (LA)**[a]

DKA: Tachypnea or slow, deep breathing, dehydration, may have acetone on breath, urine positive for glucose and acetone. Hyperglycemic, low serum bicarbonate. Arterial studies show metabolic acidosis. Serum acetoacetate-positive. Serum PO_4 and K^+ normal on admission, but fall with treatment

HHNK: Very dehydrated, may have muscle fasciculations. Urine positive for glucose and, often, acetone. Hyperglycemic, normal or borderline low serum bicarbonate. Serum acetone negative or weakly positive. Serum osmolality (mOsm/kg) high by osmometry or, as calculated by $2\,[Na^+ + K^+] + [\text{glucose}/18] + [\text{urea nitrogen}/2.8]$, will usually be over 300. Serum Na^+ low; if Na^+ normal or high suggests severe depletion of body water

LA: Very rapid, deep breathing. Patient may have known respiratory or renal failure or have acute vascular insufficiency (e.g., mesenteric artery thrombosis). Arterial studies show metabolic acidosis. Anion gap $= [Na^+] - [Cl^- + \text{serum bicarbonate}]$. A normal anion gap is <12 mEq/liter.

[a] Patients may have mixtures of each syndrome.

Table 9 **Treatment of Diabetic Emergencies: Diabetic Ketoacidosis (DKA), Hyperglycemic, Hyperosmolar, Nonketotic State (HHNK), and Lactic Acidosis (LA)**

Therapy	*Amounts for Adults*	*Comments*
Fluid	4–8 liters in first 12 hours	LA may require less than this; HHNK may require more. Monitor central venous pressure in elderly debilitated patients
Insulin (crystalline)	0.33 units/kg i.v. bolus, then 4–7 units/hr, constant i.v.	I.m. or s.c. route with similar hourly dose is acceptable. Avoid s.c. route if shock present. Increase hourly dose 30–50% if glucose decrement <60–100 mg/dl/hr HHNK should receive one-half the indicated doses to start since may be more sensitive LA may be only mildly hyperglycemic or not hyperglycemic. Insulin (0.03 unit/kg/hr) along with glucose (0.25 g/kg/hr) should keep patient's plasma glucose level constant
Glucose	As 5% glucose in normal saline	In DKA or HHNK, wait until plasma glucose approximately 250 mg/dl before beginning glucose. LA may receive higher glucose infusion rate when coinfused with insulin (see above)
Anions and cations		
Na^+	As normal saline 4–8 liters i.v. in the first 12 hours (and as bicarbonate, if required).	Half normal saline may be given in patients with high serum Na^+, for the first 1–2 liters
K^+	100–300 mEq in first 24 hours, as KCl 40 mEq/liter, alternating with potassium phosphate, 40 mEq/liter, (27 mmoles P/liter)	Do not use K^+ supplement if urine output <30 ml/hr
Cl^-	As NaCl and KCl	
PO_4^{-3}	See above. Begin phosphate as glucose falls	Do not use if uremic and hyperphosphatemic. Can lower serum calcium when given too vigorously
HCO_3^-	80–100 mEq i.v. in the first hour in patients with arterial pH < 7.1	Usually not required after first hour with proper insulin and fluid in DKA. Not required in HHNK. More HCO_3 required in LA. This condition may require replacement of urinary volume, ml for ml, with a solution of 75 mEq/liter Na HCO_3 (and 20 mEq/liter KCl) to deliver 22.5–37.5 mEq Na HCO_3/hr or 540–900 mEq/day

For elective procedures it is a good policy to have the patient's plasma glucose level under reasonable control for a few days before surgery. This can be done in an outpatient setting or, if possible, as an inpatient. Since the condition for which the patient is undergoing surgery can cause problems with control (e.g., cholecystitis), preoperative euglycemia is not a realistic goal. However, a safe and reasonable fasting blood sugar level is between 150 and 200 mg/dl. The patient's anxiety about the surgical procedure may also contribute to hyperglycemia. For emergency surgery it may be advisable to start an infusion of insulin at 1 unit/hr via a side-arm syringe to attain the plasma glucose levels indicated above by the time the patient is ready for surgery. If the plasma glucose level does not fall to 60–100 mg/dl in the first hour, the insulin infusion rate should be increased 30–50% in the subsequent hour.

Patients with inflammatory disease or under severe stress may require up to 10 units/hr for optimal control. Obviously, a means of rapid measurement of glucose should be readily available. For this reason I do not depend on hospital laboratories but utilize the Ames Glucometer (or other portable meters) or BG strips. I believe that such devices for rapid measuring of glucose levels should be available in an area very close to the operating room. Glucose levels can be measured during the surgery and should range between 150 and 250 mg/dl. Other than as a means of monitoring urinary output there is no need for catheterization of the diabetic patient.

Table 10 indicates the approaches for minor surgical procedures and elective and emergency surgery. Our surgeons use solutions containing 5% dextrose.

Under no circumstances should insulin be totally withdrawn preoperatively in a ketoacidosis-prone diabetic patient. In a number of cases in which this has been done the patient leaves the surgical procedure in ketoacidosis because of the stress and the elevated levels of counterinsulin hormones (e.g., epinephrine, glucagon, cortisol) that have been secreted during the procedure. With the insulin-treated patient who is not absolutely insulin-requiring (not ketoacidosis-prone) or in the non-insulin-requiring patient, insulin may be withheld and the decision to give insulin determined by the blood sugar level during the surgery. Crystalline (regular) insulin should be the form of intraoperative insulin. Again, this can be given subcutaneously if the patient is not in shock. If adequate monitoring is available, we have found that there is more precise control with a low-dose, constant-insulin infusion. However, in most hospitals, it is just as effective to give one-half to one-third of the usual insulin dose on call to surgery. In the postoperative period, blood glucose levels should be measured, ideally, each hour for at least 3 hours after surgery. If the patient has an infection or other postoperative surgical complication, hyperglycemia is likely to develop and close monitoring of plasma glucose levels may be required every 2–4 hours. When the patient is able to void, glycosuria will guide the physician to slow the glucose infusion or to administer insulin. When the urine is negative, beside glucose tests confirmed by the laboratory, whose results arrive later, are indicated.

Finally, some patients who never required insulin will require it during the perioperative period. This includes some obese patients who have only mild hyperglycemia. I do not hesitate to use insulin in such patients before, during, and after surgery.

Pregnancy and Delivery

Hyperglycemia occurs in pregnancy, especially in the last two trimesters, as a consequence of an increase in anti-insulin hormones, including human chorionic somatomammotropin (hCS). The objective of good control during pregnancy is euglycemia, with the plasma glucose level close to that seen in normal women undergoing pregnancy. Other factors harmful to the fetus are dehydration of the mother, ketonemia, infection, acidosis, hypertension, and noncompliance.

The goals of glucose control during pregnancy are considerably more rigid than those for the chronic diabetic patient. Excellent control is defined as a fasting plasma glucose level of

Table 10 **Guidelines for Surgical Management of the Diabetic Patient**[a]

Preoperative[b,c]

Insulin-requiring		Non-insulin-requiring	
History of hypoglycemic episodes ↓	No hypoglycemia ↓	Hyperglycemic[d] (>300 mg/dl) ↓	<300 mg/dl ↓
one-third of:	one-half of:	Defer surgery and control diabetes with insulin	Insulin not necessary preoperatively

Usual morning insulin dose (s.c.) on call to surgery

or

Begin 1.0–1.5 units i.v. regular insulin/hr on call to surgery

Intraoperative[c]

For all patients, i.v. bolus 10 units regular insulin for each 100 mg/dl blood glucose above 250 mg/dl, every 2 hours[e]

or

1.0–1.5 units i.v. regular insulin/hr with hourly blood glucose monitoring[e]

Postoperative[c]

10 units S.C. insulin for each 100 mg/dl blood glucose above 250 mg/dl[e] every 4–6 hours for at least 24 hours

or

Urine-testing method (sliding scale): 15 units s.c. for 3+ glucose, 10 units for 2+ glucose, every 4–6 hours. This method is effective if superimposed upon some intermediate-acting insulin given earlier that day. It is a poor method with wide glycemic oscillations when regular is the sole form of postoperative insulin

or

0.5–1unit/hr low dose i.v. (monitor blood glucose every 2 hours[e]).

[a] Try to have the surgery performed as first case in the morning. Patient should be well hydrated in all phases.

[b] This scheme represents elective surgery. For emergency surgery, give preoperative insulin as suggested for intraoperative patient.

[c] Fluid in 5% dextrose.

[d] Glycemia just prior to surgery should be measured in all patients using a rapid bedside test. However, an inference about the degree of control can be made from the blood glucose level of the previous morning or the night prior to surgery. If patient is hyperglycemic the night before surgery, NPH or Lente insulin, 10 units s.c. for each 100 mg/dl blood glucose above 250 mg/dl, can be given to attempt to alleviate severe hyperglycemia by the next morning. As another option, 0.5–1 unit/hr i.v. regular insulin can be started, but blood glucose level must be more closely monitored when this low-dose insulin option is used.

[e] With a rapid bedside test (see text).

100 mg/dl or less. After meals a plasma glucose level not over 130 mg/dl is considered optimal. Patients who are taking oral hypoglycemic agents and become pregnant should discontinue the oral agent and insulin may be required.

Home glucose monitoring has been an addition to pregnancy in diabetes that has led to even more favorable outcomes for the newborn than simply controlling fasting and postprandial glucose. Tables 11 and 12 deal with special aspects of managing the gestational diabetic, the diabetic patient without complications, and the diabetic with complications.

The objectives of optimal management of the diabetic are (1) reduced morbidity and mortality in the mother, (2) reduction in the occurrence of macrosomia, (3) avoidance of neonatal hypoglycemia (4) enhancement of pulmonary maturation, and (5) reduction in the occurrence of congenital anomalies.

Table 13 describes the techniques for evaluating the health of the fetus during pregnancy.

Cesarean section is indicated when there is severe systemic disease, such as toxemia, uncontrolled hypertension, or hydramnios. Also, severe microvascular disease and fetal distress are indications for cesarean section. These are diabetes-specific reason for cesarean section. Obstetric problems, such as abnormal presentation, prolonged labor, previous cesarean section, and placenta previa, are also indications for cesarean section.

Table 11 **The Diabetic Patient during Pregnancy**

Classification

Gestational diabetes—any degree of impaired carbohydrate metabolism that develops during pregnancy ranging from impaired glucose tolerance to diabetes (elevated fasting glucose level)

Diabetes in pregnancy—patients with known abnormal carbohydrate balance who become pregnant:

White's classification (Modification from Marble A et al, *Joslin's Diabetes Mellitus,* Philadelphia, Lea & Febiger 1971)

- A No symptoms. Diet results in euglycemia, though glucose tolerance test abnormal
- B Onset at over 20 years of age *and* diabetes of less than 10 years' duration. No micro- or macrovascular disease
- C Onset at 10–19 years of age *or* duration of 10–19 years. No evidence of micro- or macrovascular disease
- D Onset at <10 years of age *or* duration of over 20 years *or* evidence of nonproliferative retinopathy
- E Calcified pelvic vessels (by X-ray films)
- F Nephropathy
- R Proliferative retinopathy
- FR Both nephropathy and proliferative retinopathy
- G Multiple failures in pregnancy

Importance

To the fetus—increased fetal loss and/or congenital abnormalities or neonatal hypoglycemia, especially B–G

To the mother—some increases in the complications of diabetes, especially classes D–G

To the physician—classes C–G require team approach (internist, obstetrician, pediatrician) throughout pregnancy

Table 12 **Suggested Management of Pregnancy in Diabetic Patients**

Diagnosis

Gestational diabetes: Suggested by history, previous stillbirth or baby with congenital abnormality, macrosomia (>4,000 g), family history of diabetes, age over 25, obesity

Screening (as early in 1st trimester as possible, and again between 24 and 28 weeks and, at 32 weeks) Plasma glucose test, fasting and at 2 hours after a usual meal. If fasting >105 mg/dl or 2-hour postprandial >130, do OGTT. If fasting >135, diabetes exists and OGTT not necessary

OGTT: 100 g glucose. Abnormal if two or more specimens, taken fasting, 1-, 2-, or 3-hour plasma glucose level (mg/dl), respectively, over 105, 190, 165, and 145 mg/dl

Diabetes: Determine classification of the patient (see Table 11)

Treatment: Achieve as close to euglycemia as is possible, in both gestational diabetics and in patients with known antecedent diabetes

Diet

Avoid weight loss. Allow up to 24 lb weight gain. (Ketonemia accompanying weight loss can harm the fetus)

Calories 18–23 calories/lb (activity taken into account). 20–25% protein, otherwise similar nutrient distribution as in nonpregnant state)

Added supplements—3–4 cups milk/day, iron, and vitamins

Na^+ restriction not necessary unless hypertensive

Nausea and vomiting—ketonemia is harmful to the fetus. Inability to take food will perturb insulin schedule. Approaches include delay of insulin injection until 10–11 AM especially with morning nausea, small amounts of clear juices. Intravenous feedings may be required.

Insulin: Goal is excellent control (plasma glucose fasting level not >105; after meal 1 hour not >130, 2 hours not >120, 3 and 4 hours not >105). This may require injections 2–3 times per day, combinations of regular and intermediate-acting insulin, home blood glucose monitoring. Dosage may double (versus prepregnancy) in 3rd trimester. On day of anticipated delivery, whether by cesarean section or induction, start i.v. 5% glucose (200 ml/hr) and insulin 2–3 units/hr.

Drugs: Should be minimized. Sulfonylureas should be discontinued and insulin used for control. Diuretics should be used for hypertension but not for small to moderate dependent edema. Drugs to treat urinary infection may be required

Outpatient program

Visits: 1st trimester, every 2 weeks. Weekly in 3rd trimester. Include fasting or postmeal blood glucose test and urinalysis with microscopic

Home records: Should include written records of Q.I.D. urine (or blood) glucose and urine ketones

Physical exam should include weight and ophthalmoscopy

Upon delivery, there is often a great reduction in the requirement for exogenous insulin. The patient must have monitoring of the glucose level and receive much less insulin, and often supplemental glucose intravenously until she is able to eat.

Prevention of pregnancy is important especially in patients who have had two pregnancies that are beyond White's classification C. A properly fitting diaphragm used with a spermicidal agent is probably the first-choice preventive for the diabetic women. Intrauterine devices are

Table 13 **Fetal Surveillance during Pregnancy in Diabetic Patients**[a]

Test	*Purpose*	
Serial nonstress testing	To evaluate fetal heart rate with fetal movement along with spontaneous uterine contractions. Doppler ultrasound or fetal ECG used. During a 20-minute monitoring period, five episodes or more of accelerations of >10 beats/minute are normal. Fewer than five of such episodes are considered abnormal, and OCT should be done	Readily available. Results obtained immediately. Can be done twice weekly from weeks 32–36, then daily
Oxytocin contraction test (OCT)	I.V. oxytocin results in uterine contractions. These should be accompanied by increases in fetal heart rate (or no change). Slowing of fetal heart rate with contraction is abnormal and probably indicates need for delivery	Readily available
Real-time ultrasonagraphy	Can delineate rate of growth, head size, viability. Serial ultrasound tells actual gestational age	Readily available
Plasma unconjugated estriol (E_3)	Abnormal E_3, and a sign of compromised fetal environment is a 35% fall from the mean of 3 preceding sequential morning values (normal E_3 = 10–25 ng/ml at the 34th week)	Very few laboratories can report a value on the same day of a specimen drawn at 8:00 AM
Amniotic fluid lecithin/sphingomyelin (L/S) ratio	About 35th week, the fetal lung begins to manufacture surfactant in sufficient amounts to prevent respiratory distress syndrome, indicated by an adequate L/S ratio of at least 2:1	1–3 days may be required to receive results; 5-ml samples can be taken as early as 32 weeks
pH	Fetal acidosis is an index of deteriorated fetal environment, 7.24 is mild acidosis. 7.2 or less is severe	Readily available

[a] This is important since currently most deliveries are between 37 and 39 weeks. If evidence of fetal distress, however, delivery may be earlier. Clinical judgement applies information from the above tests to balance the chances of death in vitro from disturbed fetal environment versus neonatal death because of immaturity. Cesarean section often the method of delivery for classes D–G and/or the presence of fetal distress, obstetrical complications, toxemia, uncontrolled hypertension, ketoacidosis, or failure of induction. Induction is usual method for uncomplicated A–C.

not satisfactory because of infection and because of the inconsistency of effectiveness. Birth control pills with the lowest possible dose of estrogen, or progestins, are a second choice. Tubal ligation or, for the husband, vasectomy, should be seriously considered in patients with long-duration diabetes.

Total Parenteral Nutrition

Patients who have diabetes may have to undergo periods of total parenteral nutrition, (TPN), especially those who have undergone serious surgery. There are two major forms of TPN being given in hospitals today. The first involves classic hyperalimentation. This entails the intravenous feeding of up to 750 g of glucose per day along with essential amino acids and trace elements. Such patients are given essential fatty acids intermittently. Second, patients may receive total parenteral nutrition via a peripheral vein, in contrast to the central vein required for hyperalimentation. These patients usually receive essential amino acids and 5% dextrose in the peripheral vein. One day a week they may also receive essential fatty acids as part of the TPN solution. The goal in either type of TPN is to keep the plasma glucose between 100 and 200 mg/dl. If 15 units/8 hr (usually 1 liter is given during this time) does not keep the patient's plasma glucose in this range, insulin is increased by 30–50% at 2- to 4-hour intervals until the glucose is kept at optimal levels. For stressed, seriously infected diabetics on hyperalimentation we have used as much as 100 units of insulin per liter. For the peripheral vein form of TPN, 1–1.5 units/hr in a side-arm infusion using a pump has been most successful.

Steroid Treatment

Some known diabetic patients, or even patients not previously known to have diabetes, are put on high doses of glucocorticoids for a number of indications. In my experience, regardless of body build, hyperglycemia in such patients is best controlled with insulin. Even if the patient is obese, sulfonylureas or a diet program are not effective. Such steroid-treated diabetic patients may require much higher dosages of insulin than they took during their presteroid period.

Gangrene and Foot Ulcers

Gangrene must be considered a medical emergency and can involve a patient who 1 day before the episode was asymptomatic. The toes suddenly become cold and discolored. Gangrene can also develop in a previously infected foot in which tissue death is due to necrosis induced by the infection. In either case the blackening or putrefaction of an extremity or a digit, usually the leg, is an indication for surgery. In the infective types it is wise to culture the blood as well as the local ulcer, using both aerobic and anaerobic cultures. Anaerobic infection can frequently be the culprit and may not be cultured from the superficial portions of the ulcer. Antibiotics and local debridement may assist in managing the problem. Regional amputations or amputation of the limb provide the only definitive care in many cases.

Since the prognosis for the requirement for amputation of the ipsilateral or contralateral limb is over 40% in the 5 years following the initial amputation, means of prevention of the problem are being sought. Avoidance of smoking is recommended, but a clear implication of smoking in diabetic gangrene has not been proven. Inspection of the feet, care of the feet, and avoidance of trauma are strongly recommended. A current 10-hospital VA cooperative study is being conducted with regard to the preventive effects of asprin and dipyridamole, agents that inhibit platelet aggregation.

Management of the Complications of Diabetes

The complications of diabetes include microvascular disease (retinopathy and nephropathy), neuropathy, cataracts, and advanced macrovascular disease. Gangrene and foot ulcer are believed to be due to a combination of the above problems. Increased occurrence of certain infections, such as fungal infections, must also be included. Complications of treatment include those due to insulin, such as resistance, allergy, and hypoglycemia. Complications of sulfonylureas include hypoglycemia, allergies, liver disease, and the Antabuse-like reaction.

It is believed that meticulous control will prevent or diminish the incidence of microvascular disease, neuropathy, and cataracts. However, advanced macrovascular disease has not been shown to be prevented in animals or in epidemiologic studies in humans to be avoided by more meticulous control of the hyperglycemia.

Some recent studies have strongly indicated that control of hypertension will reduce the incidence of nephropathy and retinopathy.

Table 14 lists the complications and outlines management. The table does not deal with preventive measures which may be even more important. In addition to the control of hypertension, careful use of radiographic contrast agents should be pointed out. There is evidence that, in the attempt to find out more about a patient's coronary artery disease or about renal anatomy using a radiographic dye, acute renal failure has been induced. Factors that seems to make such patients more susceptible to contrast media-induced renal failure include dehydration, renal failure, hypotension, old age, hypertension, abnormal hepatic function, proteinuria, and hyperuricemia. For such patients, I use as a guideline the consideration of whether the contrast study will lead to something that can be done for the patient. I then make a strong effort to see that the patient is hydrated, that the diabetes is well controlled, and that the hypertension is regulated as well as possible prior to the procedure.

With regard to macrovascular disease, patients with diabetes have, in general, less success after bypass procedures, such as coronary arterial grafts or peripheral vascular arteriovenous shunts for dialysis. Successes are being reported, however, and each case must be individually evaluated.

For the treatment of diabetic complications, diabetologists often emphasize that it is important to control the diabetes as perfectly as possible. This has not been shown to reverse all the problems or to restore normal function. However, with diabetic neuropathy the disturbing tingling and numbness that occurs with the peripheral syndrome can often be helped by metabolic control. Recently, one group has even reported a change toward normal of motor nerve conduction velocity by meticulous control with an insulin infusion pump. Although it remains to be shown whether motor and/or sensory neuropathy can be corrected, it is possible that some of the neurological abnormalities can be diminished by metabolic control. I have not tabulated the multiple drugs that have been recommended for diabetic neuropathy. This is because there have been very few controlled studies evaluating the effects of various drugs in this condition, neuropathy. Mild analgesic agents may be helpful for a short time. Though success has been reported with diphenylhydantoin, tricyclic antidepressants, and various vitamins in treating the symptoms of peripheral neuropathy, it is not clear whether the remission is due to these agents. In the course of 2–6 months the condition may remit spontaneously or go to a more dangerous anesthetic stage in which the patient cannot feel a foreign body entering the foot. Though disturbing numbness, tingling, and pain may cease under such circumstances, anesthesia is an additional hazard for the patient in regard to neuropathic ulcers or infection from foreign body entry. Disturbing symptoms may remit after 3–6 months, even with evidence of recovery of sensation. However, in my experience, when the metabolic disorder is uncontrolled, the syn-

Table 14 **The Anatomic Complications of Diabetes**

Condition	*Management*[a]
Retinopathy	Control hypertension. Obtain fluorescent angiography at an early date. Effects of aspirin (antiplatelet aggregation agents) are being evaluated. Photocoagulation—indicated for proliferative retinopathy. Impedes but does not cure diabetic retinopathy. Used in certain cases for severe, nonproliferative retinopathy. Indicated for macular edemia. Contraindications to photocoagulation: (1) severe glial proliferation; (2) severe vitreoretinal traction; (3) florid, arborizing neovascularization; (4) excessive (60%) capillary closure; (5) extensive retinal edemia; (6) severe uremic retinopathy; (7) severe hypertensive retinopathy Vitrectomy—to remove blood from vitreous, improving vision in a viable eye Pituitary ablation—helpful in some cases of florid neovascularization
Nephropathy	Control hypertension. Avoid contrast media, unless some clear action might be taken as a result of the study. Treat infections and urinary tract infection. Rule out other causes of renal failure. Note reduced insulin requirements as renal failure progresses. With reduction of creatinine clearance to 20–40 ml/minute consider for dialysis (peritoneal or hemodialysis). Restrict protein to 40 g/day and dietary salt to 2 g/day. Cease cigarette smoking. Consider renal transplantation
Neuropathy	Sensory—Control glycemia, mild analgesics, proper nutrition, keep extremity clean, dry, and protected. Motor: Protect involved area; usually self-limited 3–8 weeks Autonomic: (1) Hypotension—rule out other causes. Use supportive (full leg) hosiery. Mineralocorticoids e.g., Florinef (0.1–0.3 mg/day) may relieve severe postural fall in blood pressure. (2) Gastroparesis—upright postprandially, chew food well, manual pressure on epigastrium. Cholinergic agents occasionally help. (3) Diarrhea—rule out other causes. Tetracyline 10 days, and Lomotil (10 days). (4) Neurogenic bladder—urologic consultation. Treat infection. Medical—indwelling catheter 3–4 weeks, with intermittent clamping and parasympathetic drugs, to restore tone. Remove catheter and encourage manual voiding with suprapubic pressure every 3 hours. Surgical—bladder neck resection. (5) Neuropathic impotence—counseling, penile implant
Cataracts	Surgical removal

Table 14 **(Continued)**

Condition	*Management*[a]
Accelerated macrovascular disease	No effective preventive therapy, even in diabetic animal models. Effects of exercise and control of hyperlipidemia are not yet clear. Bypass therapy (coronary arteries, peripheral vessels) effective. Suggest avoidance of smoking. Sympathectomy occasionally effective for peripheral vascular obstruction. Effect of peripheral vasodilators not clear. Caution with contrast materials. (see text)

[a] The first four conditions are believed to be preventable, to some degree, with meticulous control of glycemia. None, with the possible exception of neuropathy (see text), has been shown to be reversible in human beings with meticulous control.

drome returns or the anesthetic phase supervenes. Two pharmacologic modalities for diabetic peripheral neuropathy have been studied in a double-blind fashion. One is carbamazepine (Tegretol), which has been shown to give some relief of the pain compared to a placebo. However, since there is some risk of bone marrow supression with this drug, patients should be followed with peripheral blood counts. The syndrome may be reversed by withdrawal of the drug. Recently, we had the opportunity to use vitamin B_6 in a double-blind fashion in a small group of 19 patients. We did the study because it had been reported in the podiatric literature in a noncontrolled study that this vitamin was beneficial in relieving the symptoms of diabetic peripheral neuropathy. However, in our study an equal number of patients (about half) in the placebo group and half of the B_6 group had relief of symptoms during a 4-month course of the vitamin or a placebo.

Diabetic gangrene can come on suddenly with lack of control in someone with or without palpable pulses in the feet. The cause of this gangrene is unknown. However, it is believed that it may be related to a hypercoagulable state in the diabetic. Another way the diabetic can lose a digit or extremity is from a skin infection, usually in the foot, which can lead to osteomyelitis often due to an anaerobic organism, often accompanied by sepsis. When the infection is brought under control with antibiotics, debridement can save the limb or even the life of the patient. The most effective debridement is that which is done daily or three or four times a week. In many teaching hospitals it is often difficult to get the orthopedic or general surgical house staff to do daily debridement, and I advise our internal medicine house officers to become involved with such care. We are fortunate to have excellent podiatrists who can see patients two or three times each week. Soaks and cleansing by nurses help. The water should be just above room temperature, never hot. The foot must be dried well after soaking. In a private hospital setting, orthopedic surgeons who can visit patients three or four times a week or podiatrists have provided excellent help to patients. This can become quite expensive. I believe it is worth the expense, however, and diabetic patients should be instructed to be certain that their health insurance includes both inpatient and outpatient podiatric care.

For macrovascular complications of diabetes, as well as in diabetic retinopathy, studies are currently being conducted with aspirin with and without Persantin (dipyridamole). Until these studies are completed and show that these agents will prevent macovascular disease in diabetic patients, I would not recommend their liberal use. This is because the side effects of the medications and their expense currently do not justify their use.

The approaches to the complications of insulin and sulfonylurea drugs are listed in Table 15.

Table 15 **Complications of Sulfonylureas and Insulin**

	Type	*Management*
Sulfonylureas	Rash Nausea, vomiting, diarrhea Leukopenia Thrombocytopenia Agranulocytosis Anemia Abnormal liver function including cholestatic jaundice (especially with chlorpropamide)	Discontinue drug
	Disulfiram (Antabuse)-like reaction (mild to severe flushing)	Discontinue drug or reduce or eliminate alcohol
	Hyponatremia (Excessive ADH-like syndrome). Usually older patient, or patients with congestive failure or renal insufficiency	Discontinue drug
	Hypoglycemia (with renal or hepatic insufficiency, the former especially with chlorpropamide; or if not eating, while taking drug). Certain drugs (see below) can displace sulfonylureas from binding protein, enhancing sulfonylurea effect	Discontinue drug. Treat hypoglycemia, with i.v. glucose acutely. With chlorpropamide, especially in the presence of renal insufficiency, 1 to several days of treatment (i.v. glucose and frequent meals) is required
	Drug interaction. Certain drugs can be displaced from binding proteins by sulfonylureas, thus enhancing the effects of these drugs. These include coumarin anticoagulants, phenylbutazone, possibly propranolol, and salicylates	Readjust dosage of one or both the sulfonylurea and the interacting drug
Insulin	Allergy (urticaria, local or generalized; rarely severe systemic reaction)	Several options: (1) Use purified insulin (see Table 6), (2) change form (e.g., from NPH to Lente), (3) desensitize[a], (4) systemic antihistamines[a], (5) steroids (up to 60 g prednisone for several weeks, with slow withdrawal, (6) change species (usually from beef-pork to pork)

Table 15 **(Continued)**

	Type	*Management*
	Localized lipoatrophy (pitted area at injection site, as result of loss of fat tissue)	Purified insulin injected into involved area
	Localized lipohypertrophy (fatty swelling at injection site)	Purified insulin given other than in involved site
	Immune resistance (usually require over 200 units/day for 48 hours under professional observation, have high antibody titer)[b]	Several options: (1) increase dose, using U500 (crystalline insulin) one or two times per day[a], (2) change species (usually to porcine), (3) change to purified insulin (see Table 6)[a], (4) use steroids—up to 60 mg prednisone for several weeks with slow withdrawal, (5) use nonmammalian insulin, e.g., fish (difficult to obtain)
	Tissue destruction (destruction of insulin at injection site)	Rare. Such patients respond normally to intravenous insulin. Increase dosage and/or use aprotinin (Trasylol, a protease inhibitor). Aprotinin (4–160 KIU/unit insulin) is mixed with the patient's insulin. Aprotinin is still experimental.
	Hypoglycemia	Readjust dose by reduction or "splitting" day's dosage (see text). For acute episode, give oral juice or sugar if conscious, i.m. glucagon 1 mg can be given by spouse or other household members. i.v. glucose, usually by medical personnel, with several hours observation may be required. Secondary to exercise (glycemia usually well controlled), treat as above. Prevent with reduced insulin (20–50% less) before exercise, and/or simple sugar drink during exercise, and/or inject into least exercised portion of body (e.g., into arm if cycling)

[a] Method usually used by author.
[b] Syndrome may remit suddenly.

DISCUSSION CASES

Case 1

A 62-year-old man has taken insulin for 18 years. He now complains of tingling and burning of the feet, especially at night, for about 4 months. His diabetes was detected by routine urinalysis at the time of his discharge from the army. He reports that his control has always been "pretty good," with urine glucose tests reading negative to 2+. He tries not to overeat but follows no specific diet. He has never had an insulin reaction. He weighs 234 lb (5 ft 10 in. tall), which is about what he weighed while in the service. He feels otherwise well. Physical examination showed a blood pressure of 168/95, a few retinal microaneurysms, obesity, reduced light touch sensation in the feet, and trace patellar and Achilles reflexes. Laboratory data included a fasting plasma glucose level of 238 mg/dl and a serum creatinine level of 1.6 mg/dl; urinalysis showed 2+ protein and 2+ glucose. His current insulin dosage is 60 units of NPH in the morning and 10 units of NPH in the afternoon.

Discussion

The obese diabetic given insulin because of hyperglycemia is a real problem. This patient responded to five measures:

1. Education: He was taught the difference between type I and type II diabetes, in plain words that he could easily understand ("Type I patients have very little insulin, are lean, and require insulin injections. Type II patients have their own insulin, but it isn't working efficiently because of obesity. You have type II diabetes, and I believe you did not need insulin at the start of your problem, 18 years ago. What was really needed was a weight loss program").
2. Diet education: The physician calculated his ideal body weight (IBW) (see Table 1): IBW = 106 + 60 = 166 lb (based on medium frame); ideal caloric intake = 166 × 10 = 1660 calories; add 10% more for wide frame: 1660 + 160 = 1820 calories; no additional calories for extra activity will be given until the exercise program is initiated; then add 10% more for moderate exercise.

   Start with 1,300 calories/day. This allows 500 calories less than his weight maintenance requirements and should result in a 1- to $1\frac{1}{2}$-lb weight loss per week. A 1,300-calorie ADA diet was ordered. The patient and his wife were interviewed and trained by a dietitian, who followed them monthly for 4 months to answer questions and to assess understanding and compliance. At 2 months, high-fiber intake was added because of the laboratory follow-up (see item 5, below).
3. Exercise: Rather than initiating the program outlined in the text and in Table 2, this patient was started on a walking program, working gradually up to 2 mi/day.
4. Withdrawal from insulin: At each monthly visit, 10–15 units of insulin were subtracted from his dosage. At the fifth monthly visit, insulin was totally removed, and he was begun on tolazamide, 250 mg b.i.d., with the plan of discontinuing this medication when postprandial glycemia was optimally controlled (i.e., approached fasting values).
5. Clinical follow-up: The patient was seen at monthly intervals for 6 months.
   a. His weight at 1, 2, 3, 4, 5, and 6 months was 230, 223, 218, 216, 208, and 202 lb.
   b. His fasting plasma glucose level at months 1, 2, 3, 4, 5, and 6 was 206, 178, 108, 112, 98, and 109 mg/dl; his fasting plasma triglyceride level, initially 406 mg/dl, fell to 143 mg/dl. His cholesterol remained in the range of 200 mg/dl.
   c. His 2-hour postprandial plasma glucose level at months 3, 4, 5, and 6 was 220, 190, 245, and 216 mg/dl.

d. His urine protein level did not change; his serum creatinine fell to 1.4 mg/dl.
e. Signs and symptoms: His retinal microaneurysms remained unchanged during the 6-month period. After a few weeks of taking aspirin at bedtime, the pain and paresthesias in the feet remitted.

Comments

This patient's management focuses on a weight loss program. Surprisingly, he had never received formal instruction regarding diabetes, diet, or exercise. The patient was very well motivated and continues to lose weight. Most obese diabetic patients may seem, at first, unmotivated. However, confrontation with actuarial data (four times higher death rate in obese hyperglycemic individuals than in obese or lean nonhyperglycemic peers) often produces results. The assistance of a dietitian is essential, although the physician may have to be the professional to train the patient in an exercise program (see text).

Even patients who have received insulin for many years, if obese and non-ketosis-prone at the onset, may be candidates for insulin withdrawal.

In the laboratory, the serum triglyceride levels often reflect diabetic control; the total serum cholesterol level is usually normal. The postprandial (after usual meals) glucose level is obtained after the fasting glucose level is reasonably controlled (less than 150 mg/dl). This patient's postprandial glucose level ranged between 140 and 160 mg/dl on tolazamide, and weight loss continues at a rate of 2–4 lb/month.

Case 2

A 73-year-old man was seen in the emergency room at 3 PM, stuporous and breathing rapidly. Physical examination showed dehydration and stupor. Blood tests were obtained for a toxic drug screen and for metabolic parameters. Urinalysis showed 4+ glucose and a high level of acetone. His relatives were contacted from information found on identification cards carried by the patient. The man's daughter stated that he definitely had no history of diabetes. The laboratory data, returned at 4:30 PM, revealed a plasma glucose level of 480 mg/dl, a plasma bicarbonate concentration of 8 mEq/liter, and a BUN level of 64 mg/dl. The toxic drug screen was negative. An intravenous infusion of regular insulin, 4 units/hr, was begun, as was half-normal saline, 50 ml/hr. Within 6 hours, the plasma glucose level had fallen to 150 mg/dl. Eight hours after admission, however, he was more stuporous, and his right hand was cold and pale. Intravenous heparin was given, and he was taken to the radiology department for angiography. There he had a cardiac arrest from which he could not be resuscitated.

Discussion

Several important points should be made regarding the management of this patient with diabetic ketoacidosis. First, the laboratory data were returned before insulin therapy was started. Insulin, fluid, and electrolyte therapy should be started on the basis of bedside tests unless the laboratory can provide results within a few minutes. The bedside tests that might have been used include, for glucose, Dextrostix, with or without a Glucometer, or BG strips, and for acetoacidemia, Acetest tablets, using serial dilution of serum with water. Second, some parameter of potassium balance should have been followed. An ECG rhythm strip and an assessment of abdominal bowel sounds might help in assessing the state of total body potassium and the intracellular-extracellular potassium relationship at the start of therapy, to compare with subsequent findings. Low T waves, long Q-U intervals, prominent U waves, and reduced bowel sounds indicate hypokalemia. Potassium was not added to intravenous fluids, and with a reduction in the plasma glucose level severe hypokalemia would be likely to ensue. Serial assessment of serum potassium, EKG strips, and bowel sounds might help monitor the potassium status. As long as the urine output is at least 30 ml/hr, potassium may be given in a dose of 40 mEq added to each liter of intravenous fluid. Third, the fluid input was grossly deficient. It can be assumed that a patient with diabetic ketoacidosis has a fluid deficit of 5–8 liters at the time of diagnosis. The rapid fall in the plasma glucose level here was associated with the entry of water into cells, further depleting the circulating plasma volume and leading to hemoconcentration and thrombosis of the radial artery.

A cautious physician, however, might ask, "What if the diagnosis is wrong?" Perhaps this is simply a patient who is comatose for another reason, for example, stroke or drug ingestion. What if the glucosuria is due to "stress hyperglycemia"? Perhaps the acetonuria is due to starvation in a comatose person, and not to ketoacidosis. Should the physician wait for the laboratory results to be sure? The answer to these questions is: Treat the patient as if ketoacidosis were present, with close bedside monitoring of plasma glucose and serum acetone levels, if necessary every half-hour at first, until laboratory results return. The insulin infusion rate may be reduced to 1–2 units/hr when the plasma glucose level falls to 150 mg/dl.

Differentiation between stress–starvation syndromes and ketoacidosis may be difficult, even when the laboratory results return. Both disorders have a marked degree of prerenal azotemia, hence both may be associated with acidosis. In general, patients with diabetic ketoacidosis have more intense acetoacidemia, a lower serum bicarbonate level, and a lower arterial pH than stressed or starved patients. The degree of dehydration and the elevation of the BUN level may be similar in both situations. A stressed or starved patient may respond more promptly to intravenous fluids, with a faster fall in the blood glucose level and clearance of urine acetone than a patient with diabetic ketoacidosis.

Elderly, hypotensive, or debilitated patients should have some means of monitoring central venous pressure to be certain that a fluid input of 250–500 ml/hr for several hours can be tolerated.

The choice of fluid for replacement, 0.45% (half-normal) or 0.9% (normal) saline, has been debated. I prefer 0.9% saline. It is often hypotonic to the patient's serum; however, 0.45% (half-normal) saline is even more hypotonic, and hemolysis may result. It is true, however, that a patient with diabetic ketoacidosis has lost more water than salt. In the final analysis, the critical factor is an adequate volume of fluid and electrolyte replacement and the coordination of these factors with the effects of insulin.

The cause of death in this patient was probably a combination of volume depletion, hypokalemia, and hypoglycemia. The errors seen in the management of this man are all preventable. Physicians should also realize that insulin-dependent, type I diabetes (old term: juvenile diabetes) may be seen as the first manifestation of diabetes in patients of any age.

SUGGESTED READING

Anderson J, Ward K: Long-term effects of high carbohydrate, high fiber diets on glucose and lipid metabolism: A preliminary report on patients with diabetes. *Diabetes Care* 1:77–82, 1978.

Arky RA: Current principles of dietary therapy of diabetes mellitus. *Med Clin North Am* 62:655–662, 1978.

Davidson M: *Diabetes Mellitus: Diagnosis and Treatment*. New York, John Wiley and Sons, New York, 1981.

Galloway JA, Bressler R: Insulin treatment in diabetes. *Med Clin North Am* 62:663–680, 1978.

Krall L, Chabot V: Oral hypoglycemic agent update. *Med Clin North Am* 62:681–694, 1978.

Kreisberg RA: Diabetic ketoacidosis: New concepts and trends in pathogenesis and treatment. *Ann Intern Med* 88:681–695, 1978.

Levin SR: Diabetes mellitus and hypoglycemia, in Hershman JM (ed): *Management of Endocrine Disorders*. Philadelphia, Lea & Febiger, 1980, pp 134–173.

Levin SR: Diabetes mellitus and hypoglycemia, in Hershman JM (ed): *Practical Endocrinology*. New York, John Wiley and Sons, 1981, pp 141–188.

Olson OC: *Diagnosis and Management of Diabetes Mellitus*. Philadelphia, Lea & Febiger, 1981.

Porte D, Halter J: The endocrine pancreas and diabetes mellitus, in Williams R (ed): *Textbook of Endocrinology*. Philadelphia, WB Saunders Co, 1981, pp 715–842.

Vranic M, Horvath S, Wahren J: Conference on diabetes and exercise. *Diabetes* 28(suppl 1):1–13, 1979.

16 SEYMOUR R. LEVIN

Hypoglycemia

There are two major types of hypoglycemia: One is that seen in the fasting state, and the other is that seen after meals. The type seen in the fasting state often indicates an important organic or chemical disorder and usually a requirement for hospitalization. The type seen in the postprandial state indicates a requirement for adjustments in meals. For the latter, many drugs have been suggested. However, I have found that simple meal adjustments are more effective and accompanied by fewer problems than the various drugs that are used.

The level of glucose required to trigger hypoglycemic symptoms has not been universally agreed upon. I believe that the plasma glucose level should reach 45 mg/dl or less before the patient's symptoms are attributed to hypoglycemia.

Table 1 lists the causes of fasting hypoglycemia. Any of these may also cause postmeal hypoglycemia if one waits long enough after a meal. The important fact is that, in these conditions, after an overnight fast or after 24, 48, or 72 hours fasting is accompanied by hypoglycemia. In fact, in most of these conditions, during the glycemic nadir the patient is quite uncomfortable. The test should be stopped when the patient becomes symptomatic (irritable or irrational). Before receiving food or intravenous glucose, it is essential to obtain a plasma glucose level determination and, if insulinoma is suspected, a serum insulin level determination. Assessment of most of the causes of fasting hypoglycemia can be made from the history and by some simple laboratory tests.

The major method for diagnosis of insulinoma is a fasting test (Table 1). Provocative tests are used if the diagnosis of insulinoma is not clearly made with fasting. The tolbutamide tolerance test, the glucagon test, and the leucine test are the most frequently used. In the tolbutamide tolerance test, 1 g of tolbutamide is given intravenously over 30 seconds, and blood samples are taken every 5 minutes for 30 minutes for serum insulin and glucose. When this test is done for insulin response, patients with insulinoma will usually have plasma insulin levels over 200 μU/ml at some time during the test. Additionally there is a steep fall in the glucose level during the 30 minutes. To avoid severe hypoglycemia the test should not be continued longer than 30 minutes, and the patient should be refed orally or intravenously at that time. In the glucagon test 1 mg is given intravenously over 10 seconds. Blood is collected for the measurement of glucose and insulin levels every 5 minutes for 30 minutes, and then every 10 minutes for a

Table 1 **Fasting Hypoglycemia**[a]

Condition	*Diagnosis*	*Management*
Insulin overdose	History	See Chapter 15
Oral hypoglycemic agents	History	See Chapter 15
Alcohol	History of drinking within the past 24–48 hours, not eating, or eating poorly. Secondary to NAD utilization in alcohol metabolism. This reduces NAD available for gluconeogenesis	Intravenous and oral feeding. Prevent by discontinuing alcohol and/or eating when taking alcohol
Prolonged fasting (>48 hours)	Not really pathologic. Up to one-third of normal subjects, especially women, will develop hypoglycemia with prolonged fasting	Gradual refeeding to avoid excessive "rebound" insulin responses
Deficient insulin antagonists (pituitary or adrenal insufficiency)	See Chapters 2 and 8	
Non-islet cell tumors	Patients usually have large physically or radiographically detectable tumors: retroperitoneal sarcoma, hepatoma, adrenal. Due to either consumption of glucose by tumor or the production of insulin-like peptides (ILA). These do not assay as immunoreative insulin	Frequent feeding. Remove tumor or give appropriate chemotherapy or radiation. A few reports indicate diazoxide (Proglycem) 100 mg two to five times per day may be effective in raising plasma glucose
Glycogen storage disease (type I, Von Gierke's)	In adults, mild fasting hypoglycemia, with hyperuricemia and, often, gout, uric acid nephropathly; 1 mg glucagon i.m. results in less than normal (30 mg/dl or more) elevation of plasma glucose. These patients usually have less than a 10 mg/dl rise in the plasma glucose level	Treat the hyperuricemia. Bedtime snack might lessen morning hypoglycemia
Medications (not including usual hypoglycemia agents) given for diabetes)	Phenylbutazone, iproniazid, propranolol, pyribenzamine, and other antihistamines; propoxyphene (Darvon); pentamidine (Lomidine, used to treat pneumocystis; may later develop hyperglycemia), probably several other drugs. The drugs act by enhancing insulin secretion and/or action or	Discontinue medication or reduce drug dosage, especially if concurrently taking sulfonylurea (see Chapter 15)

	interfere with defense against hypoglycemia (e.g., glucagon secretion and action) or reduce the perception of hypoglycemia	
Severe liver necrosis	In some cases of hepatitis with severe clinical and laboratory manifestations, profound hypoglycemia can occur. Liver unable to provide glucose via gluconeogenesis	Intravenous and oral glucose
Uremia	Uremic patients may be undergoing dialysis. In part, due to defective gluconeogenesis	Intravenous and oral glucose. May require frequent feedings
Factitious hypoglycemia	Self-administration of insulin or oral agents in patients without diabetes. May be medical professionals. Insulin: serum insulin level may be high. Serum C peptide very low. Insulin antibodies present. Sulfonylureas: may detect sulfonylurea in serum, especially if hypoglycemic at the time of sampling. Serum insulin level not elevated	Psychotherapy
Insulinoma	Fasting insulin level elevated over 10–50 μU/ml when plasma glucose level is low, and glucose/insulin (mg/dl and μU/ml) ratio is usually <2.5. Provocative tests (see text). Proinsulin level (normally 10% of total insulin, may be elevated to 40–80% total insulin, especially in B-cell carcinoma. Recently, i.v. Ca^{2+} infusion, 4 mg/kg per hour for 3–5 hours has been reported to raise serum insulin level to three to five times basal in many patients with insulinoma. Normally insulin level does not rise with calcium infusion. Echogram and/or CT scan and/or angiogram can help localize lesion	Surgery. Diazoxide for metastatic B-cell carcinoma or if patient is too ill (Proglycem, 100 mg two to five times a day). May need evaluation for multiple endocrine neoplasia or secretion of ectopic hormones from B-cell carcinoma. Streptozotocin chemotherapy

[a]In all these conditions, the serum immunoreactive insulin level is very low, except in insulinoma and after excessive exogenous insulin.

total duration of 60 minutes. In the first 30 minutes normal subjects have a rise in the plasma glucose level of 20–40 mg/dl. This rise often occurs in patients with insulinoma. However, later in the test patients with insulinoma may experience profound hypoglycemia. Whereas maximal insulin levels of 120 μU/ml occur in healthy subjects (200–250 μU/ml in obese subjects) 4–15 minutes after glucagon, patients with β-cell tumors have inordinately high insulin responses (over 200–1,000 μU/ml). This may occur as late as 30 minutes after glucagon administration. In the leucine test leucine, 150 mg/kg, is administered orally and blood is collected for glucose and insulin testing every 10 minutes for 30 minutes and then every 30 minutes for the final 120 minutes. Healthy subjects do not become hypoglycemic after leucine ingestion. Insulin increases not more than 28 μU/ml in lean subjects or 50 μU/ml in obese subjects. In contrast, 40 or 50% of patients with insulinoma have hypoglycemia within 120 minutes after leucine ingestion, and high insulin levels (80–800 μU/ml) accompany this hypoglycemia.

Over 90% of patients with insulinoma have had a positive fasting test, and approximately 60% of patients have a positive tolbutamide tolerance test or a positive glucagon test. The leucine test is less frequently positive. In all the tests, the patients should be fed at the conclusion.

Table 2 classifies the reactive hypoglycemias and summarizes their management. I try to make the diagnosis in ambulatory patients by measuring the plasma glucose level $1\frac{1}{2}$, 2, $2\frac{1}{2}$, 3, 4, and 5 hours after a usual meal, which is similar to the type that induces reactive hypoglycemia at home. I avoid a glucose test as the initial study because many of the patients, especially those who have had a gastrectomy, may develop profound hypoglycemia after ingesting pure glucose. If hypoglycemia does not occur after a mixed meal containing 15% simple carbohydrates and 35% complex carbohydrates and the patient has symptoms consistent with the syndrome, an oral glucose tolerance test should be performed using 50–75 g of glucose.

In all cases, if the patient becomes extremely symptomatic, it is wise to draw a plasma glucose sample and then feed the patient intravenously or orally. If such severe symptoms are not accompanied by chemical hypoglycemia, attributing the symptoms to hypoglycemia seems unwarranted. It may help in diagnosing this syndrome to allow the patient to walk about and perform the usual activity that accompanies the symptoms at home or work. Often the testing situation, with the patient lying recumbent in the doctor's office with an indwelling needle, may not simulate the actual clinical situation.

Hypoglycemia is a diagnosis which is sometimes given to the condition experienced by patients with anxiety, fatigue, depression, or restlessness. This should be avoided, since other organic or psychogenic causes might underlie the patients' problems.

DISCUSSION CASE

Case 1

A 75-year-old man was admitted to the hospital semicomatose, with left hemiparesis. His wife stated he had been in a nursing home for 6 months and that he had been taking 750 mg chlorpropamide (Diabinese) daily for those 6 months. He had been ambulatory until the past week. He had been depressed and eating poorly in the recent past. Physical examination showed a somewhat obese patient with left hemiparesis and a positive extensor toe sign on the left.

His urine was negative for glucose and showed a moderate amount of acetone. Following the obtaining of a blood specimen for glucose determination, 25 ml of a 50% glucose solution was given intravenously. He awoke, and movement of the left extremities improved. The extensor toe sign became equivocal. He was hospitalized, and intravenous glucose (10% solution) was given at a rate of 100–150 ml/hr. His initial serum glucose level was 22 mg/dl and his serum creatinine level 1.1 mg/dl.

Table 2 **Reactive Hypoglycemia**

Condition	*Diagnosis*[a]	*Management*
Tachyalimentation	Mixed meal[b] demonstrates high (>200 mg/dl) 1 hour postprandial glucose level, and then at $1\frac{1}{2}$–2 hours hypoglycemia may occur. Patient may have a history of gastrectory, or symptoms and signs of hyperthyroidism. Due to rapid gastric emptying. May have excessive insulin discharge (>200 μU/ml) at $\frac{1}{2}$–1 hour after meal.[c] It is not necessary to obtain insulin measurements	Reduce simple carbohydrates in diet to less than 5%. Complex carbohydrate to be 50–60% of total calories. Protein can be raised to 20–25%, but not usually necessary. If possible, lie down after meals. Anticholinergic agents may slow gastric emptying. May require frequent small meals (5–6/day)
Impaired glucose tolerance with late hypoglycemia	Plasma glucose high (>150 mg/dl) during first 2 hours after mixed meal,[b] followed by hypoglycemia at 3–4 hours. Insulin may be inappropriately high (not returned to baseline of 10–15 μU/ml) at 2–3 hours. No need to obtain insulin measurements. OGTT shows abnormally high glucose levels (see Chapter 15), in the first 2 hours[c]	Reduce simple carbohydrates in meal as above. Increase fiber content of diet. May require frequent, smaller meals (5–6/day). Estimated 50% of such patients may become clinically diabetic in 10–15 years
Idiopathic	Perfectly normal plasma glucose levels after mixed meal,[b] but at 3–4 hours becomes hypoglycemic. Insulin levels normal; glucagon may fail to rise slightly later in the test (not necessary to measure either of these hormones). OGTT is normal in the first 2 hours[c]	Reduce simple carbohydrates in meals as above. May require frequent small meals (5–6/day)

[a] Author's method.
[b] 700 calories. 50% carbohydrate (includes 20% of total carbohydrate as simple sugar), 15% protein, 35% fat. May use meal which by history simulates provocative meal.
[c] If mixed meal is nondiagnostic (symptoms and glucose level >45–50 mg/dl at indicated times), perform 75-g glucose tolerance test.

Over the next 36 hours, he consumed first a liquid and then a soft diet, and the intravenous infusion was stopped after 36 hours. He again became confused, so blood was obtained for serum insulin and plasma glucose tests, and intravenous glucose was again given as a bolus. The 10% glucose infusion was resumed for two more days. Plasma glucose at the time of the confusion was 36 mg/dl. The intravenous glucose was again discontinued on the fourth hospital day, when the patient was eating well and the plasma glucose was 226 mg/dl. He was discharged, ambulatory, to the nursing home, taking tolazamide (Tolinase) 250 mg each day. Eight days later, his fasting morning glucose level was 198 mg/dl. He was eating more and was somewhat less depressed. Nine days after discharge, the test for serum insulin (drawn during the episode of confusion) was returned and was less than 5 μU/ml.

Discussion

In patients taking sulfonylurea drugs, even the shorter-acting forms, hypoglycemia can result if they are not eating well. The problem is even more severe if malignancy or liver disease exists. If the patient has renal insufficiency, even of a very mild degree (e.g., a serum creatinine level over 1.5 mg/dl), chlorpropamide should not be given. This is because a large percentage of the active drug is cleared by the kidney (about 40%). The patient had normal renal function, but he was not eating. These drugs (sulfonylureas) act by potentiating the action of endogenous insulin and can thus severely reduce the plasma glucose level in patients who are fasting or starving.

The dose of chlorpropamide, 750 mg/day, was too high, and this could be another factor in hypoglycemia. A shorter-acting sulfonylurea, at a lower dose, was substituted.

This patient tended to reduce food intake when depressed. Thus the use of oral agents or even insulin might be hazardous in a setting such as a nursing home where medications might be given on a routine basis, regardless of food intake. His physicians were correctly content with less rigid metabolic control in this particular situation.

A serum insulin determination was not really necessary in this clinical setting, unless hypoglycemia tended to recur, 7 or 8 days after discontinuing chlorpropamide. This is because there is only a very remote possibility that an insulinoma could have developed in a diabetic patient. A high insulin level (see text and Table 1) would be present during hypoglycemia if this patient had an insulin-secreting tumor.

Finally, older patients can develop hyponatremia (SIADH, see Chapter 3) as a result of the effects of chlorpropamide, so the serum sodium concentration should be checked when changes in sensorium or altered consciousness occur.

SUGGESTED READING

Bouchard P, Sai P, Reach G, et al: Diabetes mellitus following pentamidine-induced hypoglycemia in humans. *Diabetes* 31:40–45, 1982.

Fajans S, Floyd J: Fasting hypoglycemia in adults. *N Engl J Med* 294:766–772, 1976.

Hofeldt F: Reactive hypoglycemia. *Metabolism* 24:1195–1208, 1975.

Low blood sugar: Fact and fiction. *Consumer Rep* July 1971, pp 444–446.

Monnier L, Pham T, Aguirre L, et al: Influence of indigestible fibers on glucose tolerance. *Diabetes Care* 1:83–88, 1978.

Roy BK, Abuid J, Wendorff H, et al: Insulin release in response to calcium in the diagnosis of insulinoma. *Metabolism* 28:246–252, 1979.

17

HAROLD E. CARLSON

Multiple Endocrine Neoplasia

In 1954, Wermer described a syndrome of tumors involving the pituitary, pancreatic islets, and parathyroid glands, which he termed multiple endocrine adenomatosis. When separate syndromes involving the thyroid and adrenal medulla were delineated by Sipple in 1961 and Schimke in 1968, it became clear that three different disorders were involved. In present terminology, *multiple endocrine neoplasia type I* (MEN-I) designates a condition characterized by tumors primarily involving the pituitary and pancreatic islets along with parathyroid hyperplasia; MEN-IIa designates a condition involving pheochromocytoma, medullary carcinoma of the thyroid, and parathyroid hyperplasia; and MEN-IIb (sometimes called MEN-III) refers to pheochromocytoma, medullary thyroid carcinoma, and multiple mucosal ganglioneuromas. The term multiple endocrine *neoplasia* is now preferred to multiple endocrine adenomatosis, since several tumors in the syndromes may be malignant (e.g., islet cell tumors, medullary carcinoma of the thyroid, pheochromocytoma). While the syndromes are usually separate and distinct, occasional instances of overlap have been reported in which patients had features of both MEN-I and MEN-IIa or -IIb.

PATHOGENESIS—THE APUD CONCEPT

The occurrence of multiple endocrine tumors in individuals and families has raised the possibility of an underlying inherited defect in these tissues that might predispose them to neoplasia. In 1966, Pearse first proposed his hypothesis that all such tissues producing peptide hormones were derived from the embryonic neural crest and shared a common biochemical ability to take up amine precursors (dihydroxyphenylalanine and 5-hydroxytryptophan) from the circulation and decarboxylate them to neurotransmitter amines (dopamine, norepinephrine, and serotonin). The acronym APUD, applied to these cells and tissues, is derived from this action of *a*mine *p*recursor *u*ptake and *d*ecarboxylation.

Although initial studies confirmed the neural crest origin of the adrenal medulla and the parafollicular cells (C cells) of the thyroid, recent work has not supported a neural crest derivation for pancreatic islets or gut endocrine cells; additionally, an endodermal origin of the parathyroid glands remains likely. In response to these criticisms, Pearse and his colleagues have suggested that endocrine cells migrate from neuroectoderm or the even more primitive epiblast to peripheral tissues such as gut and pancreas before the appearance of the neural crest per se; experimental support for this concept is presently lacking. Furthermore, this argument can also be carried to absurdity in extrapolating further and further back into embryonic life; indeed, the epiblast is not solely a precursor of neuroectoderm but is a progenitor of mesoderm and endoderm as well. Such a derivation would be necessary to accommodate the thyroid (endoderm), adrenal cortex, and adipose tissue (mesoderm) tumors also seen in MEN-I. Only in MEN-IIb do the involved tissues all share an undisputed neuroectodermal origin. Recent demonstrations of peptide hormone production by primitive unicellular organisms and plants further suggest that hormone production may be a universal attribute of all living things, not unique to neurally derived vertebrate tissues.

Aside from the question of embryologic origin, however, tissues involved in MEN syndromes generally share APUD cytochemical characteristics and many also contain a common enzyme, neuron-specific enolase. Thus there appears to be at least a functional relationship among many of the involved organs, if not an embryologic one.

GENETICS

It has been estimated that about half of all newly discovered cases of MEN are sporadic (i.e., with no prior affected relatives); these presumably represent a new mutation in the patient concerned. In familial cases, the inheritance of all three MEN syndromes has been autosomal dominant with a high degree of penetrance. Thus 50% of the offspring of an affected individual are likely to inherit the syndrome. It is true, nevertheless, that some families or some individuals within families may not manifest the entire syndrome.

CLINICAL FEATURES

MEN-I

Hyperparathyroidism is the most common feature of MEN-I (Table 1) and is often the first component of the syndrome to develop. In most instances, there is diffuse parathyroid hyperplasia rather than a single adenoma. Tumors of the pancreatic islets are also common and are frequently multiple. The separate pancreatic tumors may produce different hormones, and each individual tumor commonly produces multiple hormones; some tumors may be nonfunctional or may produce "silent" hormones, such as pancreatic polypeptide, that have no recognizable clinical effects. Of the functioning tumors, gastrinomas are the most common, followed by insulinomas, tumors secreting vasoactive intestinal polypeptide (VIPomas), and glucagonomas. A few patients have been described with diffuse islet hyperplasia (nesidioblastosis). Although pituitary tumors are less common than parathyroid or islet involvement in MEN-I, this partly reflects the underdiagnosis of pituitary lesions in the preradioimmunoassay era; the relatively recent availability of serum prolactin (PRL) determinations has led to the recognition that PRL-producing pituitary tumors are commonly found in MEN-I. Hyperprolactinemia may be clinically silent or may produce amenorrhea and galactorrhea in women or decreased libido and impotence in men. Growth hormone (GH) and ACTH-secreting tumors of the pituitary also occur, producing acromegaly or Cushing's disease.

Table 1 **Features of Multiple Endocrine Neoplasia Syndromes**

	Percentage of patients affected
Type I	
Anterior pituitary adenomas (PRL, GH, ACTH, nonfunctioning)	50
Hyperparathyroidism (parathyroid hyperplasia)	80–90
Pancreatic islet tumors	80–90
Gastrinoma (peptic ulcer)	60
Insulinoma (hypoglycemia)	25
VIPoma (watery diarrhea, hypokalemia, achlorhydria)	5
Glucagonoma	Occasional
Thyroid tumors (benign or malignant)	20–30
Adrenal tumors	40
Carcinoid tumors of gut, bronchus, or thymus	4
Multiple lipomas	17
Gastric polyps	Rare
Schwannomas	Rare
Type IIa	
Hyperparathyroidism (parathyroid hyperplasia)	30–60
Medullary thyroid carcinoma	90–100
Pheochromocytoma	20–90
Type IIb	
Medullary thyroid carcinoma	75
Pheochromocytoma	35
Multiple ganglioneuromas (eyelids, lips, tongue)	95–100
Enlarged corneal nerves	95–100
Marfanoid appearance	95–100

It is still unclear whether tumors of the adrenals and thyroid are an integral part of the syndrome. The prevalence of involvement of these glands, however, appears to be considerably greater than the occurrence of similar abnormalities in the general population (Table 1). Some adrenal abnormalities may represent diffuse or nodular hyperplasia secondary to ACTH hypersecretion from either pituitary or islet cell tumors. Carcinoid tumors and lipomas are uncommon but apparently bona fide components of the syndrome. Other rarely reported tumors (gastric polyps and schwannomas) may represent only chance associations. In general, the islet cell tumors represent the greatest threat to the patient with MEN-I, because of the effects of their hormones and the high incidence of malignancy in these lesions.

MEN-IIa

Medullary carcinoma of the thyroid is the most common component of the syndrome (Table 1) and often the earliest to appear; the lesions are almost invariably multicentric, involving both lobes of the thyroid. The earliest lesion seen is C-cell hyperplasia, which in MEN-IIa is a premalignant condition. Although medullary carcinomas secrete calcitonin, hypocalcemia is uncommon in MEN-II patients. Diarrhea may occur, perhaps related to serotonin or prostaglandin overproduction by the tumor.

Pheochromocytomas occuring in MEN-IIa are commonly multiple and bilateral. A small number are malignant, and occasional extraadrenal tumors have been reported. In analogy to the thyroid abnormality of MEN-IIa, the early lesion in the adrenal appears to be diffuse and nodular medullary hyperplasia which progresses with age to well-defined tumors. Hyperparathyroidism, usually due to parathyroid hyperplasia, occurs less commonly in MEN-IIa than in MEN-I; it does not appear to arise in response to chronic mild hypocalcemia induced by calcitonin excess, since the hyperparathyroidism may occur in MEN-IIa in the absence of medullary carcinoma. Occasional patients may develop Cushing's syndrome secondary to ectopic ACTH production by either a medullary carcinoma or a pheochromocytoma. Morbidity and mortality in MEN-IIa are primarily related to medullary thyroid carcinoma and pheochromocytoma.

MEN-IIb

The most constant finding in MEN-IIb has been the occurrence of multiple ganglioneuromas; these firm, yellow tumors are commonly visible externally on the eyelids, lips, and tongue (Fig. 1) and are also found internally along the entire length of the gut. Autonomic function is often disrupted, frequently leading to constipation and colonic dilatation. Plaques of disorganized neural tissue may also be found overlying the spinal cord, where they may interfere with motor and sensory function. Thickened corneal nerves are a nearly uniform finding on slit-lamp examination and may diminish vision. A Marfan-like habitus is common, but ectopia lentis and cardiovascular abnormalities are not seen in MEN-IIb. Medullary carcinoma and pheochromocytoma are multiple and bilateral, as in MEN-IIa; in contrast, however, hyperparathyroidism with hypercalcemia has never been convincingly described in MEN-IIb. Although the morbidity and mortality are largely related to medullary carcinoma and pheochromocytoma, the gastrointestinal abnormalities are often disabling and may in some instances indirectly result in death.

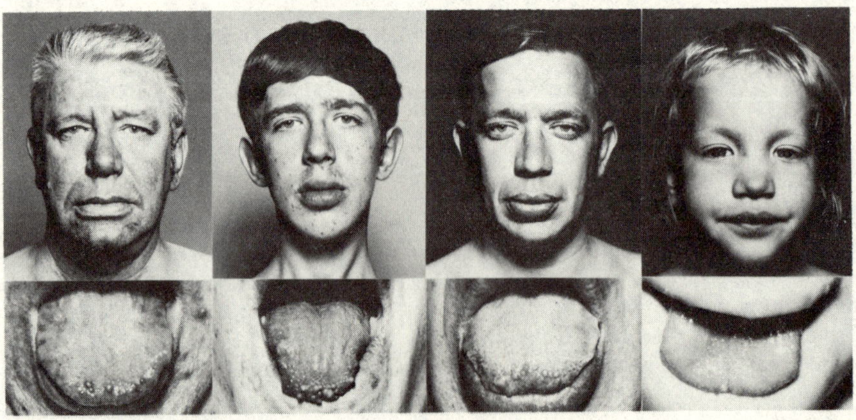

Figure 1. Abnormal facies, thickened lips, and tongue ganglioneuromas in four affected members of a family with MEN-IIb; from left to right are the grandfather, two sons, and a 2-year-old granddaughter. Reprinted by permission of Sizemore, GW, Multiple endocrine neoplasia type 2. *Clin Endocrinol Metab* 9:299–315, 1980. Copyright W. B. Saunders Co., Ltd.

TREATMENT

By and large, the individual tumors of MEN are treated as they would be in patients with only a single, isolated lesion. The major exceptions to this rule result from the multicentricity of lesions in MEN. Thus, since diffuse parathyroid hyperplasia is usually found, all four glands must be examined in any surgical procedure. The islet cell tumors in MEN-I are often multiple and frequently malignant, so pancreatic resection for cure may not be possible. The multicentric origin of medullary thyroid carcinoma mandates a total thyroidectomy in most patients. Finally, a thorough exploration of the abdomen through an anterior approach is recommended at surgery for pheochromocytoma; some authorities recommend routine bilateral adrenalectomy for patients with MEN-IIa or -IIb with pheochromocytoma.

Treatment should also focus on the detection of other components of the various syndromes, since the plan of therapy may be altered by the discovery of additional lesions. For example, finding a pheochromocytoma in a patient with medullary thyroid carcinoma will lead to resection of the pheochromocytoma first, to avoid intraoperative crises during neck surgery.

DIAGNOSIS AND SCREENING

Clinical or biochemical evidence of the MEN-I syndrome is rare before the age of 10 years. Although most affected individuals develop some evidence of disease between the ages of 10 and 30 years, the risk is lifelong. Patients may show the first manifestations of endocrine disease in late adulthood or may continue to develop new features of the syndrome well into their later years.

Although hyperparathyroidism is thought to be the earliest and most common feature of MEN-I, this may also reflect failure to apply sensitive screening tests for pituitary or pancreatic disease to families at risk. Thus normocalcemia does not exclude the presence of other features of the syndrome. A reasonable screening effort (Table 2) should be applied to all family members at risk, since intervention early in the course of pituitary disease or hyperparathyroidism may prevent later morbidity. Additionally, familial or nonfamilial patients initially having a single component of the syndrome should be screened periodically for other manifestations of MEN-I; examples include patients with the Zollinger-Ellison syndrome (about half have MEN-I), insulin-secreting islet cell tumors of the pancreas (4–10% have MEN-I), and hyperparathyroidism due to parathyroid hyperplasia (3–33% have MEN-I). Patients with apparently isolated pituitary adenomas have a very low risk of MEN-I (1–2%) and should be screened only with a personal and a family history, a physical examination, and a measurement of serum calcium levels.

In MEN-IIa and -IIb, screening is even more important in detecting medullary thyroid carcinoma and pheochromocytoma, both potentially fatal conditions. Both these lesions, especially medullary carcinoma, may be present in early childhood or infancy; thus screening for these conditions should not be delayed until the age of 10 years. A provocative test for calcitonin release using intravenous pentagastrin or combined intravenous pentagastrin and calcium is the procedure of choice for the early detection of medullary carcinoma and allows diagnosis in patients with normal basal levels of plasma calcitonin (Fig. 2). Determination of urinary catecholamine metabolites remains the mainstay of screening for pheochromocytoma. Among patients with medullary thyroid carcinoma, up to 10–20% may have MEN-IIa and 10% MEN-IIb. Similarly, in one series, 7% of patients with pheochromocytoma were found to have MEN. In families with MEN-IIb, the occurrence of ganglioneuromas and enlarged corneal nerves is such a nearly constant finding, even in childhood, that individuals without these

Table 2 **Screening for MEN Syndromes**

MEN-I	
	Serum calcium
	Serum prolactin
	Serum gastrin
	Fasting blood sugar
	Clinical assessment for nephrolithiasis, acromegaly, Cushing's syndrome, peptic ulcer disease, hypoglycemia, thyroid nodules, and lipomas
MEN-IIa	
	Serum calcium
	Plasma calcitonin, preferably after pentagastrin stimulation
	24-hour urine for VMA, catecholamines, and metanephrines *or* metanephrine/creatinine ratio in spot urine sample
	Clinical assessment for nephrolithiasis, hypertension, paroxysms, and thyroid nodules
MEN-IIb	
	Plasma calcitonin, preferably after pentagastrin stimulation
	24-hour urine test for VMA, catecholamines, and metanephrines *or* metanephrine/creatinine ratio determination in spot urine sample
	Clinical assessment for hypertension, paroxysms, thyroid nodules, ganglioneuromas, habitus, corneal nerves, and gastrointestinal function

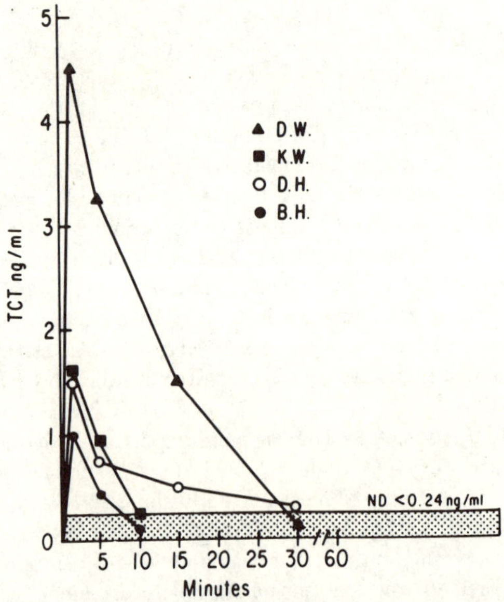

Figure 2. Thyrocalcitonin responses to pentagastrin stimulation (0.5 μg/kg body weight) in four children with a family history of multiple endocrine neoplasia type II; all were found to have medullary thyroid carcinoma at surgery. Reprinted by permission of Wells SA, The early diagnosis of medullary carcinoma of the thyroid gland in patients with multiple endocrine neoplasia type II. *Ann Surg* 182:362–370, 1975. Copyright J. B. Lippincott Co.

features probably do not require further screening other than a medical history, thyroid palpation, and a blood pressure determination.

A proposed screening program for the three syndromes is given in Table 2. Although there are no firm data on the time needed to develop new abnormalities, it is probably reasonable to repeat the screening procedure at 5-year intervals in asymptomatic individuals at risk for MEN-I, and at 1- or 2-year intervals for MEN-IIa or -IIb.

DISCUSSION CASES

Case 1

A 29-year-old man with abdominal pain was found to have a duodenal ulcer. When antacid therapy failed to control his symptoms, he underwent a vagotomy and pyloroplasty, followed 1 year later by a subtotal gastrectomy and gastrojejunostomy. Abdominal pain recurred after another 6 years and led to a third laparotomy, which revealed the presence of multiple pancreatic tumors; celiac lymph nodes contained metastatic islet cell tumor. A total gastrectomy was performed, with relief of his ulcer symptoms.

When evaluated at age 37, he complained of frequent headaches, decreased beard growth, and impotence. Physical examination showed intact visual fields and no band keratopathy. There was no gynecomastia or galactorrhea. Pubic and axillary hair was normal; the testes were soft but of normal size.

The serum calcium level ranged between 11.2 and 12.2 mg/dl; the serum parathyroid hormone level was 76 pg/ml (normal <100 pg/ml during normocalcemia). The serum prolactin level was 50 ng/ml (normal males <15 ng/ml), with no further rise after intravenous thyrotropin-releasing hormone (TRH) injection. Tomograms of the sella turcica were normal.

In light of the above findings, a neck exploration was performed. Only three parathyroid glands could be located; the two largest glands were removed, and the third biopsied and marked with surgical clips. The histologic diagnosis was parathyroid hyperplasia. The patient remained normocalcemic after surgery. Further pituitary function testing gave normal results except for persistent hyperprolactinemia. He died of unrelated causes 2 years later. Family studies uncovered a brother with pituitary-dependent Cushing's disease and hyperparathyroidism.

Comment

This patient developed all three major components of MEN-I, with involvement of the pancreatic islets, parathyroids and, in all likelihood, pituitary. The failure of his elevated serum prolactin level to rise further in response to TRH is consistent with a diagnosis of a prolactin-secreting pituitary tumor. Although his hyperparathyroidism was asymptomatic and detected only on biochemical screening, the pituitary lesion may have caused his headaches, impotence, and decreased beard growth (see Chapter 2). Present-day management might employ cimetidine rather than a total gastrectomy to control his ulcer disease, and bromocriptine to suppress the prolactin hypersecretion. Chemotherapy with streptozotocin, with or without 5-fluorouracil, may be useful in controlling the growth and spread of islet cell tumors.

Case 2

A 31-year-old man presented with a recently noticed 1-cm hard mass in the left upper pole of the thyroid. Additionally, he had recently been found to be hypertensive (160/90) without orthostatic change and complained of tachycardia, heat intolerance, nocturia, and a 20-pound weight loss over 2 months despite a good appetite and adequate food intake. No ganglioneuromas or ocular abnormalities were detected. The patient's mother had had surgery 17 years previously for medullary carcinoma of the thyroid. A thyroid scan with pertechnetate in the present patient showed the left upper pole nodule to be "cold"; fine needle aspiration biopsy revealed the presence of a carcinoma. The serum calcium level was 11.4–11.8 mg/dl, the phosphorus level 1.9 mg/dl, and the parathyroid hormone level 1,750 μlEq/ml (normal <100 μlEq/ml), suggesting the presence of hyperparathyroidism. The basal plasma calcitonin level was 3,750 pg/ml (normal <200 pg/ml), rising to 27,000 pg/ml 10 minutes after intravenous pentagastrin injection, consistent with a diagnosis of medullary thyroid cancer.

Because the patient's clinical history also suggested the presence of a pheochromocytoma, further investigation was undertaken. A 24-hour urine specimen for VMA yielded a value of 7.5 mg/24 hr (normal <10.8 mg/24 hr), while urinary catecholamine excretion was mildly elevated at 156 μg/24 hr (normal <125 μg/24 hr). An abdominal computerized axial tomography (CAT) scan suggested the presence of a possible mass in the left adrenal. Selective venous sampling from both adrenal veins was carried out; baseline plasma epinephrine and norepinephrine levels in the right adrenal vein were 18,600 and 5,890 pg/ml, respectively, rising to 115,000 pg/ml and 55,000 pg/ml after intravenous histamine injection. For the left adrenal, the baseline plasma epinephrine level was 331,000 pg/ml and the norepinephrine level zero; the posthistamine plasma epinephrine level in the left adrenal vein rose insignificantly to 337,000 pg/ml, while norepinephrine was still undetectable. The substantial response to histamine in the right adrenal vein suggested a right adrenal pheochromocytoma; after appropriate preoperative preparation with phenoxybenzamine, he was taken to surgery and a right adrenalectomy performed. Pathological examination showed a 3-cm pheochromocytoma in the excised adrenal; the left adrenal was inspected, palpated at surgery, and felt to be normal, as were the sympathetic chains bilaterally. His blood pressure returned to normal postoperatively.

One month later he underwent neck exploration and a total thyroidectomy. Pathologic examination showed a 1.5-cm medullary carcinoma in the left upper pole of the thyroid and a 0.4-cm medullary carcinoma in the right upper pole (previously undetected). Three of four excised left cervical lymph nodes were positive for carcinoma. Three large parathyroids were removed (the pathological diagnosis was parathyroid hyperplasia), and one normal-sized parathyroid was left in place. He was given L-thyroxine replacement therapy.

Five months after thyroidectomy, the serum calcium level was normal, but the plasma calcitonin level was still elevated at 380 pg/ml (normal <200 pg/ml), rising to 4,400 pg/ml after pentagastrin stimulation. A palpable left cervical node was excised and contained a medullary carcinoma; eight additional nodes were negative for carcinoma. Although he remained normotensive, the levels of 24-hour urine total metanephrines were slightly elevated (1.4 mg/24 hr; normal <0.9 mg/24 hr), as was the level of urinary norephinephrine (119 μg/24 hr; normal <81 μg/24 hr). Accordingly, he was returned to the operating room and a left adrenalectomy performed after again preparing him with phenoxybenzamine; pathological examination of the excised left adrenal revealed medullary hyperplasia. He has since been maintained on replacement hydrocortisone and mineralocorticoid. His blood pressure, serum calcium levels, and plasma calcitonin levels have all remained normal for 3 years since his last surgery.

Comment

Although this patient initially had a thyroid lesion, it was important to diagnose and remove his pheochromocytoma before proceeding with neck surgery, to avoid a hypertensive or a hypotensive crisis during the operative period. In retrospect, the high incidence of bilateral adrenal medullary involvement (70–95%) in MEN-II syndromes might have prompted a bilateral adrenalectomy at the time of the first laparotomy, sparing the patient his later surgery; such an approach would also avoid the risk and expense of extensive localization procedures, as were done in this case.

Plasma calcitonin measurements proved to be extremely helpful in detecting residual medullary thyroid carcinoma in this patient with MEN-IIa, and he may well be cured of this tumor. Since medullary cancer is nearly always bilateral and multicentric in MEN-II, a total thyroidectomy was the procedure of choice.

Continued lifelong follow-up is necessary to detect further recurrences of any of the three components of the MEN-IIa syndrome.

SUGGESTED READING

Alberts WM, McMeekin JO, George JM: Mixed multiple endocrine neoplasia syndromes. *J Am Med Soc* 244:1236–1237, 1980.

Ballard HS, Frame B, Hartsock RJ: Familial multiple endocrine adenoma-peptic ulcer complex. *Medicine* 43:481–516, 1964.

Dyck PJ, Carney JA, Sizemore GW, Okazaki H, Brimijoin WS, Lambert EH: Multiple endocrine neoplasia, type 2b: Phenotype recognition—Neurological features and their pathological basis. *Ann Neurol* 6:302–314, 1979

Khairi MRA, Dexter RN, Burzynski NJ, Johnston CC: Mucosal neuroma, pheochromocytoma and medullary thyroid carcinoma: Multiple endocrine neoplasia type 3. *Medicine* 54:89–112, 1975.

Leichter SB: Clinical and metabolic aspects of glucagonoma. *Medicine* 59:100–113, 1980.

Modlin IM: Endocrine tumors of the pancreas. *Surg Gynecol Obstet* 149:751–769, 1979.

Pearse, AGE, The APUD concept and hormone production. *Clin Endocrinol Metab* 9:211–222, 1980.

Schimke RN, Hartmann WH, Prout TE, Rimoin DL: Syndrome of bilateral pheochromocytoma, medullary thyroid carcinoma and multiple neuromas. *N Engl J Med* 279:1–7, 1968.

Schimke RN: Multiple endocrine adenomatosis syndromes. *Adv Intern Med* 21:249–265, 1976.

Sipple JH: The association of pheochromocytoma with carcinoma of the thyroid gland. *Am J Med* 31:163–166, 1961.

Sizemore GW, Heath H III, Carney JA: Multiple endocrine neoplasia, type 2. *Clin Endocrinol Metab* 9:299–315, 1980.

Steiner AL, Goodman AD, Powers SR: Study of a kindred with pheochromocytoma, medullary thyroid carcinoma, hyperparathyroidism and Cushing's disease: Multiple endocrine neoplasia, type 2. *Medicine* 47:371–409, 1968.

Veldhuis JD, Green JE, Kovacs E, Worgul TJ, Murray FT, Hammond JM: Prolactin-secreting pituitary adenomas: Association with multiple endocrine neoplasia, type I. *Am J Med* 67:830–837, 1979.

Wermer P: Genetic aspects of adenomatosis of endocrine glands. *Am J Med* 16:363–371, 1954.

Yamaguchi K, Kameya T, Abe, K: Multiple endocrine neoplasia type 1. *Clin Endocrinol Metab* 9:261–284, 1980.

18 GILDON N. BEALL

Endocrine Autoimmunity

A number of endocrine disorders are apparently caused by autoimmune mechanisms. In addition, several different endocrine diseases and immunization to different endocrine antigens often coexist. This chapter includes information that should allow clinicians to use wisely the available immunologic studies for diagnosis and assessment of endocrine disease. A brief consideration of the known and proposed immunopathologic mechanisms is also included to give the necessary background for those who must evaluate the complicated and sometimes dangerous methods being proposed for control of immune responses. With these aims, Addison's disease, diabetes mellitus, and autoimmune thyroid disease will be discussed, along with some remarks about hypoparathyroidism. Detailed information about these diseases is available in the appropriate chapters of this book. Allergic reactions to hormones and drugs used in endocrine disorders will be considered in another volume, *Allergy and Clinical Immunology for the Practicing Internist.*

ADDISON'S DISEASE

There is general agreement that autoimmunity is the major cause of idiopathic adrenal insufficiency. Tuberculosis has been declining in importance as a cause of adrenal failure, while other causes such as metastatic cancer, adrenal hemorrhage or infarction, amyloidosis, and fungal infections such as histoplasmosis are unusual.

Immunologic Findings

The most important immunologic observation made in patients with idiopathic Addison's disease has been the detection of autoantibodies to adrenal cortical cells in about 50–70% of such patients. The frequency is greatest soon after diagnosis and decreases with the passage of time. These IgG antibodies are best recognized by immunofluorescence, using freshly frozen human or primate adrenal tissue. Several different specificities of antibodies have been described based on varying staining patterns of the cytoplasm of glomerulosa and fasciculata cells. Although antibodies have been detected by complement fixation and particle agglutination with microsomal extracts of adrenal cells, such techniques are less reliable. Unlike many other autoantibodies, these adrenal autoantibodies are rarely present in either normal subjects or patients with other endocrine disorders. In fact, the detection of adrenal autoantibodies in such patients is cause for investigation and careful observation of adrenal function. Several patients have been described who have first developed adrenal antibodies and later adrenal failure.

Although evidence for cell-mediated immunity to adrenal antigens has been produced in some patients with Addison's disease, the data are insufficient to permit interpretation at present.

Histocompatibility Typing

Histocompatibility type HLA-B8 is found in 70–80% of Caucasian Addisonian patients and in only about 20% of the general population. As with most of the other endocrine autoimmune diseases, there seems to be an even better correlation of disease with the *D* locus antigen Dw3. These findings tend to support theories that an HLA-linked immune response gene is required to permit autosensitization.

Overlaps

There is a very striking clinical overlap of Addison's disease with other endocrine disorders suspected to be caused by immunologic mechanisms. Nearly 40% of patients have some type of an associated disease, including lymphocytic thyroiditis, Graves' disease, type I diabetes, pernicious anemia, and menstrual disturbances. Twenty percent of patients have some associated thyroid disease. The association of Hashimoto's disease and Addison's disease (Schmidt's syndrome) is familiar to many internists, but the association with diabetes may be even more common. Irvine has called particular attention to the association of idiopathic Addison's syndrome with amenorrhea or oligomenorrhea and has demonstrated autoantibodies to steroid-producing cells that cross-react with adrenal and ovarian tissue in many of these patients. These associations make it imperative that patients with Addison's disease be evaluated carefully and continuously for the presence of these other clinical conditions.

In addition to this clinical overlap, there is also an extensive serologic overlap. Patients with Addison's disease and their first-degree relatives have a greatly increased frequency of organ-specific autoantibodies, particularly to thyroidal and gastric parietal cell antigens.

Diagnostic Use of Immunologic Tests

Adrenal autoantibodies are not present frequently enough to be useful in diagnosis. Difficulties in obtaining suitable tissue have led most laboratories that have studied these antibodies to do a group of assays during one period of time. It is likely that laboratories performing the test irregularly will have difficulty in maintaining a similar competency in performing and interpreting these tests.

Immunopathogenesis

Association of the disease with autoantibodies supports the idea that the autoantibodies are the cause of the adrenal failure. The autoantibodies are potentially cytotoxic, since they fix complement. There is also a theoretical possibility that the autoantibodies or immune complexes derived from them might arm killer cells to damage the adrenal cells. Placental passive transfer of adrenal autoantibodies, however, apparently causes no harm.

Adrenalitis can be produced by immunization of animals. In guinea pigs the result is a cell-mediated immune reaction, while rabbits develop autoantibodies. It is uncertain whether either model is appropriate for the human disease.

HYPOPARATHYROIDISM

Idiopathic hypoparathyroidism is associated with a number of immunologic abnormalities, although there has been little definite evidence implicating immune mechanisms in pathogenesis. Patients with hypoparathyroidism frequently have other possibly immunologically mediated disorders such as diabetes, Addison's disease, pernicious anemia, and thyroid disease. Association of the parathyroids with the third and fourth pharyngeal pouches is probably related to an association of hypoparathyroidism with immunodeficiency. In the DiGeorge syndrome, disturbed cell-mediated immunity due to deficiency of thymic epithelium is found together with hypoparathyroidism and structural abnormalities of the neck. Mucocutaneous candidiasis is variably associated with disturbances of cell-mediated immunity, hypoparathyroidism, Addison's disease, and diabetes.

DIABETES MELLITUS

The current classification of diabetes is stimulated partly by immunological observations. Insulin-dependent diabetes mellitus (IDDM) is now called type I, and insulin-independent diabetes, type II. In type II diabetes there are few or no reported immunologic abnormalities and no definite linkage with HLA types, despite strong evidence of familial aggregation of the disease. Type I diabetes, on the other hand, has been associated with both immunologic abnormalities and linkage to certain histocompatibility types. A subgroup of type I diabetes is associated with other autoimmune endocrine diseases.

Immunologic Findings

Antibodies to the pancreatic islets were first discovered by Bottazzo and Doniach, and their observations have now been confirmed in many laboratories. Patients with type I, but not those with type II diabetes, have islet cell antibody (ICA) in their serum with a frequency related to the duration of their disease. Many laboratories have found frequencies of 60–70% in patients with type I diabetes within the first year of diagnosis. The frequency of detection of ICAs, however, declines rapidly, and by 10 years ICAs are found only in 10–20% of patients with IDDM (Fig. 1). The ICAs are IgG in type. They have been assayed by immunofluorescence, using fresh human pancreas from a type-O donor. ICAs are quite specific to type I diabetes, since they are found in only 1–3% of patients with other conditions, including type II diabetes. Careful examination of sera containing ICAs has revealed that the antibodies are not specific for β cells but may contain antibodies that react also with α, δ, and pancreatic polypeptide-forming cells. These antibodies, however, do not react with insulin, glucagon, or other hormone products of the cells (Fig. 2).

A second type of autoantibody, islet cell surface antibody (ICSA), reacts with islet cell surfaces. Dispersed islet cells from human or rat pancreas are used to identify this antibody by

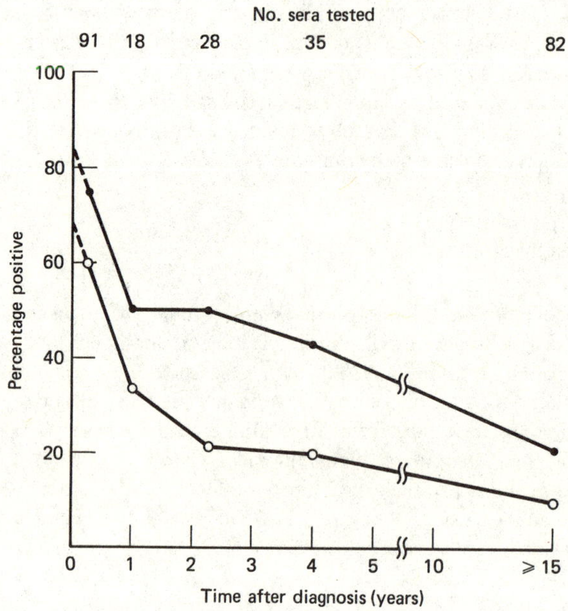

Figure 1. Prevalence of ICA-IgG in 198 insulin-dependent (type I) diabetics. Closed circles designate ICA-IgG, and open circles CF-ICA. CF-ICA disappeared from the circulation more rapidly and formed a higher proportion of the total ICAs near the time of diagnosis (78%) than after 15 or more years of insulin treatment (40%). Reprinted by permission of Bottazzo GF, Complement fixing islet cell antibodies in type I diabetes: Possible monitors of active beta-cell damage. *Lancet* 1:668–672, 1980. Copyright *The Lancet.*

fluorescence or radioisotopic means. A cytotoxic assay procedure has been developed in which cloned rat islet cells are destroyed by ICSA and complement (Fig. 3). Fixation of complement can also be demonstrated by immunofluorescence on frozen tissue sections from human pancreas (CF-ICA). ICSA and CF-ICA, presumably identical, clearly have the ability to destroy pancreatic islet cells.

Sensitization produces cell-mediated immunity to pancreatic antigens in a limited number of patients with IDDM. Immune complexes, too, have been identified with sensitive assays in patients with type I diabetes. The significance of these findings is unknown. It is entirely possible that some of the immune complexes are composed of insulin and insulin antibodies.

Histocompatibility Typing

HLA-B8 is often associated with A1 and Dw3, and this whole group of antigens is commonly found in patients with Addison's disease, Graves' disease, and type I diabetes. B8 frequencies of 19–55% have been reported in type I diabetes. These antigens may be found even more frequently in patients with both type I diabetes and other endocrine disease. Such patients have been tentatively classified as having type IB diabetes. According to Morris, Irvine, and colleagues, the incidence of HLA-B8 rises from 50% in patients with ICAs and IDDM to 70% in patients with ICAs, IDDM, and another autoimmune endocrine disease.

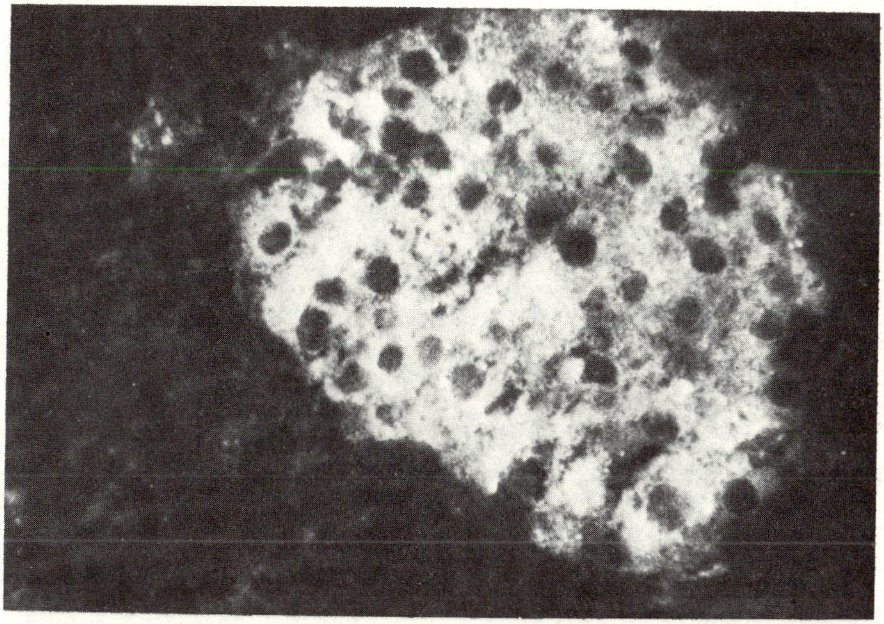

Figure 2. Human pancreas stained by immunofluorescence with serum containing ICAs, showing cytoplasmic reaction with all cells in an islet of Langerhans. Reprinted by permission of Doniach D., Autoimmunity and the endocrine pancreas, in Joachim HL (ed), *Pathobiology Annual.* New York, Appleton-Century-Crofts, 1980, vol 7, p 327. Copyright Appleton-Century-Crofts.

Unlike other endocrine diseases, type I diabetes is associated with more than one linked histocompatibility system. HLA-Bw15 has been found in 4–50% of type I patients, a definitely increased frequency. Bw15 appears to be linked with Dw4 and, again, the *D* locus antigen's presence appears to be more highly correlated with IDDM than the *B* locus antigen (Table 1). Several workers have also demonstrated a *decreased* frequency of B7 and its linked Dw2 in patients with IDDM, leading to speculation that Dw2 may be protective.

Overlaps

Careful observation of patients with IDDM for such disorders as Addison's disease, thyrotoxicosis, and pernicious anemia is appropriate, although the frequency of such occurrences is not great. Organ-specific autoantibodies to endocrine organs are also found in a few patients with type I diabetes. Patients with Graves' disease or Addison's disease have been reported to have as much as a 5 or 6% incidence of ICAs. This is, in fact, the only group where a significant number of such positive results are found other than in patients with IDDM.

Diagnostic Use of Immunologic Tests

The detection of ICAs has been a great stimulus to studies on the pathogenesis of diabetes. It is less certain that assay of these antibodies is a useful clinical tool. Some authorities have

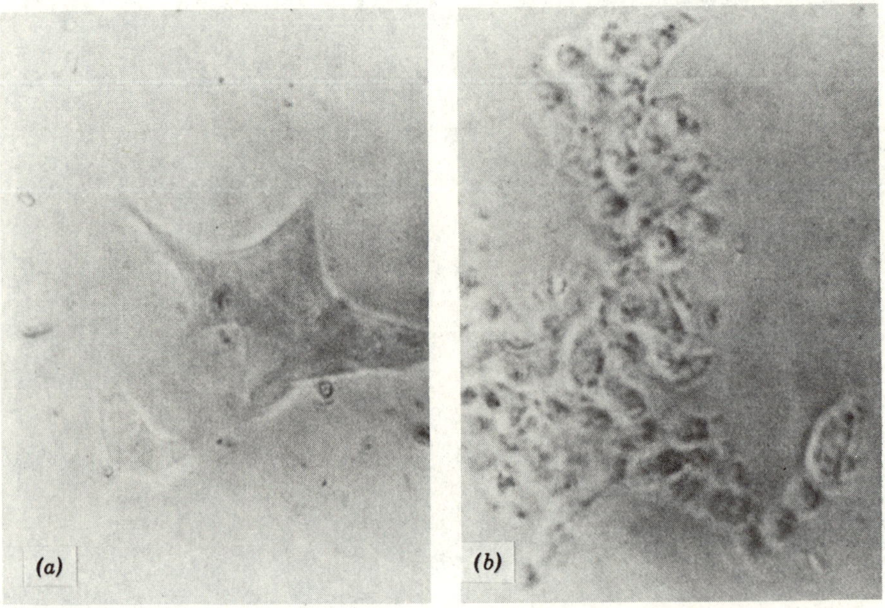

Figure 3. Phase-contrast photomicrograph of a monolayer culture of rat islet (RINm5F) cells at the completion of a cytotoxicity assay. Cells were incubated with a positive serum (^{51}Cr cytotoxicity assay) from a patient with insulin-dependent diabetes (*b*) or serum from a patient with insulin-dependent diabetes negative by the ^{51}Cr cytotoxicity assay (*a*). The antibody-positive serum has produced marked cell destruction (*b*). Reprinted by permission of Eisenbarth GS, Cytotoxic antibodies to cloned rat islet cells in serum of patients with diabetes mellitus. *J Clin Invest* 67:403–408, 1981. Copyright The American Society for Clinical Investigation, Inc.

argued that patients with newly diagnosed diabetes should have their serum assayed for ICAs and ICSAs. A positive result would suggest the eventual necessity for insulin even if the patient could be initially managed without it. This approach is difficult to justify, however, since even in the most experienced laboratories ICAs are detected in only 70–80% of newly diagnosed cases of IDDM. The difficulties in performing the test may make this figure unobtainable in many laboratories. Further simplification of some of the newer assay procedures may, however, alter this conclusion.

Immunopathogenesis

Not only are ICAs not specific for beta cells, but there has been at least one report of ICA appearing in the serum following ingestion of the rodenticide Vacor, which has toxic effects on the pancreatic islet cells. Thus it seems likely that ICA production follows antigenic release from damaged islets. This idea fits nicely with current views that much of the insulitis of type I diabetes is caused by viral agents. It is entirely possible, of course, that the antibody contributes to the pathogenesis of the disease. The disappearance of the antibody with the passage of time is consistent with the effects of the removal of the antigen with loss of the islet tissue. ICAs,

Table 1 **Classification of Diabetes Mellitus**

Type I
Insulin-dependent
Juvenile onset
Repeated episodes of ketoacidosis
Islet cell cytoplasmic and cell surface autoantibodies
Associated with HLA-B8,DW3; and HLA-B15,DW4
Type IA
Associated with and possibly caused by viral infections
Type IB
Associated with other endocrine diseases: Graves' disease, Addison's disease, thyroiditis, pernicious anemia
Frequency of HLA-B8,DW3 is greater than in type IA
Frequency of persistent islet cell antibodies is greater than in type IA
Type II
Insulin-dependent
Maturity-onset (also insulin-independent with juvenile-onset)
Rare or no islet cell antibodies
No distinctive HLA linkage
Increased incidence in certain families

not fixing complement, may not be cytotoxic, but ICSAs or CF-ICAs are antibodies that may contribute to pathogenesis by virtue of their cytotoxicity. In type IB diabetes, there is more reason to believe that the antibodies may be pathogenic, but the problem of specificity remains. Nevertheless, there may be individual susceptibility in such patients, as evidenced by the HLA linkages, so that the antibodies are more effective in producing damage.

Hypotheses attempting to explain the linkage of HLA antigens with disease evolve either from the possibility that HLA-linked immune response genes allow response to otherwise tolerated antigens or that the HLA antigen, the macrophage's recognition and communication system with other cells, predisposes to susceptibility to certain viral infections. Either or both of these concepts may be relevant to type I diabetes.

There are some opinions that complications of IDDM may be related to immune complexes either of insulin and antiinsulin or other immune reactants. There is, however, little evidence available on this subject.

There does not appear to be any current role for manipulation of the immune system in the treatment of IDDM or its complications. If the viral causes were known, vaccines might prevent the disease. Antiviral substances such as interferon may find a role in therapy in the future.

Autoantibodies to the Insulin Receptor

A small group of patients have been described who manifest extreme insulin resistance due to autoantibodies to their own insulin receptors. These patients, who have ranged considerably in age, have been predominantly female and non-Caucasian. Doses of insulin exceeding 1,000 units/day have been used in attempts to treat some of these patients. Most of them have the cutaneous disorder acanthosis nigricans, and many have other evidence of systemic disease, including typical systemic lupus erythematosus. Serologic abnormalities such as the presence of antinuclear antibodies have also been found. The autoantibody to the insulin receptor has been demonstrated by its ability to inhibit the binding of insulin to cells such as monocytes. The antibody also precipitates solubilized receptors labeled with [^{125}I]insulin. The autoantibodies appear to be mainly IgG, although some IgM has been demonstrated. Unlike the antireceptor antibodies that stimulate the thyroid in Graves' disease, the antiinsulin receptor antibodies are associated with insulin resistance. However, in vitro the same antibodies show many insulinomimetic effects. These effects apparently have also been seen in vivo in a very few patients in whom profound hypoglycemia has developed. Assays for antiinsulin receptor antibodies are practical but not widely available. The incidence of the disorder appears to be very low. In patients with profound insulin resistance who demonstrate manifestations of systemic disease other than diabetes, it is reasonable to obtain such studies.

In this disorder, the role of the autoantibody in producing insulin resistance is clear. The origin of the autoantibodies, which has not been explored, may be somehow related to a more generalized disturbance of immune function.

Treatment of the disorder has been attempted with glucocorticoids and azothioprine, with slight lowering of antibody titers and some benefit. Partial, transient remission has also been induced by plasmapheresis. The hazards of such therapeutic interventions should be carefully considered, because spontaneous remissions have also occurred in a few patients. The relative lack of effectiveness of immunosuppressive agents is not unexpected. Such agents are often effective as antagonists of the inflammatory effects of immunologic reactions, but a reduction in antibody titers is much more difficult to achieve.

AUTOIMMUNE THYROID DISEASE

Several forms of thyroid disease are probably caused by immunologic mechanisms. These include not only Hashimoto's (or lymphocytic) thyroiditis and Graves' disease but also primary myxedema. There are clinical overlaps between these disorders, suggestions that one disorder may evolve into another, and evidence of familial predisposition to autoimmune thyroid diseases without regard to the type of disease. Frequently, immunologic studies have been performed with material from patients with both Graves' disease and Hashimoto's thyroiditis, with evidence of abnormality in each condition. Despite these connections, however, there are dramatic differences in the clinical presentations of these disorders and some very distinct immunological abnormalities, which make it likely that the pathogeneses are similarly distinct. Too little is known about immunologic findings in primary myxedema to warrant discussion, but Hashimoto's thyroiditis and Graves' disease will be discussed separately.

Hashimoto's Thyroiditis

This is probably an extremely common disorder that often produces no disease. Its prevalence at autopsy is at least 1–2%, and the prevalence of thyroid autoantibodies may be 5–10%.

Immunologic Findings

Patients with mild forms of the disease, without goiter or hypothyroidism, are presumably included in normal populations used for control studies, making it extremely difficult to assess the frequency and distribution of immunologic abnormalities in patient groups as compared to normals. Clinical diagnosis usually rests on multiple criteria which may include immunologic tests. Patient selection in this way may bias the results of other immunologic studies. The diagnosis can be made with assurance on histologic examination, but there is disagreement as to whether a needle biopsy will provide this information. Lymphocytes may be aspirated and recognized from needle biopsies, but it may not be possible to detect colloid depletion, germinal center formation, or fibrosis. Comments about the frequency of immunologic changes in Hashimoto's thyroiditis are subject to these conditions.

The first autoantibody demonstrated in patients with Hashimoto's thyroiditis was antithyroglobulin (anti-Tg). Although anti-Tg was originally recognized by its ability to precipitate thyroglobulin, such precipitating activity is distinctly unusual and the precipitin assay is no longer clinically useful. Anti-Tg can be detected by agglutination of tanned red cells coated with thyroglobulin or by several types of radioassay procedures. Most anti-Tg's are IgG, although IgA anti-Tg activity occurs rarely. The antibodies do not fix complement.

Antimicrosomal antibodies (anti-M) are also found with considerable frequency in patients with Hashimoto's thyroiditis. These antibodies react with a microsomal antigen specific to thyroid cells. The antigen is present in increased amounts at the epithelial margin of the cell and in thyrotoxic thyroid glands. Anti-M, which was detected by immunofluorescence for many years, is currently assayed by hemagglutination of microsomal-coated erythrocytes. Radioassays are also practical. Anti-M fixes complement and appears to be responsible for the ability of thyroiditis serum to exhibit complement-mediated thyroid cytolysis in vitro.

Cell-mediated immunity to thyroidal antigens has been demonstrated in some patients with Hashimoto's thyroiditis. Peripheral blood mononuclear cells (PBMCs) of Hashimoto's thyroiditis but not of normal subjects will produce migration inhibition factor or proliferate and incorporate tritiated thymidine when exposed to thyroidal homogenates. Although the frequency of positive results in such assays is usually less than that for autoantibody detection, this may be due to insensitivity of the assays. Immune complexes have been found in many patients with Hashimoto's thyroiditis and Graves' disease. In some instances, thyroglobulin–anti-Tg immune complexes have been described, although most of the immune complexes found are not related to a specific thyroidal immunologic system. The theoretical ability of such immune complexes to arm killer cells provides one nominee for the agent involved in destruction of the thyroid cells. Electron micrographs have revealed electron-dense deposits in the thyroid follicular basement membrane of patients with Hashimoto's thyroiditis, and it has been postulated that these deposits are immune complexes. These findings are difficult to interpret at present, since only a minority of patients with either Hashimoto's thyroiditis or Graves' disease have been found to have immune complexes in their serum and the frequency has varied greatly from laboratory to laboratory.

Histocompatibility Typing

Alone among the endocrine disorders suspected to be caused by immune mechanisms, Hashimoto's thyroiditis has no known association with histocompatibility type. It is possible, however, that more testing of larger numbers of patients for *D* and *DR* locus antigens may yet reveal such a link.

Overlaps

Many physicians interested in the subject have noted the concurrence of Hashimoto's thyroiditis with endocrine or nonendocrine diseases of putatively autoimmune origin, and a large literature of case reports has recorded these observations. Despite this, an epidemiologic study on a large number of patients with autopsy-diagnosed Hashimoto's thyroiditis showed only a slightly increased incidence of rheumatoid arthritis. Nonetheless, the inferences drawn from uncontrolled observations are probably correct, since many of these diseases are too uncommon to detect in an epidemiologic study of reasonable size.

Patients with other forms of immunologic disturbance are frequently found to have antithyroid antibodies, albeit in low titer. About 30% of patients with Graves' disease and Hashimoto's thyroiditis have antibodies to gastric parietal cells. Another interesting facet of Hashimoto's thyroiditis that is unexplained is the association of both antithyroid antibodies and Hashimoto's thyroiditis with Down's syndrome and some other forms of mental retardation.

Diagnostic Use of Immunologic Tests

Only anti-Tg and anti-M determination are helpful in diagnosis of Hashimoto's thyroiditis. Assays for both anti-Tg and anti-M should be obtained initially and at periodic reevaluations. Significant anti-Tg titers (≥1:10) can be found in about 80% of patients with Hashimoto's thyroiditis. At this level of sensitivity only 2–3% of the normal population is found to have such antibodies. Of more concern is the fact that about 20% of patients with other thyroid diseases, including cancer, will also have significant anti-Tg titers. Thus discrimination of thyroiditis from cancer may still require biopsy.

With radioassay techniques, it is possible to increase the sensitivity so that all patients with Hashimoto's thyroiditis have detectable anti-Tg, but assays at this sensitivity will detect anti-Tg in approximately 20% of what appears to be a normal population.

Elevated serum concentrations of thyroglobulin, found in many thyroid diseases, can interfere with radioassay procedures for anti-Tg unless precautions are taken. Also, a serum inhibitor of hemagglutination found in rare cases can invalidate such assays.

Doniach has reported that anti-M hemagglutinating antibodies at titers ≥1:100 are present in approximately 95% of patients with Hashimoto's thyroiditis and in 5% of normal persons. This excellent discriminating ability, again, must be tempered by knowledge of a higher false-positive rate in patients with other forms of thyroid disease. Radioassays for anti-M are positive in virtually all patients with autoimmune thyroid disease. The false positive rate in normal persons is probably about 15%.

Fortunately, the data obtained from immunological tests need not be interpreted as simply positive or negative. Most false positives have very low antibody titers. High titers of antithyroid antibodies (anti-Tg ≥1:640 or anti-M ≥1:6400) are almost never found in patients other than those with Hashimoto's thyroiditis or Graves' disease.

Immunopathogenesis

It is difficult to ignore the frequency of high titers of anti-Tg and anti-M when theorizing about the pathogenesis of Hashimoto's thyroiditis. Anti-Tg antibodies or antibodies associated with them seem to be the cause of at least some forms of experimentally induced thyroiditis in animals. If anti-Tg is to be regarded as pathogenic, one must also hypothesize a means by which this pathogenicity can be expressed. Since anti-Tg does not fix complement, it is not cytotoxic to thyroid cells in vitro. Thyroglobulin–anti-Tg immune complexes could arm K cells and damage thyroid cells by this means. Immune complexes of thyroglobulin and anti-Tg, if deposited in the thyroid basement membrane as has been hypothesized, could possibly promote similar activity. Recent studies have indicated that peripheral blood lymphocytes can produce anti-Tg in vitro when stimulated with either pokeweed mitogen or antigen. Intrathyroidal production of anti-Tg by immunocompetent cells might account for a major portion of the anti-Tg found in the serum as well as the pathologic effects on the tissues.

Anti-Tg synthesis occurs as the result of a failure to regulate B cells normally. A lack of T-cell suppression might account for such an abnormality, and studies on cell-mediated immunity have supported this possibility, but in vitro studies on anti-Tg synthesis by human lymphoid cells have not demonstrated a T-cell defect.

Cell-mediated immunity causes the thyroidal damage in some types of experimental thyroiditis in animals. Although the histologic findings of lymphocytic infiltration and fibrosis in the human disease are suggestive, the evidence for cell-mediated immunity to thyroidal antigens in patients with thyroiditis is not sufficiently striking or frequent to suggest cell-mediated immunity as a common form of pathogenesis.

Immunotherapy

To be useful in the treatment of Hashimoto's thyroiditis a procedure would have to be extremely nontoxic and would have to be applied to patients before thyroid destruction and fibrosis. These conditions cannot be met at present. Presumably, fibrosis in the gland might be delayed or altered by the administration of antiinflammatory agents or corticosteroids, but the risks of such procedures would exceed any possible benefit.

GRAVES' DISEASE

Immunologic Findings

Thyroid-Stimulating Immunoglobulins

Patients with Graves' hyperthyroidism possess immunoglobulins capable of stimulating the thyroid gland. The first demonstration of one of these factors was by Adams and Kennedy who found that a γ-globulin in the serum of patients with Graves' hyperthyroidism was capable of stimulating guinea pig and mouse thyroid. It was soon demonstrated that the long-acting thyroid stimulator (LATS), as this substance was called, was a serum IgG, but it was present in only about 60% of patients with the disease and was occasionally found in euthyroid patients. This led to the general conclusion that antibodies that stimulate the mouse thyroid may not necessarily stimulate the human thyroid. Evidence that LATS was indeed an antibody was provided by studies showing that it could be removed from serum by absorption with thyroid tissue and could be eluted from the thyroid tissue with procedures appropriate for dissolving antigen–antibody complexes. The ability of thyroid antigens to remove LATS from the serum provided the basis for demonstration by Adams of "LATS protector." This IgG substance in the serum of patients with Graves' hyperthyroidism blocks thyroid homogenates so that they are then incapable of absorbing LATS. LATS protector does not stimulate the mouse thyroid, but detection of the substance correlates extremely well with Graves' hyperthyroidism. Other workers have demonstrated immunoglobulin substances in the serum of patients with Graves' hyperthyroidism that stimulate colloid droplet formation in human thyroid slices (human thyroid stimulator, HTS) or stimulate adenyl cyclase in homogenates or (better) slices of human thyroid (human thyroid adenyl cyclase stimulator, HTACS; thyroid-stimulating antibody, TSAb). For some time, many investigators had felt that the actions of these thyroid-stimulating immunoglobulins (TSIs) were best explained by a hypothesis that the antibody reacts at or near the thyroid-stimulating hormone (TSH) receptor. Smith and Hall developed this idea into an assay system for the measurement of antibodies that prevent TSH from binding to its thyroidal receptor. The assay involves preincubation of TSH-receptor-rich thyroidal membranes with immunoglobulin followed by [^{125}I]TSH. Immunoglobulins that inhibit TSH binding have been referred to by various names, TSAb's, TSH-inhibiting activity, TSH-blocking antibodies, thyroid-stimulating immunoglobulin, and TSH-binding inhibitor (TBI). It is clear that the assay system measures inhibition of TSH binding and not stimulation, so terminology indicating this appears to be preferable. TBI is present not only in patients with Graves' hyperthyroidism but also in some patients with Hashimoto's thyroiditis without hyperthyroidism. This is probably best explained as a result of antibodies capable of blocking in vitro TSH binding but not capable of fitting tightly enough with the receptor to stimulate thyroidal activity.

TSIs have been found in culture supernatants of patient's lymphocytes stimulated by mitogen or antigen. An intriguing observation has recently been made that antithyroid drugs are capable of inhibiting this lymphocytic activity, thus suggesting that part of the effect of carbimazole and propylthiouracil in Graves' disease may be due to immunosuppression.

Other Immunologic Findings

As mentioned earlier in the section on Hashimoto's thyroiditis, serum from patients with Graves' disease often contains anti-M and, less commonly, anti-Tg. Approximately 80% of patients will possess significant titers of one or both of these antibodies, using standard hemagglutination test kits.

Cell-mediated immunity to thyroidal antigens as evidenced by migration inhibition or lymphocyte proliferation has also been described in a smaller proportion of patients with Graves' disease.

Histocompatibility Types

Approximately 50% of Caucasian women with Graves' disease possess HLA-B8. In studies in which *D* locus typing has been performed, the linked gene, *Dw3*, is present with even greater frequency. A similarly strong relationship with an B antigen exists between Bw35 and Graves' disease in Japanese women.

Overlaps

In addition to the coexistence of Graves' disease with other endocrine disorders, as mentioned previously, Graves' disease is associated with myasthenia gravis.

Practical Use of Immunologic Tests

Immunologic findings have not proven particularly valuable in the diagnosis of Graves' disease. Contentions, too, that the results of assays for TSI could be used to predict response to antithyroid drugs have not been confirmed. As will be mentioned below, Graves' ophthalmopathy can present a difficult problem in diagnosis, particularly when unilateral. In such instances, detection of TSI would heavily tip the diagnostic balance toward Graves' ophthalmopathy over pseudotumor or an infectious or neoplastic cause of the exophthalmos. It is probably not practical, however, to maintain one of these assay procedures for such narrowly defined clinical purposes.

Immunopathogenesis

TSIs are surely the cause of Graves' hyperthyroidism, but there is less certainty as to which of the various assays being used is the most successful in measuring such immunoglobulins. There are probably several autoantibodies specific for thyroidal membrane antigens, reactions with which have varying effects on the TSH receptor. The clinical effects of these antibodies may be related not only to their specificity but conceivably to coordination of the effects of two or more antibodies.

Although there seems to be little reason to hypothesize a role for cell-mediated immunity as a cause of thyroid stimulation in Graves' disease, evidence of abnormal effector function of T cells in Graves' disease may indicate that T-cell regulation of antibody synthesis is also deranged, although other possibilities exist. In particular, there is a possibility that an HLA-linked immune response gene, possibly operating through macrophage control of antibody response, allows autosensitization.

Immunotherapy

Although destruction or removal of the thyroid gland is not an entirely satisfactory form of treatment for Graves' hyperthyroidism, it appears preferable to the currently available forms of immunosuppression. Perhaps in the future it will be possible to manipulate the immune system by specifically altering reactivity to thyroidal antigens.

Extrathyroidal Manifestations of Graves' Disease

Immunological Findings and Possible Immunopathogenesis

Ophthalmopathy, dermopathy (pretibial myxedema), and vitiligo are commonly found in Graves' disease. Vitiligo, which may also be associated with a number of other disorders, is commonly associated with antimelanocyte antibodies. Several investigations of Graves' dermopathy have not produced any evidence for deposition of immunoglobulins in the affected tissues. Local administration of corticosteroids is helpful in dermopathy. Such effects could be due to interference in an immunologic process, but other explanations are possible.

Few patients with euthyroid ophthalmopathy possess thyroid-stimulating antibodies or anti-Tg, but anti-M is reasonably common. Other immunologic investigations, however, have detected a number of abnormalities leading to some interesting theories about the causation of the disorder.

Sera from patients with euthyroid Graves' ophthalmopathy are said to stimulate protrusion of the eyes of the Atlantic minnow. A factor in such sera binds selectively to human eye muscle membranes, binding that is enhanced by an accompanying immunoglobulin. The factor is thought to be derived from the pituitary, possibly a fragment of TSH.

A second group of observations has emphasized that serum factors from patients with ophthalmopathy can stimulate incorporation of ^{35}S in the mucopolysaccharides of the Harderian gland, a retro-orbital structure in the guinea pig that may be analogous to human retro-orbital connective tissue. Another group of investigators has found that lymphatic flow from the thyroid to the orbit is possible. They have demonstrated a selective affinity of eye muscle membranes for thyroglobulin–anti-Tg immune complexes capable of cell-dependent cytotoxicity and postulate that these or other immune complexes cause the disease. Finally, others have demonstrated evidence of inhibition of cell migration by eye muscle antigens, but no convincing theory implicating cell-mediated immunity has been put forward. It has not been possible to find serum antibodies directly capable of binding to eye muscle membrane or retro-orbital structures.

The theories of pathogenesis provide interesting points of departure for further studies but leave many aspects of the disorder unexplained. Particularly intriguing is the mucinous infiltrate found in the retro-orbital tissues. There does not seem to be any counterpart to this in immunologically mediated inflammation in other diseases.

Immunotherapy

Although spontaneous resolution occurs frequently, the disorder may progress with great rapidity and cause loss of vision. In Graves' ophthalmopathy some therapeutic risks are warranted. Conventional treatment has usually included large doses of corticosteroids, often for months or years. This seems to have been successful in some patients, and such improvement could be attributed to an immunosuppressive effect, possibly inhibition of antibody synthesis since such large doses are needed. Cyclophosphamide has also been given with what was thought to have been some benefit. Plasmapheresis coupled with immunosuppression has also been used, and a few anecdotes have reported dramatic changes in rapidly progressive endocrine exophthalmos. The reasons for this remain uncertain. Plasma and lymphopheresis are capable of removing antibodies and immune complexes and also removing or interfering with cellular functions, such as that of macrophages. In addition, plasma or albumin solutions used for plasma replacement may have therapeutic effects.

DISCUSSION CASES

Case 1

Description

R.F. is a 22-year-old woman with a history of IDDM diagnosed at age 5, Hashimoto's thyroiditis diagnosed at age 11, and amenorrhea since age 20.

History

Problem 1: IDDM. The patient has had numerous admissions to hospital for ketoacidosis, hypoglycemia, and recurrent episodes of massive hepatomegaly. She has been very poorly compliant in her diabetic regimen. She frequently omits or alters her insulin dosage and usually does not follow a diabetic diet, preferring to skip meals and eat candy bars for the subsequent hypoglycemic reactions. Many insulin preparations and combinations have been used without success in regulating her blood sugar. She requires about 30 units of Lente insulin and 15–30 units of Semi-Lente for moderate control when she is hospitalized or is complying with her regimen. Liver biopsy has revealed massive fat and glycogen infiltration.

Problem 2: Hasimoto's Thyroiditis. At age 11 she was admitted to a hospital for headaches. An enlarged thyroid and a serum cholesterol level of 554 mg/100 ml were detected. Her serum thyroxine (T_4) level was 4.0 μg/dl and her serum TSH level was 40 μU/ml. Anti-Tg hemagglutinins were present, 1:640. Antibodies to thyroid cytoplasm and gastric parietal cells were detected by immunofluorescence. Antimitochondrial, antismooth muscle, and antinuclear antibodies were absent. Radioiodine uptake was 18.8% at 24 hours and was not increased by preliminary administration of TSH. A thyroid scan showed slightly uneven distribution of isotope with no nodules in a normal-shaped thyroid. A perchlorate dumping test was markedly positive (RAI 39–14%). A needle biopsy of the thyroid revealed small acini, increased fibrous tissue, and lymphocytic infiltration. She is now euthyroid on 0.2 mg of L-thyroxine each day.

Problem 3: Amenorrhea. Although her menarche was at age 12, the patient has had no menses for the past 2 years. She reported no bleeding in response to two separate 5-day courses of medroxyprogesterone (Provera). Hormonal assays: LH 7.8 and 10.9 mIU/ml; FSH 2.3 and 3.4 mIU/ml.

Problem 4: Poor Appetite and Nutrition. A diagnosis of anorexia nervosa has been entertained in the past, but the patient did not complete a psychiatric evaluation.

A physical examination revealed the following: weight $81\frac{1}{2}$ lb, height $56\frac{3}{4}$ in., blood pressure 100/70, pulse 80. Well developed, thin, quiet, female. There were a few microaneurysms in the optic fundi; no hemorrhages or exudates were seen. The thyroid gland was small and finely nodular; the estimated weight was 10 g. The heart and lungs were not remarkable. The breasts were small, with no galactorrhea. The abdomen was soft. There was minimal tenderness to palpation in the right upper quadrant. The liver was palpated 3 cm below the costal margin and the percussed span was 11 cm. There was no splenomegaly. There was normal pubic and axillary hair. On neurologic examination, the ankle jerks were present. Sensation was slightly decreased in the feet. Laboratory results were as follows: creatinine 0.7 mg/dl; BUN 21 mg/dl; hematocrit 39%, hemoglobin 12.8 gm/dl; ACTH stimulation test, cortisol 21 μg/dl before and greater than 50 μg/dl 1 hour after ACTH; L-dopa test, growth hormone rises to 10.5 ng/dl at 90 minutes; metyrapone test, compound S 19.8 μg/dl.

Question

1. Should the patient have HLA typing performed? What would you expect the results to be?

Answer

HLA typing probably has no clinical usefulness in these disorders. The studies are expensive and, although some tissue types are much more frequent in such patients, their frequency is not great enough to add to diagnosis or prognosis. If it were desired to type this patient as part of a research protocol, it is likely that she would be found to be HLA-B8,Dw3, since these antigens are very common in patients with IDDM who have other endocrine disorders.

Question

2. What are the possible causes of the patient's amenorrhea?

Answer

Amenorrhea is not uncommon in patients with poorly controlled diabetes or hypothyroidism. The patient has also been chronically undernourished, which also could contribute to amenorrhea. It is also possible that the patient's amenorrhea may be a result of autosenitization to steroid-producing cells; her normal, rather than elevated, serum LH and FSH make this improbable, however. It is not likely that assays for autoantibodies to steroid-producing cells would be helpful.

Question

3. In addition to caring for the patient's hypothyroidism and type I diabetes, what other endocrinological evaluations should be performed in the future?

Answer

Patients with multiple autoimmune endocrine disorders have a greatly increased frequency of both adrenal insufficiency and pernicious anemia. Regular follow-ups should keep these possibilities in mind, and periodic functional assessments should be performed.

Case 2

Description

R.P., a 14-year-old girl, was quite normal except for mild asthma until age 10, when a goiter was first noted. At age 11, she began to have weight loss, nervousness, fatigue, and hair loss. She sought medical advice after several months of these symptoms.

A physical examination revealed the following: pulse 120, blood pressure 100/70. In general, she was a well-developed well-nourished, prepubertal female with a tremor of her outstretched hands. Her thyroid gland was symmetrically enlarged to about 30–35 g, with a firm, nodular texture. There was no proptosis, lid lag, or lymphadenopathy. Laboratory results showed a corrected T_4 level of 11.9 μg/dl (normal 5–11 μg/dl) and a ^{131}I uptake of 57% at 24 hours, which was not suppressible by exogenous triiodothyronine. Perchlorate discharge test positive. A thyroid scan showed uneven uptake. Anti-Tg by hemagglutination 1:2560; antinuclear factor, positive, anti-M 1:6400.

The patient was considered to have "Hashitoxicosis" and was treated with propylthiouracil. She developed polyarthritis after several months, and the medication was changed to methimazole. On this drug she remains euthyroid clinically and chemically at age 14.

The patient's mother, 35, had had a partial thyroidectomy for hyperthyroidism at age 22 and is now euthyroid clinically and by laboratory testing; a thyroid scan shows no tissue on the left. Anti-Tg <1:10, anti-M 1:1600. A 16-year-old sister of the patient has a thyroid that is twice the normal size, which on scan shows irregular uptake. Her T_4 level is 5.8 μg/dl, her TSH level 12.8 μU/ml, and her ^{131}I uptake 30% at 24 hours. Anti-M 1:6400; anti-Tg <1:10; antinuclear factor, positive. She is currently being treated with T_4, 0.2 mg daily. An 18-year-old sister is clinically normal but had a positive antinuclear factor and an anti-Tg of 1:640. Two normal brothers have anti-Tg of 1:40 and 1:80.

Questions

1. Can a diagnosis be made of the disorder in the patient's 16-year-old sister?

Answer

Although euthyroid (the T_4 is normal) in a technical sense, the increased level of TSH indicates that the level of T_4 in the pituitary is inadequate, so TSH secretion is increased. This latent hypothyroidism together with high titers of anti-M and a goiter with irregular iodine uptake is quite characteristic of Hashimoto's thyroiditis.

Question

2. What, if any, follow-up should be planned for the 18-year-old sister?

Answer

Her high titers of anti-Tg suggest that she is likely to have Hashimoto's thyroiditis. Follow-up examinations once or twice a year should include palpation of the neck and assay of T_4 and TSH in order to detect hypothyroidism in its early stages.

SUGGESTED READING

Craighead JE: Current views on the etiology of insulin-dependent diabetes mellitus. *N Engl J Med* 299:1439–1445, 1978.

Dobersen MJ, Scharff JE, Ginsberg-Fellner F, Notkins AL: Cytotoxic autoantibodies to beta cells in the serum of patients with insulin-dependent diabetes mellitus. *N Engl J Med* 303:1493–1498, 1980.

Doniach D, Bottazzo GF: Autoimmunity in the endocrine pancreas, in Joachim HL (ed): *Pathobiology Annual.* New York, Appleton-Century-Crofts, 1977, vol 7, p 327.

Doniach D, Bottazzo GF, Russell RCG: Goitrous autoimmune thyroiditis (Hashimoto's disease). *Clin Endocrinol Metab* 8:63–80, 1979.

Irvine WJ: Autoimmunity in endocrine disease. *Recent Prog Hormone Res* 36:509, 1980.

Neufeld M, Maclaren NK, Blizzard RM: Two types of autoimmune Addison's disease associated with different polyglandular autoimmune (PGA) syndromes. *Medicine* 60:355–362, 1981.

Pinchera A, Doniach D, Fenzi GF, Baschieri L: *Autoimmune Aspects of Endocrine Disorders.* New York, Academic Press, 1980.

Tattersall R, Pyke D, Nerup J: Genetic patterns in diabetes mellitus. *Hum Pathol* 11:273–283, 1980.

Index